NURSING PHARMACOLOGY

NURSING PHARMACOLOGY

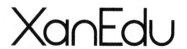

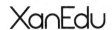

4750 Venture Drive, Suite 400
Ann Arbor, MI 48108
800-562-2147
www.xanedu.com

CONTENTS

INTRODUCTION

This open access Nursing Pharmacology textbook is designed for entry-level undergraduate nursing students. It explains basic concepts of pharmacology and describes common medication classes. This book is not intended to be used as a drug reference book, but direct links are provided to DailyMed, which provides trustworthy information about marketed drugs in the United States.

This textbook is aligned with the Wisconsin Technical College System (WTCS) statewide nursing curriculum for the Nursing Pharmacology course (543-103). The project is supported by a $2.5 million grant from the Department of Education and is licensed under a Creative Commons Attribution 4.0 International License.

This book is available for download in multiple formats, but the online version is required for interaction with the adaptive learning activities included in each chapter.

The following video provides a quick overview of how to navigate the online version.

 An interactive or media element has been excluded from this version of the text. You can view it online here: https://wtcs.pressbooks.pub/pharmacology/?p=4

PREFACE

This open access Nursing Pharmacology textbook is designed for entry-level undergraduate nursing students. It may also be a helpful resource for students in other health programs. It explains basic concepts of pharmacology and describes common medication classes. This book is not intended to be used as a drug reference book, but it does provide direct links to DailyMed, a trustworthy U.S. National Library of Medicine website, that contains information about marketed drugs in the United States.

This textbook is aligned with the Wisconsin Technical College System (WTCS) statewide nursing curriculum for the Nursing Pharmacology course (543-103). Online learning activities are provided in each chapter using the free H5P software platform (https://h5p.org/). This textbook will also be uploaded to LibreTexts (https://libretexts.org/) for easy remixing by faculty. The project is supported by a $2.5 million grant from the Department of Education and is licensed under a Creative Commons Attribution 4.0 International License.

More information about the Open RN grant can be found at: cvtc.edu/OpenRN.

ABOUT THIS BOOK

Editors

This book was edited by:

- Kimberly Ernstmeyer, *MSN, RN, CNE, CHSE, APNP-BC*
- Elizabeth Christman, *MSN, RN, CNE*

Developing Authors

Developing authors remix existing open educational resources and build content from evidence-based sources that is aligned with the Wisconsin Technical College Nursing Curriculum.

- Elizabeth Christman, *MSN, RN, CNE, Chippewa Valley Technical College*
- Kim Ernstmeyer, *MSN, RN, CNE, CHSE, APNP-BC, Chippewa Valley Technical College*
- Chelsea Gonyer, *MSN, RN, Chippewa Valley Technical College*
- Dr. Julie Teeter, *DNP, RN, CNE, Gateway Technical College*
- Jamie Zwicky, *MSN, RN, Moraine Park Technical College*

Contributors

Contributors to the development of this OER textbook include educators, librarians, and staff from a variety of Wisconsin Technical Colleges:

- Nic Ashman, *Librarian, Chippewa Valley Technical College*
- Tara Basu, *MSN, RN, Madison Area Technical College*
- Emily Ernster, *PharmD, Chippewa Valley Technical College*
- Jane Flesher, *MST, Proofreader, Chippewa Valley Technical College*
- Bruce Foraciea, *PhD, Anatomy and Physiology Instructor, Moraine Park Technical College*
- Chelsea Gonyer, *MSN, RN, Chippewa Valley Technical College*
- Kim LaPlante, *Research and Library Services Manager, Northeast Technical College*
- Vince Mussehl, *Open RN Lead Librarian, Chippewa Valley Technical College*
- Joshua Myers, *Web Developer, Chippewa Valley Technical College*
- Barbara Peters, *MSN, RN, Northeast Technical College*
- Gail Powers-Schaub, *Librarian, Madison Area Technical College*
- Rorey Pritchard, *EdS, MEd, MSN, RN-BC, CNOR(E), CNE, Senior RN Clinical Educator, Allevant Solutions, LLC*
- Lauren Richards, *Graphic Designer, Chippewa Valley Technical College*
- Dominic Slauson, *Technology Professional Developer, Chippewa Valley Technical College*
- Lee Wagner, *Librarian, Gateway Technical College*

Advisory Committee

The Open RN Advisory Committee provided input on this book and contains industry members, nursing associate deans, and nursing students:

- Jenny Bauer, *Mayo Clinic Health System Northwest*
- Angela Branum, *Western Wisconsin Health*
- Lisa Cannestra, *Eastern Wisconsin Healthcare Alliance*
- Travis Christman, *HSHS Sacred Heart Hospital*
- Sheri Johnson, *UW Population Health Institute*
- Vicki Hulback, *DNP, RN, Gateway Dean of Nursing*
- Megan Kimber, *CVTC Grants Specialist*
- Brian Krogh, *MSN, RN, NWTC Associate Dean – Health Sciences*
- Pam Maxwell, *SSM Health*
- Mari Kay-Nobozny, *NW Wisconsin Workforce Development Board*
- Ernise Watson, *PhD, RN, MATC Associate Dean – Nursing*
- Sherry Willems, *HSHS St. Vincent Hospital*
- Kristen Bowman & Amanda Swope, *CVTC Nursing Students and Student Nurse Club Leaders*

Peer Review

The Peer Reviewer process was completed February–March 2020 by the following reviewers:

- LaRae Alcidor, *Instructional Designer, San Jacinto College, LaPorte, TX*
- Sarah Babini, *MSN, RN, Grossmont Community College Nursing, El Cajon, CA*
- Jenny M. Bauer, *MSN, RN, NPD-BC, Mayo Clinic Health System Northwest Wisconsin, Eau Claire, WI*
- Gina Bloczynski, *MSN, RN, Chippewa Valley Technical College, Eau Claire, WI*
- Nancy Bonard, *MSN, RN-BC, St. Joseph's College of Maine, Standish, ME*
- Joan Buckley, *PhD, RN, Nassau Community College, Garden City, NY*
- Travis Christman, *BSN, RN, HSHS Sacred Heart Hospital, Eau Claire, WI*
- Dr. Catina Davis, *DNP, MSN, RN, Tidewater Community College, Portsmouth, VA*
- Dr. Andrea Dobogai, *DNP, RN, Moraine Park Technical College, Fond du Lac, WI*
- Dr. Rachael Farrell, *EdD, RN, CNE, Howard Community College, Columbia, MD*
- Samantha Fisher, *MSN, RN, Lakeshore Technical College, Cleveland, WI*
- Dr. Jaime Hannans, *PhD, RN, CNE, California State University Channel Islands, Camarillo, CA*
- Camille Hernandez, *MSN, APRN, ACNP, FNP, Hawaii Community College, Hilo, HI*
- Jenna Julson, *MSN, RN, NPD-BC, Mayo Clinic Health System Northwest Wisconsin, Eau Claire, WI*
- Dr. Andrew D. Kehl, *DNP, MSN, MPH, APRN, RN, FNP-BC, CCRN, NRP, Vermont Technical College, Randolph Center, VT*

- Tamella Livingood, *MSN, FNP-BC, Northwestern Michigan College, Traverse City, MI*
- Dr. Jennifer Lucas, *PharmD, Gateway Technical College, Elkhorn, WI*
- Dawn M. Lyon, *MSN, RN, St. Clair County Community College, Port Huron, MI*
- Sandra Moorman, *MSN, RN, Frederick Community College, Frederick, MD*
- Jody Myhre-Oechsle, *MS, CPhT, Chippewa Valley Technical College, Eau Claire, WI*
- Angela Ngo-Bigge, *MSN, FNP-C, Grossmont College, El Cajon, CA*
- Dr. Colleen Nevins, *DNP, RN, CNE, California State University Channel Islands, Camarillo, CA*
- Dr. Stacey Nseir, *PhD, RN, University of Arizona, Tucson, AZ*
- Dr. Amy I. Olson, *DNP, RN, Mayo Clinic Health System, Eau Claire, WI*
- Marcia M. Osborne, *MSN, FNP B-C, APNP, Northeast Wisconsin Technical College, Green Bay, WI*
- Dr. Grace Paul, *DNP, MPhil, MSN, RN, CNE, Glendale Community College, Glendale, AZ*
- Cassandra Porter, *MSN, RN, Lake Land College, Mattoon, IL*
- Amber J. Price, *MSN-Ed, RN, University of Arizona, Tucson, AZ*
- Dr. Regina Prusinski, *DNP, APRN, Otterbein University, Westerville, OH*
- Dr. Debbie Rickeard, *DNP, MSN, BscN, BA, RN, CNE, CCRN, University of Windsor, Ontario, Canada*
- Kelly Wenzel, *MSN, RN, Chippewa Valley Technical College, River Falls, WI*
- Vanora Taylor Wilmott, *MSN, RN, CWCN, Lyme, NH, Vermont Technical College*

Note to Those Using This Resource: Usage Data

We encourage you to use this resource and would love to hear if you have integrated some or all of it into your curriculum. If you are utilizing this OER book, please submit usage information every semester for grant reporting purposes to the Department of Education using this short usage survey.

Customization/Terms of Use

This textbook is licensed under a Creative Commons Attribution 4.0 International (CC-BY) license unless otherwise indicated, which means that you are free to:

- SHARE – copy and redistribute the material in any medium or format
- ADAPT – remix, transform, and build upon the material for any purpose, even commercially

Licensing Terms

The licensor cannot revoke these freedoms as long as you follow the license terms.

- Attribution: You must give appropriate credit, provide a link to the license, and indicate if any changes were made. You may do so in any reasonable manner, but not in any way that suggests the licensor endorses you or your use.
- No Additional Restrictions: You may not apply legal terms or technological measures that legally restrict others from doing anything the license permits.

- Notice: You do not have to comply with the license for elements of the material in the public domain or where your use is permitted by an applicable exception or limitation.

- No Warranties are Given: The license may not give you all of the permissions necessary for your intended use. For example, other rights such as publicity, privacy, or moral rights may limit how you use the material.

Attribution

Some of the content for this textbook was adapted from the following open educational resources. For specific reference information about what was used and/or changed in this adaptation, please refer to the footnotes at the bottom of each page of the book.

- *Anatomy and Physiology* by OpenStax is licensed under CC BY 4.0.

- *Daily Med* by U.S. National Library of Medicine available in the public domain.

- *Digesting Food* by Stanford School of Medicine and Khan Academy is licensed under CC BY-NC-SA 3.0.

- *Medication Safety in High Risk Situations* by World Health Organization is licensed under CC BY-NC-SA 3.0.

- *Medication Safety in Polypharmacy* by World Health Organization is licensed under CC BY-NC-SA 3.0.

- *Medication Safety in Transition of Care* by World Health Organization is licensed under CC BY-NC-SA 3.0.

- *Medicines by Design* by US Department of Health and Human Services, National Institute of Health, National Institute of General Medical Sciences is licensed under CC BY 4.0.

- *Microbiology* by Open Stax is licensed under CC BY 4.0.

- *Pharmacology Notes: Nursing Implications for Clinical Practice* by Gloria Velarde is licensed under CC BY-NC-SA 4.0.

- *Principles of Pharmacology* by LibreTexts licensed under CC BY-NC-SA 4.0.

- *The Scholarship of Writing in Nursing Education* (1st Canadian Edition) is licensed under CC BY-SA 4.0.

- *Supporting Individuals with Intellectual Disability and Mental Illness* by Sheri Melrose is licensed under CC BY 4.0.

Suggested Attribution Statement for this Book

Content that is not taken from the above OER should include the following attribution statement:

Ernstmeyer, K. and Christman, E. (Eds.). (2020). *Nursing Pharmacology by Chippewa Valley Technical College* licensed under CC BY 4.0.

References

This Preface chapter is a derivative of *The Scholarship of Writing in Nursing Education*, 1st Canadian Edition licensed under CC BY-SA 4.0.

Chapter I

Kinetics and Dynamics

1.1   PHARMACOLOGY BASICS INTRODUCTION

Learning Objectives

- Discuss the processes of pharmacokinetics
- Use multiple professional resources including technology to identify pertinent information related to drugs
- Describe the processes of pharmacodynamics
- Consider pharmacodynamic differences across the life span
- Differentiate among prescription drugs, over-the-counter drugs, herbals, and dietary supplements

Safe medication administration is a vital component of the nursing role. Each day it is common for nurses to make critical decisions regarding the safety, appropriateness, and effectiveness of the medications administered to their patients. Examples of decisions that a nurse might make during patient care include:

- Is my patient's heart rate within the correct range to receive this beta-blocker medication?
- Does my patient have adequate renal function prior to administering this dose of antibiotic?
- Is this pain medication effective in controlling my patient's discomfort?

In order to make safe medication administration decisions, the nurse must have a strong understanding of **pharmacology**. Symptom management, physical recovery, and individual well-being can be strongly connected to the use of medications in a patient's treatment plan. Before a student nurse reviews a medication order, checks a medication administration record, or removes a medication from a dispensing machine, it is important to have a foundational understanding of how medications work within the human body. Let's take a deeper look at the science of pharmacokinetics.

1.2   PHARMACOKINETICS

Pharmacokinetics—Examining the Interaction of Body and Drug

Overview

Pharmacokinetics is the term that describes the four stages of absorption, distribution, metabolism, and excretion of drugs. **Drugs** are medications or other substances that have a physiological effect when introduced to the body. There are four basic stages for a medication to go through within the human body: absorption, distribution, metabolism, and excretion. This entire process is sometimes abbreviated **ADME**. **Absorption** occurs after medications enter the body and travel from the site of administration into the body's circulation. **Distribution** is the process by which medication is distributed throughout the body. **Metabolism** is the breakdown of a drug molecule. **Excretion** is the process by which the body eliminates waste. Each of these stages is described separately later in this chapter.

Research scientists who specialize in pharmacokinetics must also pay attention to another dimension of drug action within the body: time. Unfortunately, scientists do not have the ability to actually see where a drug is going or how long it is active. To compensate, they use mathematical models and precise measurements of blood and urine to determine where a drug goes and how much of the drug (or breakdown product) remains after the body processes it. Other indicators, such as blood levels of liver enzymes, can help predict how much of a drug is going to be absorbed.

Principles of chemistry are also applied while studying pharmacokinetics because the interactions between drug and body molecules are really just a series of chemical reactions. Understanding the chemical encounters between drugs and biological environments, such as the bloodstream and the oily surfaces of cells, is necessary to predict how much of a drug will be metabolized by the body.

Pharmacodynamics refers to the effects of drugs in the body and the mechanism of their action. As a drug travels through the bloodstream, it will exhibit a unique **affinity** for the drug-receptor site, meaning how strongly it will bind to the site. Examination of how drugs and receptor sites create a lock and key system (see Figure 1.1[1]) is helpful to understand how drugs work and the amount of drug that may be left circulating within the bloodstream. This concept is broadly termed as drug **bioavailability**. The bioavailability of drugs is an important feature that chemists and pharmaceutical scientists keep in mind when designing and packaging medicines. Unfortunately, no matter how effectively a drug works in a laboratory simulation, the performance in the human body will not always produce the same results, and individualized responses to drugs have to be considered. Although many responses to medications may be anticipated, one's unique genetic makeup may also have a significant impact on one's response to a drug. **Pharmacogenetics** is defined as the study of how people's genes affect their response to medicines.[2]

---

1   "Drug and Receptor Binding" by Dominic Slausen at Chippewa Valley Technical College is licensed under CCBY 4.0.

2   This work is a derivative of *Medicines by Design* by U.S. Department of Health and Human Services, National Institute of Health, National Institute of General Medical Sciences and is available in the public domain.

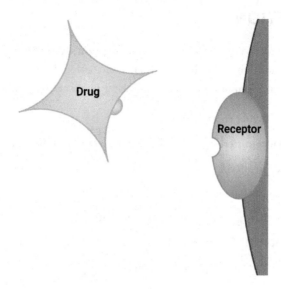

Figure 1.1 Pharmacodynamics: Drug and Receptor Binding

1.3   ABSORPTION

The first stage of pharmacokinetics is known as **absorption**. Absorption occurs after drugs enter the body and travel from the site of administration into the body's circulation. Medications can enter the body through various routes of administration. Common routes to administer medications include the following examples:

- oral (swallowing an aspirin tablet)

- enteral (administering to the GI tract such as via a NG tube)

- rectal (administering an acetaminophen [Tylenol] suppository)

- inhalation (breathing in medication from an inhaler)

- intramuscular (getting a flu shot in the deltoid muscle)

- subcutaneous (injecting insulin in to the fat tissue beneath the skin)

- transdermal (wearing a nicotine patch)

When a medication is administered orally or enterally, it faces its biggest hurdle during absorption in the gastrointestinal (GI) tract. Medications made of protein that are swallowed or otherwise absorbed in the GI tract may quickly be deactivated by enzymes as they pass through the stomach and duodenum. If the drug does get into the blood from the intestines, part of it will be broken down by liver enzymes, known as the **first pass effect,** and some of it will escape to the general circulation to either become protein-bound (inactive) or stay free (and create an action at a receptor site). These metabolic effects are further described in the "Metabolism" section later in this chapter. Thus, providers who prescribe medications, as well as nurses, understand that several doses of an oral medication may be needed before enough free drug stays active in the circulation to exert the desired effect.

What to do?

A workaround to the first pass effect is to administer the medication using alternate routes such as dermal, nasal, inhalation, injection, or intravenous. Alternative routes of medication administration bypass the first pass effect by entering the bloodstream directly or via absorption through the skin or lungs. Medications that are administered directly into the bloodstream (referred to as intravenous medications) do not undergo absorption and are fully available for distribution to tissues within the body.

Alternative routes of medication have other potential problems to consider. For example, injections are often painful and cause a break in the skin, an important barrier to infection. They can also be costly and difficult to administer daily, may cause localized side effects, or contribute to unpredictable fluctuations in medication blood levels.

Transdermal application of medication is an alternate route that has the primary benefit of slow, steady drug delivery directly to the bloodstream—without passing through the liver first. (See Figure 1.21[3] for an image of applying a transdermal patch.) Drugs delivered transdermally enter the blood via a meshwork of small arteries, veins, and capillaries in the skin. This makes the transdermal route of drug delivery particularly useful when a medication must be administered over a long period of time to control symptoms. For example, transdermal application of fentanyl, a pain medication, can provide effective pain management over a long period of time; the scopolamine patch can control motion sickness over the duration of a cruise ship vacation; and the nitro glycerin

---

3   "Applying transdermal patch.jpg" by British Columbia Institute of Technology (BCIT) is licensed under CCBY 4.0.

patch is used to control chronic chest pain. Despite their advantages, skin patches have a significant drawback in that only very small drug molecules can enter the body through the skin, making this application route not applicable for all types of medications.

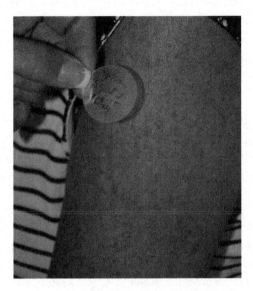

Figure 1.2 Applying Transdermal Patch

Inhaling drugs through the nose or mouth is another alternative route for rapid medication delivery that bypasses the liver (see Figure 1.3).[4] Metered-dose inhalers have been a mainstay of asthma therapy for several years, and nasal steroid medications are often prescribed for allergy and sinus problems.

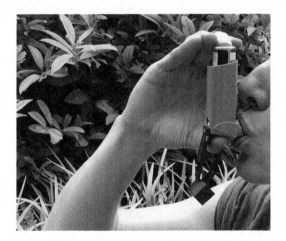

Figure 1.3 Adult using inhaler

---

4 "Adult Using Asthma Inhaler" by NIAID is licensed under CCBY 2.0.

Emerging Discoveries and Recent Developments

Researchers are currently exploring alternative methods of drug delivery such as the use of inhaled insulin powders. Afrezza® is an example of an inhaled insulin approved by the Food and Drug Administration (FDA) to assist with blood sugar control. This technology stems from novel uses of chemistry and engineering to manufacture insulin particles of just the right size for absorption. If too large, the insulin particles could lodge in the lungs; if too small, the particles will be exhaled.[5]

Life Span Considerations

Neonate and Pediatric: Gastric absorption in neonate and pediatric patients varies from that of their adult counterparts. In neonate and pediatric patients, the acid-producing cells of the stomach are immature until around the age of one to two years. Additionally, gastric emptying may be decreased because of slowed or irregular peristalsis (forward bowel movement). The liver of a neonatal or pediatric patient continues to mature, experiencing a decrease in first-pass elimination, resulting in higher drug levels in the bloodstream.[6]

Older Adult: As a natural result of aging, older adults will experience decreased blood flow to tissues within the GI tract. In addition, there maybe changes in the gastric (stomach) pH that may alter the absorption of certain medications. Older adult patients may also experience variations in available plasma proteins, which can impact drug levels of medications that are highly protein-bound. Consideration must also be given to the use of subcutaneous and intramuscular injections in older patients experiencing decreased cardiac output. Decreased drug absorption of medications can occur when peripheral circulation is decreased. Finally, as adults age, they often have less body fat, resulting in decreased absorption of medication from transdermal patches that require adequate subcutaneous fat stores for proper absorption.[7]

Table 1 summarizes route considerations that a nurse should consider when administering medication.

---

5   This work is a derivative of *Medicines by Design* by U.S. Department of Health and Human Services, National Institute of Health, National Institute of General Medical Sciences and is available in the public domain.

6   Fernandez, E., Perez, R., Hernandez, A., Tejada, P., Arteta, M., and Ramos, J. T. (2011). Factors and mechanisms for pharmacokinetic differences between pediatric population and adults. *Pharmaceutics*, 3(1), 53–72. https://doi.org/10.3390/pharmaceutics3010053.

7   Fernandez, E., Perez, R., Hernandez, A., Tejada, P., Arteta, M., and Ramos, J. T. (2011). Factors and mechanisms for pharmacokinetic differences between pediatric population and adults. *Pharmaceutics*, 3(1), 53–72. https://doi.org/10.3390/pharmaceutics3010053.

Table 1: Route Considerations

Oral (PO) or Enteral (NGT, GT, OGT) Ingestion

- Oral route is a convenient route for administration of solid as well as liquid formulations.

- Additional variables that may influence the rate and extent of absorption include enteric coating or extended-release formulations, acidity of gastric contents, gastric emptying rate, dietary contents, and presence of other drugs.

- First pass effect: Blood containing the absorbed drug passes through the liver, which can deactivate a substantial amount of the drug and decrease its bioavailability (the percentage of dose that reaches the systemic circulation).

Parenteral Injection

- Subcutaneous and intramuscular administration: Injections can be difficult for patients to self-administer at home or to administer on a daily basis. They can be costly and painful. Injections also cause a break in skin that is an important barrier to infection, can cause fluctuation in drug levels, and can cause localized side effects to skin.

- Intravenous (IV): IV drugs are fully available to tissues after administration into the bloodstream, offering complete bioavailability and an immediate effect. However, this route requires intravenous access that can be painful to the patient and also increases risk for infection. Medications must be administered in sterile fashion, and if two products are administered simultaneously, their compatibility must be verified. There is also an increased risk of toxicity.

Pulmonary Inhalation

- Inhalation allows for rapid absorption of drugs in gaseous, vaporized, or aerosol form.

- Absorption of particulates/aerosols depends on particle/droplet size, which influences depth of entry through the pulmonary tree to reach the alveoli.

- The ability of the patient to create successful inhalation, especially in the presence of bronchospasm, may also influence depth of entry in the pulmonary tree.

Topical and Transdermal Application

- Topical creams, lotions, and ointments are generally used for local effect; transdermal patch formulations are used for systemic effect.

- Absorption through the buccal or sublingual membranes may be rapid.

- Absorption through skin is generally slower but produces steady, long-term effect that avoids the first pass effect. However, absorption of medication is affected by blood flow to the skin.[8]

---

8   This work is a derivative of *Principles of Pharmacology* by Libre Texts licensed under CC BY-NC-SA 4.0.

Interactive Activity

 An interactive or media element has been excluded from this version of the text. You can view it online here: https://wtcs.pressbooks.pub/pharmacology/?p=192

1.4   DISTRIBUTION

The second stage of pharmacokinetics is the process known as drug **distribution**. Distribution is the process by which medication is dispersed throughout the body via the bloodstream. Once a drug enters into systemic circulation by absorption or direct administration, it must be distributed into interstitial and intracellular fluids to get to the target cells. The distribution of a drug throughout the body is dependent on common factors such as blood flow, plasma protein binding, lipid solubility, the blood-brain barrier, and the placental barrier. Other factors include capillary permeability, differences between blood/tissue, and volume of distribution.

Distribution of a medication can also cause unintended adverse or side effects. Drugs are designed to primarily cause one effect, meaning they bind more strongly to one specific receptor site and predictably cause or block an action. However, side effects can occur when the drug binds to other sites in addition to the target tissue, causing secondary side effects. These side effects can range from tolerable to unacceptable resulting in the discontinuation of the medication. For example, a person might take the pain reliever ibuprofen (Advil) to treat a sore leg muscle, and the pain may be subsequently relieved, but there may also be stomach irritation as a side effect that may cause the person to stop taking ibuprofen.

Blood Flow

The bloodstream carries medications to their destinations in the body. Many factors can affect the blood flow and delivery of medication, such as decreased flow (due to dehydration), blocked vessels (due to atherosclerosis), constricted vessels (due to uncontrolled hypertension), or weakened pumping by the heart muscle (due to heart failure). As an example, when administering an antibiotic to a patient with diabetes with an infected toe, it may be difficult for the antibiotic to move through the blood vessels all the way to the cells of the toe that is infected.

Once the drug is in the bloodstream, a portion of it may exist as free drug, dissolved in plasma water. Some of the drug will be reversibly taken up by red cells, and some will be reversibly bound to plasma proteins. For many drugs, the bound forms can account for 95–98% of the total. This is important because it is the free drug that traverses cell membranes and produces the desired effect. It is also important because a protein-bound drug can act as a reservoir that releases the drug slowly and thus prolongs its action. With drug distribution, it is important to consider both the amount of free drug that is readily available to tissues, as well as the potential drug reserve that may be released overtime.

Protein-Binding

A common factor impacting distribution of medication is plasma protein in the blood. Albumin is one of the most important proteins in the blood. Albumin levels can be decreased by several factors such as malnutrition and liver disease. A certain percentage of almost every drug gets bound to plasma proteins when it initially enters the bloodstream and starts to circulate. The portion of the drug that gets "protein-bound" is inactive while it is bound, but the portion of the drug that escapes initial protein binding becomes immediately "free" to bind to the target tissue and exert or block an action.

A patient taking several highly protein-bound medications often experiences greater side effects. Some drugs are able to competitively grab (or bind to) plasma proteins more easily than other drugs, thus taking up the available protein molecules first. This prevents secondary medications from binding strongly to protein and the intended target site. Instead, these medications float freely in the circulation without exerting action and increase the risk of side effects and toxicities.

My Notes

Think of protein binding like a bus stop (see Figure 1.4[9]). Many passengers (or medication molecules) want to take a ride on the bus. Everyone is eager to get to their destination and interested in finding a seat. Some passengers are stronger and will get in the seats first (like drug molecules with greater protein-binding ability bind to the protein). Sometimes, there may not be enough seats on the bus, and some passengers are left at the bus stop. The passengers (medication molecules) who were left behind are "free" to move around and walk to their destination. They may strike out on their own and get "snatched" (connected to a target receptor site) while on foot. In a similar way, "free" drug particles that are not protein-bound are circulating in the bloodstream and connecting in a pre-dictable fashion to receptor sites that have an affinity for that particular drug. These active drug molecules that did not bind to the protein (like those passengers that were unable to get a seat on the bus) will produce the first effect in the body. Over time, the medication molecules that are bound to the protein (like the passengers with seats on the bus) will get off the bus, start walking around, and get "snatched" to the receptor site that has affinity for them.

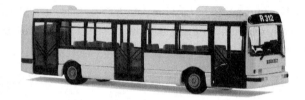

Figure 1.4 Protein binding is like available seats on a bus

Blood-Brain Barrier

Medications destined for the central nervous system (the brain and spinal cord) face an even larger hurdle than protein-binding; they must also pass through an early impenetrable barricade called the **blood-brain barrier**. This blockade is built from a tightly woven mesh of capillaries that protect the brain from potentially dangerous substances, such as poisons or viruses. Only certain medications made of lipids (fats) or have a "carrier" can get through the blood-brain barrier.

Research scientists have devised ways for certain medications to penetrate the blood-brain barrier. An example of this is the brand-named medication Sinemet®, which is a combination of two drugs: carbidopa and levadopa. Carbidopa is designed to carry the levadopa medication across the blood-brain barrier, where it enters the brain and is converted into dopamine to exert its effect on Parkinson's disease symptoms.

Some medications inadvertently bypass the blood-brain barrier and impact an individual's central nervous system function. For example, diphenhydramine (Benadryl®) is an antihistamine used to decrease allergy symptoms. However, it can also cross the blood-brain barrier, depress the central nervous system, and cause the side effect of drowsiness. In the case of a person who has difficulty falling asleep, this drowsy side effect may be useful, but for another person it may be problematic, as they try to safely carry out daily activities.

Placental Barrier

It is always important to consider the effects of medication during pregnancy or for patients who may become pregnant. The placenta is permeable to some medications, while others have not been specifically studied in

---

9   "Renault Type R321 Service Bus" by Emslichteris licensed under CC0 1.0.

pregnant patients. Some drugs can cause harm to the unborn fetus during any trimester. Therefore, it is imperative to always consult a healthcare provider regarding the safety of medications for use during pregnancy. This imperative is assumed in the remaining chapters discussing medication classes, and nurses should always check the most recent, evidence-based drug references before administering medications during pregnancy.[10]

Life Span Considerations

Neonate and Pediatric: Fat content in young patients is decreased because of greater total body water. Additionally, for the growing pediatric patient, the liver is still forming, and protein binding capacity is decreased and the developing blood-brain barrier allows more drugs to enter the brain.[11]

Older Adult: The aging adult patient will experience a decrease in total body water and muscle mass. Body fat may increase and subsequently result in a longer duration of action for many medications. Serum albumin often also decreases, resulting in more active free drug within the body. This is one reason why many older adult patients require lower levels of medication.[12]

Table 1.2 describes other factors that impact drug distribution.

Table 1.2: Other Factors that Impact Drug Distribution

1. Tissue differences in rates of uptake of drugs.

   - Blood flow: distribution occurs most rapidly into tissues with a greater number of blood vessels that allow high blood flow (lungs, kidneys, liver, brain) and least rapidly in tissues with fewer numbers of blood vessels resulting in low blood flow (fat).

   - Capillary permeability: permeability of capillaries is tissue-dependent. Distribution rates are relatively slower or non-existent into the CNS because of the tight junction between capillary endothelial cells and the blood-brain barrier. Capillaries of the liver and kidney are more porous, allowing for greater permeability.

2. Differences in tissue/blood ratios at equilibrium

   - Dissolution of lipid-soluble drugs in adipose tissue

   - Binding of drugs to intracellular sites

   - Plasma protein-binding

---

10   This work is a derivative of *Principles of Pharmacology* by Libre Texts licensed under CC BY-NC-SA 4.0.

11   Fernandez, E., Perez, R., Hernandez, A., Tejada, P., Arteta, M., and Ramos, J. T. (2011). Factors and mechanisms for pharmacokinetic differences between pediatric population and adults. *Pharmaceutics,* 3(1), 53–72. https://doi.org/10.3390/pharmaceutics3010053.

12   Fernandez, E., Perez, R., Hernandez, A., Tejada, P., Arteta, M., and Ramos, J. T. (2011). Factors and mechanisms for pharmacokinetic differences between pediatric population and adults. *Pharmaceutics,* 3(1), 53–72. https://doi.org/10.3390/pharmaceutics3010053.

3. Apparent Volume of Distribution

- Fluid compartments: plasma, extracellular water, total body water.

- The plasma half-life of a drug

  - **Half-life** is the amount of time it takes for half of the medication to be eliminated in the body. Half-life directly correlates to the duration of the therapeutic effect of the medication. Many factors can influence half-life, for example, liver disease or kidney dysfunction.[13]

  - Information about half-life of a medication can be found in evidence-based medication references. For example, in the "Clinical Pharmacology" section of the *Daily Med* reference for *furosemide*, the half-life is approximately 2 hours.

13 This work is a derivative of *Principles of Pharmacology* by Libre Texts licensed under CC BY-NC-SA 4.0.

1.5   METABOLISM

Once a drug has been absorbed and distributed in the body, it will then be broken down by a process known as metabolism. The breakdown of a drug molecule usually involves two steps that take place primarily in the body's chemical processing plant: the liver. (See Figure 1.5[14] for an image of a human liver.) Everything that enters the bloodstream—whether swallowed, injected, inhaled, absorbed through the skin, or produced by the body itself—is carried to this largest internal organ.

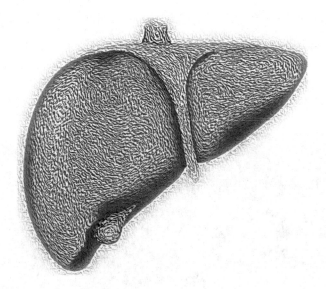

Figure 1.5 Liver

The biotransformations that take place in the liver are performed by the liver enzymes. Every one of your cells has a variety of enzymes, and each enzyme specializes in a particular job. Some enzymes break molecules apart, while others link small molecules in to long chains. With drugs, the first step in metabolizing occurs through a process known as the **first pass effect**, in which orally administered drugs are broken down in the liver and intestines. This makes the substance easier to excrete in the urine. Medications made of protein that are swallowed or otherwise absorbed in the GI tract may quickly be deactivated by enzymes as they pass through the stomach and duodenum. If the drug enters the blood from the intestines, part of it will be broken down by liver enzymes, known as the first pass effect, and some of it will escape to the general circulation to either be protein-bound (inactive) or stay free (and create an action at a receptor site). Thus, several doses of an oral medication may be needed to maintain enough active free drug in the circulation to exert the desired effect.

Many of the products of enzymatic breakdown, which are called metabolites, are less chemically active than the original molecule. For this reason, scientists refer to the liver as a "detoxifying" organ. However, rather than being destroyed by liver enzymes, a few drugs are metabolized into an active form of an intended drug called a "pro-drug." Prodrugs have chemical activities of their own—sometimes as powerful as those of the original drug. When prescribing certain drugs, healthcare providers must take into account these added effects. Once liver enzymes

---

14   "Liver Hepatic Organ Jaundice Bile Fatty Liver-Liver" by VSRao is licensed under CC0.

My Notes

are finished working on a medicine, the now-inactive drug undergoes the final stage of its time in the body—excretion—as it exits via the urine or feces.[15]

Life Span Considerations

Neonate and Pediatric: The developing liver in infants and young children produces decreased levels of microsomal enzymes. This may result in a decreased ability of the young child or neonate to metabolize medications. In contrast, older children may experience increased metabolism and require higher doses of medications once the hepatic enzymes are fully produced.[16]

Older Adult: Hepatic metabolism may experience a significant decline in the older adult. As a result, dosages should be adjusted according to the patient's liver function and anticipated metabolic rate. First-pass metabolism is also decreased with aging; therefore, older adults may have higher "free" circulating drug concentrations and be at higher risk for side effects and toxicities.[17]

Critical Thinking Activity

Metabolism can be influenced by many factors within the body. If a patient has liver damage, the patient may not be able to breakdown (metabolize) medications as efficiently. Dosages are calculated according to the liver's ability to metabolize and the kidney's ability to excrete.

When caring for a patient with cirrhosis, how does this condition impact the dosages prescribed for the patient?

Note: Answers to the Critical Thinking activities can be found in the "Answer Key" sections at the end of the book.

15   This work is a derivative of *Medicines by Design* by U.S. Department of Health and Human Services, National Institute of Health, National Institute of General Medical Sciences and is available in the public domain.

16   Fernandez, E., Perez, R., Hernandez, A., Tejada, P., Arteta, M., and Ramos, J. T. (2011). Factors and mechanisms for pharmacokinetic differences between pediatric population and adults. *Pharmaceutics, 3*(1), 53–72. https://doi.org/10.3390/pharmaceutics3010053.

17   Fernandez, E., Perez, R., Hernandez, A., Tejada, P., Arteta, M., and Ramos, J. T. (2011). Factors and mechanisms for pharmacokinetic differences between pediatric population and adults. *Pharmaceutics, 3*(1), 53–72. https://doi.org/10.3390/pharmaceutics3010053.

Did you know the power of grapefruit juice?

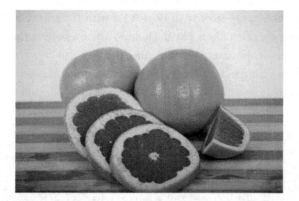

A Juicy Story[18]

Did you know that, in some people, a single glass of grapefruit juice can alter levels of drugs used to treat allergies, heart diseases, and infections? Fifteen years ago, pharmacologists discovered this "grapefruit juice effect" by luck, after giving volunteers grapefruit juice to mask the taste of a medicine. Nearly a decade later, researchers figured out that grapefruit juice affects the metabolizing rates of some medicines by lowering levels of a drug-metabolizing enzyme, called CYP3A4 (part of the CYP450 family of drug-binding enzymes), in the intestines.

More recently, Paul B. Watkins of the University of North Carolina at Chapel Hill discovered that other juices like Seville (sour) orange juice—but not regular orange juice—have the same effect on the liver's ability to metabolize using enzymes. Each of ten people who volunteered for Watkins' juice-medicine study took a standard dose of felodopine (Plendil), a drug used to treat high blood pressure, diluted in grapefruit juice, sour orange juice, or plain orange juice. The researchers measured blood levels of Plendil at various times afterward. The team observed that both grapefruit juice and sour orange juice increased blood levels of Plendil, as if the people had received a higher dose. Regular orange juice had no effect. Watkins and his coworkers have found that a chemical common to grapefruit and sour oranges, dihydroxybergamottin, is likely the molecular culprit. Thus, when taking medications that use the CYP3A4 enzyme to metabolize, patients are advised to avoid grapefruit juice and sour orange juice.[19]

1.6   EXCRETION

Excretion is the final stage of a medication interaction within the body. The body has absorbed, distributed, and metabolized the medication molecules—now what does it do with the leftovers? Remaining parent drugs and metabolites in the bloodstream are often filtered by the kidney, where a portion undergoes reabsorption back into the bloodstream, and the remainder is excreted in the urine. The liver also excretes byproducts and waste into the bile. Another potential route of excretion is the lungs. For example, drugs like alcohol and the anesthetic gases are often eliminated by the lungs.[20]

Critical Thinking Activity

When providing care for a patient who has chronic kidney disease, how does this disease impact medication excretion?

Note: Answers to the Critical Thinking activities can be found in the "Answer Key" sections at the end of the book.

Routes of Excretion

Now let's further discuss the various routes of excretion from the body.

Kidney

The most common route of excretion is the kidney. As the kidneys filter blood, the majority of drug byproducts and waste are excreted in the urine. The rate of excretion can be estimated by taking into consideration several factors: age, weight, biological sex, and kidney function. Kidney function is measured by lab values such as serum creatinine, glomerular filtration rate (GFR), and creatinine clearance. If a patient's kidney function is decreased, then their ability to excrete medication is affected and drug dosages must be altered for safe administration.

Liver

As the liver filters blood, some drugs and their metabolites are actively transported by the hepatocytes (liver cells) to bile. Bile moves through the bile ducts to the gallbladder and then on to the small intestine. During this process, some drugs may be partially absorbed by the intestine back into the bloodstream. Other drugs are biotransformed (metabolized) by intestinal bacteria and reabsorbed. Unabsorbed drugs and byproducts/metabolites are excreted via the feces. If a patient is experiencing decreased liver function, their ability to excrete medication is affected and drug dosages must be decreased. Lab studies used to estimate liver function are called liver function tests and include measurement of the ALT and AST enzymes that the body releases in response to damage or disease.

Other Routes to Consider

Sweat, tears, reproductive fluids (such as seminal fluid), and breast milk can also contain drugs and byproducts/metabolites of drugs. This can pose a toxic threat, such as the exposure of an infant to breast milk containing drugs

---

20   This work is a derivative of *Principles of Pharmacology* by Libre Texts licensed under CC BY-NC-SA 4.0.

or byproducts of drugs ingested by the mother. Therefore, it is vital to check all medications with a healthcare provider before administering them to a mother who is breastfeeding.[21]

Putting It All Together . . .

Prescribing and administering medications in a safe manner to patients is challenging and requires a team effort by pharmacists, healthcare providers, and nurses. In addition to the factors described in this chapter, there are many other considerations for safe medication administration that are further explained in the "Legal/Ethical" chapter.

Life Span Considerations

Neonate and Pediatrics: Young patients have immature kidneys with decreased glomerular filtration, resorption, and tubular secretion. As a result, they do not clear medications as efficiently from the body. Dosing for most medications used to treat infants and pediatric patients is commonly based on weight in kilograms, and a smaller dose is usually prescribed. In addition, pediatric patients may have higher levels of free circulating medication than anticipated and may become toxic quickly. Therefore, frequent assessment of infants and children is vital for early identification of drug toxicity.[22]

Older Adult: Kidney and liver function often decrease with age, which can lead to decreased excretion of medications. Subsequently, medication may have a prolonged half-life with a greater potential for toxicity due to elevated circulating drug levels. Smaller doses of medications are often recommended for older patients due to these factors, which is commonly referred to as "Start low and go slow."[23]

Interactive Activity

 An interactive or media element has been excluded from this version of the text. You can view it online here: https://wtcs.pressbooks.pub/pharmacology/?p=199

---

21 This work is a derivative of *Principles of Pharmacology* by Libre Texts licensed under CC BY-NC-SA 4.0.

22 Fernandez, E., Perez, R., Hernandez, A., Tejada, P., Arteta, M., and Ramos, J. T. (2011). Factors and mechanisms for pharmacokinetic differences between pediatric population and adults. *Pharmaceutics*, 3(1), 53–72. https://doi.org/10.3390/pharmaceutics3010053.

23 Fernandez, E., Perez, R., Hernandez, A., Tejada, P., Arteta, M., and Ramos, J. T. (2011). Factors and mechanisms for pharmacokinetic differences between pediatric population and adults. *Pharmaceutics*, 3(1), 53–72. https://doi.org/10.3390/pharmaceutics3010053.

1.7   PHARMACODYNAMICS

Complex Interactions

So far, we have learned the importance of pharmacokinetics in describing how the body absorbs, moves, processes, and eliminates a medication. Now let's consider a drug's impact on the body, a series of complex interactions known as **pharmacodynamics**.

When considering how the cells of the body respond to medications, it is important to remember that the majority of drugs bind to specific receptors on the surface or interior of cells. However, there are many other cellular components and non-specific sites that can serve as receptor sites where drugs can bind to create a response. For example, did you know that an osmotic laxative like magnesium citrate attracts and binds with water? This medication works to pull water content into the bowel and increases the likelihood of a bowel movement.

Other medications may inhibit specific enzyme binding sites in order to impact the functionality of a cell or tissue. For example, antimicrobial and antineoplastic drugs commonly work by inhibiting enzymes that are critical to the function of the cell. With blockage of the enzyme binding site, the cell microbe or neoplastic cell is no longer viable and cell death occurs.

Agonist and Antagonist Actions

Understanding the **mechanism of action**,[24] or how a medication functions within the body, is essential to understanding the processes medications go through to produce the desired effect (see Figure 1.6). Drugs have agonistic or antagonistic effects. A drug **agonist** binds tightly to a receptor to produce a desired effect. A drug **antagonist** competes with other molecules and blocks a specification or response at a receptor site. For example, the cardiac medication atenolol (Tenormin) is a Beta-1 receptor antagonist used to treat patients with hypertension or heart disease. Beta-1 receptor antagonist medications like atenolol produce several effects by blocking Beta-1 receptors: a negative inotropic effect occurs by weakening the contraction of the heart, thus causing less work oft he heart muscle;a negative chronotropic effect occurs when the heart rate is decreased; and a negative dromotropic effect occurs when the conduction oft he electrical charge in the heart is slowed. Understanding the effects of a Beta-1 antagonist medication allows the nurse to anticipate expected actions of the medication and the patient response. Agonistic and antagonistic effects on receptors are further discussed in the "Autonomic Nervous System" chapter.[25]

---

24   "Mechanism of Action" by Dominic Slausen at Chippewa Valley Technical College is licensed under CCBY 4.0.

25   This work is a derivative of *Principles of Pharmacology* by Libre Texts licensed under CC BY-NC-SA 4.0.

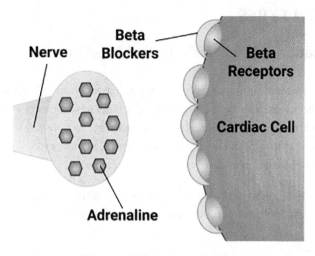

Figure 1.6 Mechanism of Action

Critical Thinking Activity

Atenolol (Tenormin) is a beta-1 antagonist with a negative inotropic and chronotropic effects. What should a nurse assess before administration?

Note: Answers to the Critical Thinking activities can be found in the "Answer Key" sections at the end of the book.

1.8   MEDICATION TYPES

Prescription Medications, OTCs, Herbals, and Supplements

There are a variety of drug types and substances patients may utilize for symptom management or to enhance wellness. Having an accurate record and knowledge of the different types of substances a patient is taking is important to the patient's medical and nursing plan of care. It is also important to note any substances that are prescribed, over-the-counter, or herbal that have been taken in the past month, as some medications have a long half-life and still be in the body with the potential to interact with new medications.

A variety of substances available to the public include (but are not limited to) prescription medications (including brand name and generic drugs), over-the-counter medications, and herbals and supplements.

Prescription Medications

Drugs are prescribed by a licensed prescriber for a specific person's use and regulated through the United States Food and Drug Administration (FDA). More information about FDA approval of medications is described in the "Legal/Ethical" chapter. Prescription medications include brand-name medications and generic medications.[26]

Generic Medications

Generic medications can be safe and effective alternatives to their brand-name counterparts and often at a reduced cost. By FDA law, generic medications must have the same chemically active ingredient in the same dose (i.e., they must be "bio-equivalent"). However, the excipients (the base substance that holds the active chemical ingredient into a pill form (such as talc) or the flavoring can be different. Some patients do not tolerate these differences in excipients very well. When prescribing a medication, the provider must indicate that a generic substitution is acceptable. Nurses are often pivotal in completing insurance paperwork on the patient's behalf if the brand-name medication is more effective or better tolerated by that particular patient. When studying medications in nursing school, it is important to know medications by their generic name, since the NCLEX exam does not currently include brand-name medications in their question format.[27]

Over-the-Counter Medications

Over-the-counter (OTC) medications do not require a prescription. They can be bought at a store and may be used by multiple individuals. OTC medications are also regulated through the FDA. Some prescription medications are available for purchase as OTC in smaller doses. For example, diphenhydramine (Benadryl) is commonly prescribed as 50 mg every 6 hours, and the prescription strength is 50 mg. However, it can also be purchased OTC in 25 mg doses (or less for children.)[28]

---

26   U.S. Food and Drug Administration. (2017, Nov. 13). *Prescription drug and over the counter drugs: Questions and answers.* https://www.fda.gov/drugs/questions-answers/prescription-drugs-and-over-counter-otc-drugs-questions-and-answers.

27   U.S. Food and Drug Administration. (2018, Jun. 19). *Patient education.* https://www.fda.gov/drugs/generic-drugs/patient-education.

28   U.S. Food and Drug Administration. (2017, Nov. 13). *Prescription drug and over the counter drugs: Questions and answers.* https://www.fda.gov/drugs/questions-answers/prescription-drugs-and-over-counter-otc-drugs-questions-and-answers.

Herbals and Supplements

Herbs and supplements may include a wide variety of substances including vitamins, minerals, enzymes, and botanicals. Supplements such as "protein powders" are marketed to build muscle mass and can contain a variety of substances that may not be appropriate for all individuals. These herbal and supplement substances are not regulated by the FDA and most have not undergone rigorous scientific testing for safety for the public. While patients may be tempted to try these herbals and supplements, there is no guarantee that they contain the ingredients listed on the label. It is also important to remember that there is a potential for adverse effects or even overdose if the herbal or supplement contains some of the same drug that was also prescribed to a patient.[29]

---

29 U.S. Food and Drug Administration. (2017, Nov. 13). *What are dietary supplements?* https://www.fda.gov/food/information-consumers-using-dietary-supplements/tips-older-dietary-supplement-users#what.

1.9   EXAMINING EFFECT

Onset, Peak, and Duration

Dosing considerations play an important role in understanding the effect that a medication may have on a patient. During administration, the nurse must pay close attention to the desired effect and therapeutic patient response, as well as the safe dose range for any medication. The nurse should have an understanding of medication **efficacy** in order to ensure its appropriateness. If a nurse is provided different medication choices according to a provider's written protocol, the nurse should select the option with the anticipated desired therapeutic response. Additionally, the nurse must be aware of the overall **dose-response** based on the dosage selected.

Three additional principles related to the effect of a medication on a patient are onset, peak, and duration.

Onset: the onset of medication refers to when the medication first begins to take effect.

Peak: the peak of medication refers to the maximum concentration of medication in the body, and the patient shows evidence of greatest therapeutic effect.

Duration: the duration of medication refers to the length of time the medication produces its desired therapeutic effect.

Consider this patient care example and apply the principles of onset, peak, and duration: A 67-year-old female post-operative patient rings the call light to request medication for pain related to the hip replacement procedure she had earlier that day. She notes her pain is "excruciating, a definite 9 out of 10." Her brow is furrowed, and she is grimacing in obvious discomfort. As the nurse providing care for the patient, you examine her post-operative medication orders and consider the pain medication options available to you. In reviewing the various options, it is important to consider how quickly a medication will work (onset), when the medication will reach maximum effectiveness (peak), and how long the pain relief will last (duration). Understanding these principles is important in effectively relieving the patient's pain and constructing an overall plan of care.

Critical Thinking Activities

1. At 0500, your patient who had a total knee replacement yesterday rates his pain while walking as 7 out of 10. Physical therapy is scheduled at 0900. The patient has acetaminophen (Tylenol) 625 mg ordered every four hours as needed for discomfort. What should you consider in relation to the administration and timing of the patient's pain medication?

2. Your patient is prescribed NPH insulin to be given at breakfast and supper. As a student nurse, you know that insulin is used to decrease blood sugar levels in patients with diabetes mellitus. During report, you hear that the patient has been ill with GI upset during the night, and the nursing assistant just informed you he refused his breakfast tray. While reviewing this medication order, you consider the purpose of the medication and information related to the medication's onset, peak, and duration. When reviewing the drug reference, you find the NPH insulin has an onset of about 1–3 hours after medication administration. What should you consider in relation to the administration and timing of the patient's insulin?

Note: Answers to the Critical Thinking activities can be found in the "Answer Key" sections at the end of the book.

Duration and Dosing

Now let's consider the implication of duration and dosing. Remember the duration of medication is correlated with the elimination. If a medication has a short half-life (and thus eliminated more quickly from the body), the therapeutic effect is shorter. These medications may require repeated dosing throughout the day in order to achieve steady blood levels of active free drug and a sustained therapeutic effect. Other medications have a longer half-life (and thus longer therapeutic duration) and are only given once or twice per day. For example, oxycondone immediate release is prescribed every 4 to 6 hours for the therapeutic effect of immediate relief of severe pain, whereas oxycodone ER (extended release) is prescribed every 12 hours for the therapeutic effect of sustained relief of severe pain.

1.10 MEDICATION SAFETY

Now that the basic concepts of medication onset, peak, and duration have been discussed, it is important to understand the value of the therapeutic window and therapeutic index in medication administration.

Therapeutic Window

For every drug, there exists a dose that is minimally effective (the Effective Concentration) and another dose that is toxic (the Toxic Concentration). Between these doses is the **therapeutic window**, where the safest and most effective treatment will occur (see Figure 1.7).[30] Think of this area as the dosing "sweet spot."

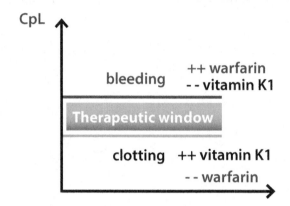

Figure 1.7 Therapeutic Window

For example, warfarin (Coumadin) is a medication used to prevent blood clotting and is monitored using a blood test called INR. Too high of a dose of warfarin would cause the INR to increase above the therapeutic window and put the patient at risk of bleeding. Conversely, too low of a dose of warfarin would cause the INR to be below the therapeutic window and put the patient at risk of clotting. It is vital that the nurse frequently monitors INR levels for a patient receiving warfarin to ensure the dosage appropriately reaches the therapeutic window and does not place the patient at risk for bleeding or clotting.

Peak and Trough Levels

Now let's apply the idea of therapeutic window to the administration of medications requiring the monitoring of peak and trough levels, which is required in the administration of some IV antibiotics. It is important for the dosage of these medications to be **titrated** to achieve a desired therapeutic effect for the patient. Titration is often accomplished by closely monitoring the blood levels of the medication. A drug is said to be within the "therapeutic window" when the serum blood levels of an active drug remain consistently above the level of effective concentration (so that the medication is achieving its desired therapeutic effect) and consistently below the toxic level (so that no toxic effects are occurring). A **peak** drug level is drawn at the time when the medication is being administered and is known to be at the highest level in the bloodstream. A **trough** level is drawn when the drug is at its lowest in the bloodstream right before the next dose is given. Medications have a predicted reference range of normal values for peak and trough levels. These numbers assist the pharmacist and provider in gauging how the

---

30   "Therapeutic Window" by Shefaa Alasfoor is licensed under CCBY-SA 3.0.

body is metabolizing, protein-binding, and excreting the drug, and assist in the adjustment of the prescribed drug doses to keep the medication within the therapeutic window. When administering IV medications that require peak or trough levels, it is vital for the nurse to time the administration of the medication according to the timing of these blood draws.[31]

Therapeutic Index

Therapeutic Index is a quantitative measurement of the relative safety of a drug. It is a comparison of the amount of drug that produces a therapeutic effect versus the amount of drug that produces a toxic effect.

- A large (or high) therapeutic index number means there is a large therapeutic window between the effective concentration and the toxic concentration of a medication, so the drug is relatively safe.

- A small (or low) therapeutic index number means there is a small therapeutic window between the effective concentration and the toxic concentration. A drug with a narrow therapeutic range (i.e., having little difference between toxic and therapeutic doses) often has the dosage titrated according to measurements of the actual blood levels of the person taking it. For example, patients who start taking phenytoin to control seizures have the drug levels in their blood stream measured frequently.

Critical Thinking Activity

Mr. Parker has been receiving gentamicin 80 mg IV three times daily to treat his infective endocarditis. He has his gentamicin level checked one hour after the end of his previous gentamicin infusion was completed. The result is 30 mcg/ml. Access the link below to determine the nurse's course of action.

View information on Therapeutic Drug Levels (Within the activity link, be sure to select "click to keep reading" in order to view drugs that are commonly checked, their target levels,and what abnormal results mean).

Based on the results in the above patient scenario, what action will the nurse take based on the result of the gentamicin level of 30 mcg/ml?

Note: Answers to the Critical Thinking activities can be found in the "Answer Key" sections at the end of the book.

---

31   This work is a derivative of *Principles of Pharmacology* by Libre Texts licensed under CC BY-NC-SA 4.0.a.

1.11 PREPARING FOR ADMINISTRATION

Monitoring the Effects

As medications are administered, the nurse should perform careful patient assessments, trend the assessment results, and monitor for side effects or toxic adverse effects. Drug dosages should be evaluated for potency in action. **Potency** refers to the amount of the drug required to produce the desired effect. A drug that is highly potent may require only a minimal dose to produce a desired therapeutic effect, whereas a drug that has low potency may need to be given at much higher concentrations to produce the same effect. Consider the example of opioid versus non-opioid medications for pain control. Opioid medications often have a much higher potency in smaller doses to produce pain relief; therefore, the overall dose required to produce a therapeutic effect maybe much less than for other analgesics.

The nurse preparing to administer medications must also be cognizant of drugs electivity and monitor for potential side effects and adverse effects. The **selectivity** of a drug refers to how readily the drug targets specific cells to produce an intended therapeutic effect. Drugs that are selective will search out target sites to create a drug action, whereas non-selective drugs may impact many different types of cells and tissues, thus potentially causing side effects. A **side effect** occurs when the drug produces effects other than the intended effect. A side effect, although often undesirable, is generally anticipated by the provider and is a known unintended consequence of the medication therapy. Conversely, there are occasional occurrences of unanticipated effects that are dangerous to the patient. These dangerous occurrences are known as **adverse effects**. Adverse effects are relatively unpredictable, severe, and are reason to discontinue the medication.[32]

---

32 This work is a derivative of *Principles of Pharmacology* by Libre Texts licensed under CC BY-NC-SA 4.0.

1.12   MODULE LEARNING ACTIVITIES

Within this unit, you have been introduced to many concepts related to pharmacokinetics and pharmacodynamics. These basic concepts are important to understand as we move our study into closer examination of various medication classes, principles of administration, and consideration of how medications can be safely incorporated into the patient's plan of care.

> *Interactive Activity*
>
> An interactive or media element has been excluded from this version of the text. You can view it online here: https://wtcs.pressbooks.pub/pharmacology/?p=237

Light Bulb Moment

Test your knowledge and application. Use the information in the text above, as well as the link to the *Daily Med* resource, to read more about the medications included in the patient scenarios. Additional pharmacokinetics information can be found under the "Clinical Pharmacology" section of each drug in *Daily Med*.

1. You are working in a nursing home caring for an 86-year-old stroke patient who complains of left knee pain secondary to arthritis. The patient has right-sided weakness and difficulty swallowing with no gag reflex. You review the patient's MAR, and note the provider has prescribed acetaminophen 325 mg either per oral or per rectal route. Which route would you choose and why?

2. Mr. Johnson is a 92-year-old male admitted to the medical-surgical unit for severe pneumonia, and the provider prescribed gentamicin antibiotic therapy. Upon review of the order, you notice the initial dose is ordered at less than the standard recommended dose. What is the rationale behind the decreased starting gentamicin dose for this patient?

3. Sara is a nurse working on the medical-surgical floor. She is reviewing her patient's chart and notes her patient has a 0600 vancomycin infusion; however, the trough level is not available. The nurse phones the lab, and they state they will not be available to draw the trough level for an hour. What actions should the nurse take?

4. Sam is a nurse working on the cardiology floor. He has an order to administer a dose of atenolol (a beta-blocker medication) to a patient at 0800. What actions should the nurse take prior to administering the medication? What is the anticipated therapeutic effect of this medication?

5. Julia is a 56-year-old patient admitted to the cardiology unit with new-onset atrial fibrillation. She has been prescribed amiodarone for her irregular heartbeat and is set to receive her first dose with her morning breakfast tray. When you arrive in the room, you notice that she has grapefruit juice on her breakfast meal tray. Is this a concern? Why? What is the nurse's next action?

6. A nurse is caring for a 55-year-old male who recently was admitted to the medical-surgical unit for a total knee replacement. He is prescribed hydrocodone/acetaminophen 5/325 mg (Norco) every 6 hours for moderate

My Notes

pain. The patient complains of pain in the knee, rating it at a "6." Review the "Clinical Pharmacology" section for this medication using the *Daily Med* link, and answer the following questions:

- When does the nurse anticipate the medication will peak in action?
- When does the nurse anticipate another dose will be needed due to the half-life of this drug?

Note: Answers to the light bulb moments can be found in the "Answer Key" sections at the end of the book.

Glossary

Absorption: The first stage of pharmacokinetics: medications enter the body and travel from site of administration into the body's circulation.

Adverse Effect: An unintended and potentially dangerous pharmacological effect that occurs when a medication is administered correctly.

Affinity: The strength of binding between drug and receptor.

Agonist: A drug that binds to a "receptor" and produces an effect.

Antagonist: A molecule that prevents the action of other molecules, often by competing for a cellular receptor; opposite of agonist.

Bioavailability: The presence of a drug in the bloodstream after it is administered.

Blood-Brain Barrier: A nearly impenetrable barricade that is built from a tightly woven mesh of capillaries cemented together to protect the brain from potentially dangerous substances such as poisons or viruses.

Distribution: The second stage of pharmacokinetics; the process by which medication is distributed throughout the body.

Dose-Response: As the dose of a drug increases, the response should also increase. The slope of the curve is characteristic of the particular drug-receptor interaction.

Duration: The length of time that a medication is producing its desired therapeutic effect.

Efficacy: The maximum effect of which the drug is capable.

Excretion: The final stage of pharmacokinetics; the process whereby drug byproducts and metabolites are eliminated from the body.

First Pass Effect: The inactivation of orally or enterally administered drugs in the liver and intestines.

Mechanism of Action: How a medication works at a cellular level within the body.

Metabolism: The break down of a drug molecule via enzymes in the liver (primarily) or intestines (secondarily).

Onset: When a medication first begins to work and exerts a therapeutic effect.

Peak: When the maximum concentration of a drug is in the bloodstream.

Pharmacodynamics: The study of how drugs act at target sites of action in the body.

Pharmacogenetics: The study of how a person's genetic make-up affects their response to medicines.

Pharmacokinetics: The study of how the body absorbs, distributes, metabolizes, and eliminates drugs.

Pharmacology: The science dealing with actions of drugs on the body.

Pharmacy: The science of the preparation of drugs.

Potency: The drug dose required to produce a specific intensity of effect.

Selectivity: A "selective" drug binds to a primary and predictable site creating one desired effect. A "non-selective" drug can bind to many different and unpredictable receptor sites with potential side effects.

Side Effect: Effect of a drug, other than the desired effect, sometimes in an organ other than the target organ.

Therapeutic Index: A quantitative measurement of the relative safety of a drug that compares the amount of drug that produces a therapeutic effect versus the amount of drug that produces a toxic effect. Medication with a large therapeutic index is safer than a medication with a small therapeutic index.

Therapeutic Window: The dosing window in which the safest and most effective treatment will occur.

Chapter II

Legal/Ethical

2.1   LEGAL/ETHICAL INTRODUCTION

Learning Objectives

- Identify drug administration guidelines within the State Nurse Practice Act

- Identify nursing responsibilities to prevent and respond to medication errors

- Identify nursing responsibilities associated with controlled substances

- Identify ethical responsibilities as they relate to medication errors

- Explain how nursing response reflects respect for a patient's rights and responsibilities with drug therapy

- Outline nursing actions within the scope of nursing practice as they relate to the administration of medication

- Demonstrate patient-centered care during medication administration by respecting a patient's gender and psychosocial and cultural needs

- Identify nursing responsibilities associated with safe medication administration

- Identify nursing responsibilities associated with patient medication education

Medication administration is an essential task nurses perform while providing patient care. However, safe medication administration is more than just a nursing task; it is a process involving several members of the health care team, as well as legal, ethical, social, and cultural issues. The primary focus of effective medication administration by all health professionals is patient safety. Although many measures have been put into place over the past few decades to promote improved patient safety, medication errors, and adverse effects continue to be a common event. The World Health Organization (WHO) estimates, "Unsafe medication practices and medication errors are a leading cause of injury and avoidable harm in health care systems across the world. Globally, the cost associated with medication errors has been estimated at $42 billion USD annually."[1] This chapter will examine the legal and ethical foundations of medication administration by nurses, as well as the practice standards and cultural and social issues that must be considered to ensure safe and effective administration of medication.

---

1   World Health Organization. (2019). *Patient safety.* https://www.who.int/patientsafety/medication-safety/en/.

2.2 ETHICAL AND PROFESSIONAL FOUNDATIONS OF SAFE MEDICATION ADMINISTRATION BY NURSES

ANA Code of Ethics for Nurses

The **American Nurses Association (ANA)** is a professional organization that represents the interests of the nation's 4 million registered nurses and is at the forefront of improving the quality of health care for all. The ANA developed the **Code of Ethics for Nurses** as a guide for carrying out nursing responsibilities in a manner consistent with quality in nursing care and the ethical obligations of the profession.[2] Several provisions from the Code of Ethics impact how nurses should administer medication in an ethical manner. A summary of each provision from the Code of Ethics and how it affects medication administration is outlined below.

- **Provision 1** focuses on respect for human dignity and the right for self-determination: "The nurse practices with compassion and respect for the inherent dignity, worth, and unique attributes of every person."

- **Provision 2** states, "The nurse's primary commitment is to the patient . . ."[3] In health care settings, nurses often experience several competing loyalties, such as to their employer, to the doctor(s), to their supervisor, or to others on the health care team. However, the patient should always receive the primary commitment of the nurse. Additionally, the patient has the right to accept, refuse, or terminate any treatment, including medications.

- **Provision 3** states, "The nurse promotes, advocates for, and protects the rights, health, and safety of the patient . . ."[4] This provision includes a nurse's responsibility to promote a culture of safety for patients. If errors occur, they must be reported, and nurses should ensure responsible disclosure of errors to patients. This also includes proper disclosure of questionable practices, such as **drug diversion** or impaired practice by any professional.

- **Provision 4** involves authority, accountability, and responsibility by a nurse to follow legal requirements, such state practice acts and professional standards of care.

- **Provision 5** includes the responsibility of the nurse to promote health and safety.

- **Provision 6** focuses on virtues that make a nurse a morally good person. For example, nurses are held accountable to use their clinical judgment to avoid causing harm to patients (**maleficence**) and to do good (**beneficence**). When administering medications, nurses should validate the medication is doing more "good" than "harm" (adverse or side effects).

- **Provision 7** focuses on a nurse practicing within the professional standards set forth by their **state nurse practice act**, as well as standards established by professional nursing organizations.

- **Provision 8** explains that a nurse must address the **social determinants of health,** such as poverty, education, safe medication, and healthcare disparities.[5]

---

2   American Nurses Association. (2019). About ANA. https://www.nursingworld.org/ana/about-ana/.

3   American Nurses Association. (2015). Code of ethics for nurses with interpretive statements. https://www.nursingworld.org/coe-view-only.

4   American Nurses Association. (2015). Code of ethics for nurses with interpretive statements. https://www.nursingworld.org/coe-view-only.

5   American Nurses Association. (2015). Code of ethics for nurses with interpretive statements. https://www.nursingworld.org/coe-view-only.

Whenever a nurse provides patient care, the ANA Code of Ethics should be kept in mind.

> ## Critical Thinking Activity
>
> A nurse is preparing to administer medications to a patient. While reviewing the chart, the nurse notices two medications with similar mechanisms of action have been prescribed by two different providers.
>
> What is the nurse's best response?
>
> *Note:* Answers to the Critical Thinking activities can be found in the "Answer Key" sections at the end of the book.

ANA Professional Standards and Scope of Practice

The American Nurses Association (ANA) publishes the *Nursing: Scope and Standards of Practice.* This resource is updated regularly and outlines professional nursing performance according to national standards.[6] The ANA defines **nursing** as "the protection, promotion, and optimization of health and abilities, prevention of illness and injury, facilitation of healing, alleviation of suffering through the diagnosis and treatment of human response, and advocacy in the care of individuals, families, groups, communities, and populations." A **registered nurse (RN)** is defined as an individual who is educationally prepared and licensed by a state to practice as a registered nurse. Nursing practice is characterized by the following tenets:

- Caring and health are central to the practice of the registered nurse.
- Nursing practice is individualized to the unique needs of the healthcare consumer.
- Registered nurses use the nursing process to plan and provide individualized care for healthcare consumers.
- Nurses coordinate care by establishing partnerships to reach a shared goal of delivering safe, quality health care.[7]

State nurse practice acts further define the scope of practice of RNs and Licensed Practical Nurses (LPNs) within each state. The Wisconsin Nurse Practice Act is further discussed in the "Legal Foundations" section.

ANA Standards of Practice

ANA Standards of Practice are authoritative statements of duties that all registered nurses, regardless of role, population, or specialty, are expected to perform competently. **Standards of Practice** include assessment, diagnosis, outcome identification, planning, implementation, and evaluation (ADOPIE) components of providing patient care. Implementation also includes the components of health promotion and health teaching. Medication administration should include all components of ADOPIE.

---

6   American Nurses Association. (2015). *Nursing : scope and standards of practice* (3rd ed.). Available for all Chippewa Valley Technical College students and employees through OneSearch.

7   American Nurses Association. (2015). *Nursing : scope and standards of practice* (3rd ed.). Available for all Chippewa Valley Technical College students and employees through OneSearch.

Health Promotion and Patient Teaching

The ANA standards for patient teaching state, "The registered nurse employs strategies to promote health and a safe environment."[8] Specific behaviors related to patient teaching about medication include:

- Use health promotion and health teaching methods in collaboration with the patient's values, beliefs, health practices, developmental level, learning needs, readiness and ability to learn, language preference, spirituality, culture, and socioeconomic status.

- Provide patients with information about intended effects and potential adverse effects of the plan of care.

- Provide anticipatory guidance to patients to promote health and prevent or reduce the risk of negative health outcomes.[9]

In the book *Preventing Medication Errors* by the Institute of Medicine (2007), additional key actions to include when teaching patients about safe use of their medications are:

- Patients should maintain an active list of all prescription drugs, over-the-counter (OTC) drugs, and dietary supplements they are taking, the reasons for taking them, and any known drug allergies. Every provider involved in the medication-use process for a patient should have access to this list.

- Patients should be provided information about side effects, contraindications, methods for handling adverse reactions, and sources for obtaining additional objective, high-quality information.[10]

ANA Standards of Professional Performance

ANA Standards of Professional Performance describe a competent level of behavior in the professional role, including activities related to ethics, culturally congruent practice, communication, collaboration, leadership, education, evidence-based practice, and quality of practice.[11] Available for all Chippewa Valley Technical College students and employees through OneSearch.

Cultural Congruent Practice

The ANA defines **culturally congruent practice** as the application of evidence-based nursing that is in agreement with the preferred cultural values, beliefs, worldview, and practices of the healthcare consumer and other stakeholders. **Cultural competence** represents the process by which nurses demonstrate culturally congruent practice. Nurses must assess the cultural beliefs and practices of their patients and implement culturally congruent interventions when administering medications and teaching about them.

---

8   American Nurses Association. (2015). *Nursing : scope and standards of practice* (3rd ed.). Available for all Chippewa Valley Technical College students and employees through OneSearch.

9   American Nurses Association. (2015). *Nursing : scope and standards of practice* (3rd ed.). Available for all Chippewa Valley Technical College students and employees through OneSearch.

10   Institute of Medicine. (2007). *Preventing medication errors.* The National Academies Press. https://doi.org/ 10.17226/11623.

11   American Nurses Association. (2015). *Nursing: scope and standards of practice* (3rd ed.).

Additional information about cultural implications for medication administration is further discussed in the "Cultural and Social Determinants Related to Medication Administration" section later in this chapter.

Critical Thinking Activity 2.2b

A nurse is preparing to administer metoprolol, a cardiac medication, to a patient and implements the nursing process:

ASSESSES the vital signs prior to administration and discovers the heart rate is 48.

DIAGNOSES that the heart rate is too low to safely administer the medication per the parameters provided. Establishes the **OUTCOME** to keep the patient's heart rate within normal range of 60-100.

PLANS to call the physician, as well as report this incident in the shift handoff report.

Implements **INTERVENTIONS** by withholding the metoprolol at this time, documenting the incident that the medication is withheld, and notifying the provider.

Continues to **EVALUATE** the patient status throughout the shift after not receiving the metoprolol.

The nurse is providing patient teaching to a patient about the medication before discharge. The nurse provides a handout with instructions, as well as a list of the current medications.

What other information should be provided to the patient?

Note: Answers to the Critical Thinking activities can be found in the "Answer Key" sections at the end of the book.

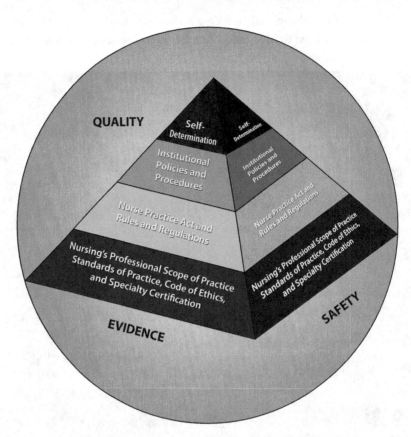

Figure 2.1 ANA Model of Professional Nursing Practice Regulation

Figure 2.1 is an image from *Nursing: Scope and Standards of Practice* by the ANA (2015).[12] It explains how professional scope of practice, standards, and code of ethics are the "base" of nursing practice. Nursing practice is further defined by the State's Nurse Practice Act, rules and regulations, institutional policies and procedures, and self-determination by the individual nurse. All these components are required to provide quality, safe patient care that is evidence-based.

---

12   American Nurses Association. (2015). *Nursing : scope and standards of practice* (3rd ed.) Available for all Chippewa Valley Technical College students and employees through OneSearch.

2.3   LEGAL FOUNDATIONS AND NATIONAL GUIDELINES FOR SAFE MEDICATION ADMINISTRATION

There are many federal and state laws, as well as national guidelines, that have been established to protect public health and safety. This section will explain how the FDA, DEA, Joint Commission, CMS, a State's Nurse Practice Act, State Boards of Nursing, and state legislatures protect the consumer from medication harm.

Food and Drug Administration

To protect the public, the U.S. Food and Drug Administration (FDA) is responsible for protecting the public health by ensuring the safety, efficacy, and security of human and veterinary drugs, biological products, and medical devices; and by ensuring the safety of our nation's food supply, cosmetics, and products that emit radiation.[13] Some of the ways that the FDA protects the public health regarding medications are by enforcing an official drug approval process based on evidence-based research; issuing Black Box Warnings for medications with serious adverse reactions; and regulating over-the-counter (OTC) medications. Each of these actions are further explained below.

Developing New Drugs

American consumers benefit from having access to the safest and most advanced pharmaceutical system in the world. The main consumer watchdog in this system is the FDA's Center for Drug Evaluation and Research (CDER).

The center's best-known job is to evaluate new drugs before they can be sold. CDER's evaluation not only prevents quackery, but also provides doctors and patients the information they need to use medicines wisely. The center ensures that drugs, both brand-name and generic, work correctly and that their health benefits outweigh their known risks.

🔗 Development and Approval Process of Drugs by the FDA

Drug companies conduct extensive research and work to develop and test a drug. The company then sends CDER the evidence from these tests to prove the drug is safe and effective for its intended use. Before the drug is approved as safe for use in the United States, a team of CDER physicians, statisticians, chemists, pharmacologists, and other scientists reviews the company's data and proposed labeling. If this independent and unbiased review establishes a drug's health benefits outweigh its known risks, the drug is approved for sale. Before a drug can be tested in people, the drug company or sponsor performs laboratory and animal tests to discover how the drug works and whether it's likely to be safe and work well in humans. Next, a series of clinical trials involving volunteers is conducted to determine whether the drug is safe when used to treat a disease and whether it provides a real health benefit.

FDA Approval: What it Means

FDA approval of a drug means that data on the drug's effects have been reviewed by CDER, and the drug is determined to provide benefits that outweigh its known and potential risks for the intended population. The drug approval process takes place within a structured framework that includes:

---

13   U.S. Food and Drug Administration. (2019) https://www.fda.gov.

- **Analysis of the target condition and available treatments:** FDA reviewers analyze the condition or illness for which the drug is intended and evaluate the current treatment landscape, which provide the context for weighing the drug's risks and benefits. For example, a drug intended to treat patients with a life-threatening disease for which no other therapy exists may be considered to have benefits that outweigh the risks even if those risks would be considered unacceptable for a condition that is not life threatening.

- **Assessment of benefits and risks from clinical data:** FDA reviewers evaluate clinical benefit and risk information submitted by the drug maker, taking into account any uncertainties that may result from imperfect or incomplete data. Generally, the agency expects that the drug maker will submit results from two well-designed clinical trials to be sure the findings from the first trial are not the result of chance or bias. In certain cases, especially if the disease is rare and multiple trials may not be feasible, convincing evidence from one clinical trial may be enough. Evidence that the drug will benefit the target population should outweigh any risks and uncertainties.

- **Strategies for managing risks:** All drugs have risks. Risk management strategies include an FDA-approved drug label, which clearly describes the drug's benefits and risks and information pertaining to the detection and management of any risks. Sometimes, more effort is needed to manage risks. In these cases, a drug maker may need to implement a Risk Management and Mitigation Strategy (REMS).

Although many of the FDA's risk-benefit assessments and decisions are straightforward, sometimes the benefits and risks are uncertain and may be difficult to interpret or predict. The agency and the drug maker may reach different conclusions after analyzing the same data, or there may be differences of opinion among members of the FDA's review team. As a science-led organization, the FDA uses scientific and technological information to make decisions through a deliberative process.[14]

Black Box Warnings

The Food and Drug Administration (FDA) approves a drug for marketing after determining that the drug's benefits of use outweigh the risks for the condition that the drug will treat. However, even with the rigorous FDA evaluation process, some safety problems surface only after a drug has been on the market and has been used in a broader population. If a safety problem surfaces, **Black Box Warnings** are issued by the FDA and appear on a prescription drug's label. The purpose is to call attention to serious or life-threatening risks.[15]

Critical Thinking Activity 2.3a

Levofloxacin is an antibiotic that received FDA approval. However, after the drug was on the market, it was discovered that some patients who took levofloxacin developed serious, irreversible adverse effects such as tendon rupture. The FDA issued a Black Box Warning with recommendations to reserve levofloxacin

14 U.S. Food and Drug Administration. (2018, June 13). *Developing new drugs.* https://www.fda.gov/drugs/development-approval-process-drugs.

15 U.S. Food and Drug Administration. (2012, November). *Consumer health information.* https://www.fda.gov/ media/74382/download.

for use in patients who have no alternative treatment options for certain indications: uncomplicated UTI, acute exacerbation of chronic bronchitis, and acute bacterial sinusitis.[16]

A nurse is preparing to administer medications to a patient and notices that levofloxacin has been prescribed for the indication of pneumonia. There is no other documentation in the provider's notes related to the use of this medication.

What is the nurse's best response?

Note: Answers to the Critical Thinking activities can be found in the "Answer Key" sections at the end of the book.

U.S. Drug Enforcement Agency (DEA)

The U.S. Drug Enforcement Agency (DEA) enforces the controlled substances laws and regulations of the United States. This includes enforcement of the Controlled Substances Act (CSA) that pertains to the manufacture, distribution, and dispensing of legally produced controlled substances that nurses administer to patients.[17]

Because controlled substances have a greater chance of being misused and abused, there are additional laws and procedures that must be followed when working with these medications. The federal government administers some laws regarding controlled substances. The DEA is responsible for enforcing these laws, and many federal laws are summarized in a document called the *Pharmacist's Manual*.[18] Most controlled substance laws, however, come from the state governments. Health care professionals are responsible for following the most stringent of the two laws, whether it be state law or federal law.

Federal Laws

The following are excerpts of federal laws that are applicable to professional nursing.

Prescriptions: A prescription for a controlled substance may be written only by a provider (physician or mid-level provider like a nurse practitioner) that has a DEA registration number.

A prescription for a Schedule II (most controlled class of medications, like opioids) must be written or electronically sent to the pharmacy through DEA approved software. Prescriptions over the phone or fax are not accepted.

It is then up to state law to decide how long a written Schedule II prescription is valid and if there are any limits on the quantity of medication that can be dispensed.

Refilling a Schedule II medication is not allowed. Schedule III or IV medications may be refilled only 5 times.

Records: There is a "closed system" for record keeping of controlled substances to prevent diversion.

To maintain a "closed system" of record keeping for controlled substances, hospitals, clinics, and pharmacies must maintain records on the whereabouts of the medication from manufacturing the medication, receipt by the pharmacy, distribution to the patient, to disposal of waste. What does this look like in practice? Inventory counts of

---

16   This work is a derivative of *Daily Med* by U.S. National Library of Medicine in the public domain.

17   U.S. Department of Justice - Drug Enforcement Administration. (n.d.). *Drug scheduling.* https://www.dea.gov/.

18   https://www.deadiversion.usdoj.gov/pubs/manuals/pharm2/index.html.

My Notes

controlled medications occur frequently, controlled substance access by individual employees is audited often, detailed records are kept for all transactions, and waste is often disposed of differently than other pharmaceuticals.

Wisconsin State Laws

Prescriptions: A Schedule II prescription is only good for 60 days after it is written.

Pharmacies and practitioners are required to participate in a prescription drug monitoring program when dispensing or prescribing a monitored prescription drug (most often opioid pain medications).

Wisconsin State Law Regarding Controlled Substance[19]

Scheduled Medications

The Controlled Substances Act (CSA) places all substances that are regulated under existing federal law into one of five schedules. This placement is based on the substance's medical use, potential for abuse, and safety or dependence liability. Schedule I drugs have a high potential for abuse and the potential to create severe psychological and/or physical dependence, whereas Schedule V drugs represent the least potential for abuse. An alphabetic listing of drugs and their schedule are located on the DEA website at "CSA Scheduling by Alphabetical Order."[20, 21] Sample medications for each schedule are included in Figure 2.2.[22]

Figure 2.2: Definitions and Sample Medications for Each Type of Scheduled Medication

Schedule	Definition	Examples
Schedule I	No currently accepted medical use and a high potential for abuse.	Heroin, LSD, and marijuana
Schedule II	High potential for abuse, with use potentially leading to severe psychological or physical dependence. These drugs are also considered dangerous.	Vicodin, cocaine, methamphetamine, methadone, hydromorphone (Dilaudid), meperidine (Demerol), oxycodone (OxyContin), fentanyl, Dexedrine, Adderall, and Ritalin
Schedule III	Moderate to low potential for physical and psychological dependence. Abuse potential is less than Schedule I and Schedule II drugs but more than Schedule IV.	Tylenol with codeine, ketamine, anabolic steroids, testosterone
Schedule IV	Low potential for abuse and low risk of dependence.	Xanax, Soma, Valium, Ativan, Talwin, Ambien, Tramadol

19 Wisconsin Administrative Code (2020). Unform Controlled Substances Act. https://docs.legis.wisconsin.gov/code/admin_code/phar/8.pdf.

20 U.S. Department of Justice - Drug Enforcement Administration.(n.d.). *Drug scheduling.*https://www.dea.gov/drug.-scheduling.

21 U.S. Department of Justice - Drug Enforcement Administration.(2019, August 21). *Controlled substances.*https://www..deadiversion.usdoj.gov/schedules/orangebook/c_cs_alpha.pdf.

22 U.S. Department of Justice - Drug Enforcement Administration.(n.d.). Drug scheduling. https://www.dea.gov/.

Schedule V	Lower potential for abuse than Schedule IV and consist of preparations containing limited quantities of certain narcotics. Generally used for antidiarrheal, antitussive, and analgesic purposes.	Robitussin AC with codeine, Lomotil, Lyrica

Drug overdoses are still a public health crisis in the United States, and the misuse of prescription opioids, which are scheduled medications, continue to contribute to a large percentage of overdose deaths. Many problems associated with drug abuse are the result of legitimately made controlled substances being diverted from their lawful purpose into illicit drug traffic. The mission of DEA's Diversion Control Division is to prevent, detect, and investigate the diversion of controlled pharmaceuticals from legitimate sources while ensuring an adequate and uninterrupted supply for legitimate medical, commercial, and scientific needs. The DEA provides education regarding related topics that apply to nurses such as drug diversion, state prescription drug monitoring systems, current drug trends, telemedicine, and proper drug disposal.[23]

Drug Diversion

Drug diversion involves the transfer of any legally prescribed controlled substance from the individual for whom it was prescribed to another person for any illicit use. The most common drugs diverted from the health care facility setting are opioids. Diversion of controlled substances is not uncommon and can result in substantial risk not only to the individual who is diverting the drugs but also to patients, coworkers, and employers. Impaired providers can harm patients by providing substandard care, denying medications to patients, or exposing patients to tainted substances. Tampering is the riskiest and most harmful type of diversion. Commonly, the diverter removes medication from a syringe, vial, or other container and injects himself or herself with the medication. The diverter then replaces the stolen medication with saline or sterile water or another clear medication or liquid. The "replacement liquid" is later used on the patient by an unaware provider. When tampering, the diverter may rarely use sterile technique. Ultimately the patient doesn't receive the required medication and may be exposed to the diverter's blood.[24,25,26]

🔗 DEA at Rx Abuse Online Reporting[27]

23 U.S. Department of Justice - Drug Enforcement Administration.(2019, August 21). *Controlled substances.* https://www.deadiversion.usdoj.gov/schedules/orangebook/c_cs_alpha.pdf.

24 New, K. (2014, June 3). *Drug diversion defined: a patient safety threat.* Centers for Disease Control and Prevention. https://web.archive.org/web/20150716073835/http://blogs.cdc.gov/safehealthcare/2014/06/03/drug-diversion-defined. -a-patient-safety-threat/.

25 Berge, K. H., Dillon, K. R., Sikkink, K. M., Taylor, T. K., and Lanier, W. L. (2012). Diversion of drugs within health care facilities, a multiple-victim crime: patterns of diversion, scope, consequences, detection, and prevention. *Mayo Clinic Proceedings, 87*(7), 674–682. https://www.ncbi.nlm.nih.gov/pubmed/22766087.

26 U.S. Department of Justice - Drug Enforcement Administration. (2019). https://www.deadiversion.usdoj.gov/prog_dscrpt/index.html.

27 U.S. Department of Justice - Drug Enforcement Administration. (n.d.). *RX abuse online reporting: report incident.* https://apps2.deadiversion.usdoj.gov/rxaor/spring/main?execution=e1s1.

The National Council of State Boards of Nursing (NCSBN) created a *Substance Abuse Disorder in Nursing* brochure.

🔖 Substance Abuse Disorder in Nursing Brochure[28]

The brochure states, "Many nurses with substance use disorder (SUD) are unidentified, unreported, untreated, and may continue to practice where their impairment may endanger the lives of their patients. SUD among health care providers also creates significant legal and ethical responsibilities for colleagues who work with these individuals. You have a professional and ethical responsibility to report a colleague's suspected drug use to your nurse manager or supervisor and, in some states or jurisdictions, to the board of nursing. You have a vital role in helping to identify nurses with SUD, so it is necessary for you to be aware of the indicators that may signal that a nurse has a problem.

It can be hard to differentiate between the subtle signs of impairment and stress-related behaviors, but there are three areas to watch: behavior changes, physical signs, and drug diversion. Behavioral changes can include changes or shifts in job performance; absences from the unit for extended periods; frequent trips to the bathroom; arriving late or leaving early; and making an excessive number of mistakes, including medication errors. Behavioral changes can be physical, including subtle changes in appearance that may escalate over time; increasing isolation from colleagues; inappropriate verbal or emotional responses; and diminished alertness, confusion, or memory lapses. When nurses are using drugs and unable to obtain them from a treating health care provider, they may turn to the workplace for access or diversion, often causing narcotic discrepancies, such as incorrect narcotic counts, large amounts of narcotic wastage, numerous corrections of medication records, frequent reports of ineffective pain relief from patients, offers to medicate coworkers' patients for pain, altered verbal or phone medication orders, and variations in controlled substance discrepancies among shifts or days of the week.

The earlier an SUD in a nurse is identified and treatment is started, the sooner patients are protected and the better the chances are of the nurse safely returning to work. You need to acknowledge that health care professionals are not immune to developing an SUD, and you should ignore stereotypes of what a "typical" person with a SUD looks like. It is important for nurses to not only be aware of the warning signs of SUD, but also be cognizant that SUD is a disease that can affect anyone regardless of age, occupation, economic circumstances, ethnic background, or gender. This will help you to identify issues in a coworker or colleague because you will be able to see behaviors and performance without the notion of "nurses wouldn't do that" or "someone like this would never have an SUD." In most states, a nurse may enter a nondisciplinary alternative-to-discipline program, which is designed to refer nurses for evaluation and treatment, monitor the nurse's compliance with treatment and recovery recommendations, monitor abstinence from drug or alcohol use, and monitor the practice upon return to work. You need to acknowledge that health care professionals are not immune to developing an SUD. When a colleague treated for an SUD eventually returns to work, it is important that you help to create a supportive environment that encourages continued recovery.[29]

Prescription Drug Monitoring Programs (PDMP)

In addition to drug diversion programs, prescription drug monitoring programs (PDMP) have been established in several states to address prescription drug abuse, addiction, and diversion. A PDMP is a statewide electronic database that collects designated data on substances dispensed in the state. By providing valuable information about controlled substance prescriptions that are dispensed in the state, it aids healthcare professionals in their

---

28 National Council State Board of Nursing. *Substance Abuse Disorder in Nursing brochure.* https://www.ncsbn.org/SUD_Brochure_2014.pdf.

29 National Council of State Boards of Nursing (NCSBN). (2018, July). *A nurse's guide to substance use disorder in nursing.* https://www.ncsbn.org/SUD_Brochure_2014.pdf.

prescribing and dispensing decisions. The PDMP also fosters the ability of pharmacies, healthcare professionals, law enforcement agencies, and public health officials to work together to reduce the misuse, abuse, and diversion of prescribed controlled substance medications.[30]

🔗 Wisconsin Prescription Drug Monitoring Program[31]

Proper Drug Disposal

The Secure and Responsible Drug Disposal Act of 2010 allows users to dispose of controlled substances in a safe and effective manner. A Johns Hopkins study on sharing of medication found that 60% of people had left-over opioids they hung on to for future use; 20% shared their medications; 8% would likely share with a friend; 14% would likely share with a relative; and only 10% securely locked their medication.[32] This act has resulted in "National Take Back Days" in all 50 states, as well as new collection receptacles.[33] Nurses should teach patients who are prescribed controlled substances how to dispose of them properly so that they don't end up being abused or overdosed by another person. Figure 2.3[34] shows an example of a controlled substances collection receptacle to prevent drug diversion.[35]

---

30   U.S. Department of Justice - Drug Enforcement Administration. (2016, June 2). *State prescription drug monitoring programs.* https://www.deadiversion.usdoj.gov/faq/rx_monitor.htm.

31   Wisconsin ePDMP. (2019). https://pdmp.wi.gov/.

32   U.S. Department of Justice - Drug Enforcement Administration. (2017, December 13). *Federal regulations and the disposal of controlled substances.* https://www.deadiversion.usdoj.gov/mtgs/drug_chemical/2017/wingert.pdf#search=drug%20disposal.

33   U.S. Department of Justice - Drug Enforcement Administration. (2017, December 13). *Federal regulations and the disposal of controlled substances.* https://www.deadiversion.usdoj.gov/mtgs/drug_chemical/2017/wingert.pdf#search=drug%20disposal.

34   "MedRx box.JPG" by York Police is licensed under CC0.

35   U.S. Department of Justice - Drug Enforcement Administration. (2017, December 13). *Federal regulations and the disposal of controlled substances.* https://www.deadiversion.usdoj.gov/mtgs/drug_chemical/2017/wingert.pdf#search=drug%20disposal.

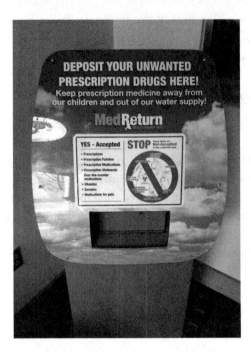

Figure 2.3 Controlled Substances Collection Receptacle to help prevent drug diversion

Critical Thinking Activity 2.3b

A nurse is providing discharge education to a patient who recently had surgery and has been prescribed hydrocodone/acetaminophen tablets to take every four hours as needed at home. The nurse explains that when the medication is no longer needed when the post-op pain subsides, it should be dropped off at a local pharmacy for disposal in a collection receptacle. The patient states, "I don't like to throw anything away. I usually keep unused medication in case another family member needs it."

1. What is the nurse's best response?

A nurse begins a new job on a medical surgical unit. One of the charge nurses on this unit is highly regarded by her colleagues and appears to provide excellent care to her patients. The new nurse cares for a patient that the charge nurse cared for on the previous shift. The new nurse asks the patient about the effectiveness of the pain medication documented as provided by the charge nurse during the previous shift. The patient states, "I didn't receive any pain medication during the last shift." The nurse mentions this incident to a preceptor who states, "I have noticed the same types of incidents have occurred with previous patients, but didn't want to say anything."

2. What is the new nurse's best response?

Note: Answers to the Critical Thinking activities can be found in the "Answer Key" sections at the end of the book.

Joint Commission

The **Joint Commission** is a national organization that accredits and certifies over 20,000 health care organizations in the United States. The mission of the Joint Commission is to continuously improve health care for the public by inspiring health care organizations to excel in providing safe and effective care of the highest quality and value.[36] Some of the initiatives that the Joint Commission supports for promoting the safe use of medications include the development of a Safety Culture and associated root cause analyses, the Speak Up Campaign, National Patient Safety Goals, and a Do Not Use List of Abbreviations. Each of these initiatives is further explained below.

Joint Commission Do Not Use List of Abbreviations

Safety Culture

The Joint Commission Center for Transforming Healthcare develops effective solutions for health care's most critical safety and quality problems with a goal to ultimately achieve zero harm to patients. Some of the projects the Center have developed include improved hand hygiene,[37] effective handoff communications,[38] and safe and effective use of insulin.[39]

The Center has also been instrumental in creating a focus on a "Safety Culture" in health care organizations. A **safety culture** empowers staff to speak up about risks to patients and to report errors and near misses, all of which drive improvement in patient care and reduce the incident of patient harm. It has been estimated that the average cost of a medical error is $11,366, resulting in approximately $17.1 billion in costs in 2008. According to the Institute of Medicine, "The biggest challenge to moving toward a safer health system is changing the culture from one of blaming individuals for errors to one in which errors are treated not as personal failures, but as opportunities to improve the system and prevent harm."[40]

Creating A Safety Culture

As a result of the focus on creating a safety culture, whenever a medication error or a "near miss" occurs, nurses should submit an incident report according to their institution's guidelines. The incident report triggers a **root cause analysis** to help identify not only what and how an event occurred, but also why it happened. When investigators are able to determine why an event or failure occurred, they can create workable corrective measures that prevent future errors from occurring.[41]

An example of safety culture in action is from 2006, when three babies died after receiving incorrect heparin doses to flush their vascular access devices. A root cause analysis found that pharmacy technicians accidentally placed

---

36   The Joint Commission. (n.d.). https://www.jointcommission.org/.

37   Joint Commission Center for Transforming Healthcare (2020). *Hand Hygiene.* https://www.centerfortransforminghealthcare.org/improvement-topics/hand-hygiene.

38   Joint Commission Center for Transforming Healthcare (2020.) *Effective Hand-off Communications.* https://www.centerfortransforminghealthcare.org/improvement-topics/hand-off-communications.

39   Joint Commission Center for Transforming Healthcare (2020). *Safe and Effective Use of Insulin.* https://www.centerfortransforminghealthcare.org/improvement-topics/safe-and-effective-use-of-insulin.

40   The Joint Commission. (2014, November). *Facts about the safety culture project.* https://www.centerfortransforminghealthcare.org/-/media/cth/documents/improvement-topics/ cth_sc_fact_sheet.pdf.

41   Patient Safety Network. (2019). *Root cause analysis.* https://psnet.ahrq.gov/primer/root-cause-analysis.

My Notes

vials containing more concentrated heparin (10,000 units/mL) in storage locations in patient care areas designated for less concentrated heparin vials (10 units/mL). Additionally, the heparin vials were similar in appearance, so the nurses did not notice the incorrect dosage until after it was administered. In response to the root cause analysis, the hospital no longer stocks heparin 10 units/mL vials in pediatric units and uses saline to flush all peripheral lines. In the pharmacy, 10,000 units/mL heparin vials were separated from vials containing other strengths. Workable corrective measures were thus implemented to prevent future tragedies from occurring as a result of incorrect doses of heparin.[42]

Speak Up

The goal of the Joint Commission Speak Up™ initiative is to help patients become more informed and involved in their health care to help prevent medication errors. Speak Up™ materials are intended for the public and have been put into a simplified, easy-to-read format to reach a wider audience.[43]

🔗 Joint Commission Patient Speak Up Brochure

National Patient Safety Goals

The **National Patient Safety Goals (NPSG)** were established by the Joint Commission in 2002 to help accredited organizations address specific areas of concern related to patient safety. Annually, the Joint Commission determines the current highest priority patient safety issues with input from practitioners, provider organizations, purchasers, consumer groups, and other stakeholders and develops National Patient Safety Goals.

Use the link below to read more information about the current NPSG for hospitals.[44] Two of the current National Patient Safety Goals relate specifically to medication administration: Patient ID and Use Medicines Safely.

🔗 National Patient Safety Goals for Hospitals[45]

Patient ID

Use at least two ways to identify patients. For example, use the patient's name and date of birth. This is done to make sure that each patient gets the correct medicine and treatment.

Use Medicines Safely

Before a procedure, label medicines that are not labeled. For example, medicines in syringes, cups, and basins should be labeled in the area where medicines and supplies are set up.

Take extra care with patients who take medicines to thin their blood (anticoagulants).

---

42 Institute for Safe Medication Practices. (2007, November 29). *Another heparin error: learning from mistakes so we don't repeat them.* https://www.ismp.org/resources/another-heparin-error-learning-mistakes-so-we- dont-repeat-them.

43 The Joint Commission. (2019). *Speak up: take medication safely.* https://www.jointcommission.org/assets/1/6/ 2019_HAP_NPSGs_final2.pdf.

44 The Joint Commission. (2019). *2019 hospital national patient safety goals.* https://www.jointcommission.org/assets/1/6/2019_HAP_NPSGs_final2.pdf.

45 The Joint Commission. (2019). *2019 hospital national patient safety goals.* https://www.jointcommission.org/assets/1/6/2019_HAP_NPSGs_final2.pdf.

Record and pass along correct information about a patient's medicines. Find out what medicines the patient is taking. Compare those medicines to new medicines given to the patient. Make sure the patient knows which medicines to take when they are at home. Tell the patient it is important to bring their up-to-date list of medicines every time they visit a doctor.

Joint Commission Official Do Not Use List

The Joint Commission maintains an Official Do Not Use List of abbreviations. These abbreviations have been found to commonly cause errors in patient care. Accredited agencies are expected to not use these abbreviations on any written or pre-printed materials.

This list does not currently apply to preprogrammed health information technology systems (i.e., electronic medical records or CPOE systems), but it remains under consideration for the future.[46]

🔎 Official Do Not Use List

CMS: Centers for Medicare and Medicaid Services

The Centers for Medicare & Medicaid Services (CMS) is a federal agency within the United States Department of Health and Human Services (HHS) that administers the Medicare program and works in partnership with state governments to administer Medicaid. The CMS establishes and enforces regulations to protect patient safety in hospitals that receive Medicare and Medicaid funding.[47]

CMS regulations related to medication administration include identifying what should be included in a prescription for the administration of medication, using the "five rights" when administering medications, reporting concerns about a medication order, assessing and monitoring patients receiving medications, and documenting medication administration. Each of these regulations is further discussed below.

Medication Orders

Medications must be administered in response to an order from a practitioner or on the basis of a standing order that is appropriately authenticated subsequently by a practitioner. All practitioner orders for the administration of drugs and biologicals must include at least the following:

- Name of the patient
- Age and weight of the patient to facilitate dose calculation when applicable. Policies and procedures must address weight-based dosing for pediatric patients as well as in other circumstances identified in the hospital's policies. (Note that dose calculations are based on metric weight (kg, or g for newborns)
- Date and time of the order
- Drug name

46   The Joint Commission. (2019, June 28). *Facts about the official "do not use" list of abbreviations.* https://www.jointcommission.org/facts_about_do_not_use_list/.

47   U.S. Department of Health and Human Services, Centers for Medicare and Medicaid Services. (2014). *Memo: requirements for hospital medication administration, particularly intravenous (IV) medications and post- operative care of patients receiving IV opioids.* https://www.cms.gov/Medicare/Provider-Enrollment-and- Certification/SurveyCertificationGenInfo/Downloads/Survey-and-Cert-Letter-14-15.pdf.

My Notes

- Dose, frequency, and route
- Dose calculation requirements, when applicable
- Exact strength or concentration, when applicable
- Quantity and/or duration, when applicable
- Specific instructions for use, when applicable
- Name of the prescriber[48]

Basic Safe Practices for Medication Administration: The Five Rights

CMS states that hospitals' policies and procedures must reflect accepted standards of practice that require the following information is confirmed prior to each administration of medication. This is often referred to as the "five rights" of medication administration practice.[49]

Interactive Activity

 An interactive or media element has been excluded from this version of the text. You can view it online here: https://wtcs.pressbooks.pub/pharmacology/?p=1016

Note: Recent literature has identified up to nine "rights" of medication administration, including Right patient, Right drug, Right route, Right time, Right dose, Right documentation, Right action (appropriate reason), Right form, and Right response. However, there does not (yet) appear to be consensus about expanding beyond the 5 "rights."[50]

Many agencies have implemented bar code medication scanning to improve safety during medication administration. Bar code scanning systems reduce medication errors by electronically verifying the "5 rights" of medication administration. For example, when a nurse scans a bar code on the patient's wristband and on the medication to be administered, the data is delivered to a computer software system where algorithms check various databases and generate real-time warnings or approvals. Research studies have shown that bar code scanning reduces errors resulting from administration of a wrong dose or wrong medication, as well as errors involving medication being given by the wrong route. However, it is important to remember that bar code scanning should be used in addition to performing the five rights of medication administration, not in place of this important safety process. Additionally, nurses should carefully consider their actions when errors occur during the bar code scanning process. Although it may be tempting to quickly dismiss the error and attribute it to a technology glitch, the error

48   U.S. Department of Health and Human Services, Centers for Medicare and Medicaid Services. (2014). *Memo: requirements for hospital medication administration, particularly intravenous (IV) medications and post- operative care of patients receiving IV opioids.* https://www.cms.gov/Medicare/Provider-Enrollment-and- Certification/SurveyCertificationGenInfo/Downloads/Survey-and-Cert-Letter-14-15.pdf.

49   Elliott M, and Liu Y. (2010). The nine rights of medication administration: an overview. *British Journal of Nursing, 19*(5), 300–305.

50   Elliott M, and Liu Y. (2010). The nine rights of medication administration: an overview. *British Journal of Nursing,* 19(5), 300–305.

may have been triggered due to a patient safety concern that requires further follow-up before the medication is administered. It is important for nurses to investigate errors that occur during the bar code scanning process just as they would do if an error is discovered during the traditional five rights of medication process.

Concerns About Medication Orders

CMS encourages hospitals to promote a culture in which it is not only acceptable, but also strongly encouraged, for staff to bring to the attention of the prescribing practitioner questions or concerns they have regarding medication orders.[51]

Assessment/Monitoring of Patients Receiving Medications

CMS states that observing the effects medications have on the patient is part of the multifaceted medication administration process. Patients must be carefully monitored to determine whether the medication results in the therapeutically intended benefit and to allow for early identification of adverse effects and timely initiation of appropriate corrective action. Depending on the medication and route/delivery mode, monitoring may need to include assessment of:

- Clinical and laboratory data to evaluate the efficacy of medication therapy to anticipate or evaluate toxicity and adverse effects. For some medications, including opioids, this may include clinical data such as respiratory status, blood pressure, and oxygenation and carbon dioxide levels.

- Physical signs and clinical symptoms relevant to the patient's medication therapy, such as confusion, agitation, unsteady gait, pruritus, etc.

- Factors contributing to high risk for adverse drug events. Although mistakes may or may not be more common with these drugs, the consequences of errors are often harmful, sometimes fatal, to patients. In addition, certain factors place some patients at greater risk for adverse effects of medication. Factors include, but are not limited to, age, altered liver and kidney function, drug-to-drug interactions, and first-time medication use may contribute to increased risk.

The nurse should consider patient risk factors, as well as the risks inherent in a medication, when determining the type and frequency of monitoring. It is also essential to communicate information regarding patients' medication risk factors and monitoring requirements during hand-offs of the patient to other clinical staff. Adverse patient reactions, such as anaphylaxis or opioid- induced respiratory depression, require timely and appropriate intervention per established protocols and should be reported immediately to the practitioner responsible for the care of the patient. An example of vigilant post-medication administration monitoring would be for post-surgical patient who is receiving pain medication via a patient controlled analgesia (PCA) pump. Narcotic medications are often used to control pain but also have a sedating effect. Patients can become overly sedated and suffer respiratory depression or arrest, which can be fatal. In addition, the patient and/or family members should be educated

---

51   U.S. Department of Health and Human Services, Centers for Medicare and Medicaid Services. (2014). *Memo: requirements for hospital medication administration, particularly intravenous (IV) medications and post- operative care of patients receiving IV opioids.* https://www.cms.gov/Medicare/Provider-Enrollment-and- Certification/SurveyCertificationGenInfo/Downloads/Survey-and-Cert-Letter-14-15.pdf.

to notify nursing staff promptly when there is difficulty breathing or other changes that might be a reaction to medication.[52]

Documentation

CMS regulations require that the documentation record of medication administration contain all practitioners' orders, nursing notes, reports of treatment, medication records, radiology and laboratory reports, vital signs, and other information necessary to monitor the patient's condition. Documentation is expected to occur after actual administration of the medication to the patient; advance documentation is not only inappropriate, but may result in medication errors. Proper documentation of medication administration actions taken and their outcomes is essential for planning and delivering future care of the patient.[53, 54]

Critical Thinking Activity 2.3c

A nurse is preparing to administer morphine, an opioid, to a patient who recently had surgery.

1. Explain the 5 rights that the nurse will check prior to administering this medication to the patient.

2. Outline 3 methods the nurse can confirm patient identification.

3. What should the nurse assess prior to administering this medication to the patient?

4. What should be monitored after administering this medication?

5. What should the nurse teach the patient (and/or family member) about this medication?

6. What information should be included in the shift handoff report about this medication?

Note: Answers to the Critical Thinking activities can be found in the "Answer Key" sections at the end of the book.

---

52   U.S. Department of Health and Human Services, Centers for Medicare and Medicaid Services. (2014). *Memo: requirements for hospital medication administration, particularly intravenous (IV) medications and post- operative care of patients receiving IV opioids.* https://www.cms.gov/Medicare/Provider-Enrollment-and- Certification/SurveyCertificationGenInfo/Downloads/Survey-and-Cert-Letter-14-15.pdf.

53   U.S. Department of Health and Human Services, Centers for Medicare and Medicaid Services. (2014). *Memo: requirements for hospital medication administration, particularly intravenous (IV) medications and postoperative care of patients receiving IV opioids.*https://www.cms.gov/Medicare/Provider-Enrollment-andCertifcation/SurveyCertifcationGenInfo/Downloads/Survey-and-Cert-Letter-14-15.pd.

54   American Society of Health-System Pharmacists (Ed.). (2018). ASHP guidelines on preventing medication errors in hospitals. *American Journal of Health-System Pharmacy, 75,* 1493–1517. https://www.ashp.org/-/media/assets/policy-guidelines/docs/guidelines/preventing-medication-errors-hospitals.ashx.

Wisconsin State Statutes, Nurse Practice Act, and Board of Nursing

In additional to federal laws, national regulations, guidelines, and initiatives, there are state laws that govern nursing. For regulations specific to nursing, the Wisconsin state legislature enacts a Nurse Practice Act and delegates authority to the Wisconsin State Boards of Nursing to enforce the Nursing Practice Act.[55]

The purpose of the Wisconsin Board of Nursing is to protect the public through licensure, education, legislation, and discipline. The Nurse Practice Act (NPA), as stated in Wisconsin Statutes Chapter 440 (Department of Safety and Professional Services) and 441 (Board of Nursing), grants the Board of Nursing the authority to regulate education as well as the licensure and practice of registered nurses (RNs), licensed practical nurses (LPNs), and advanced practice nurse prescribers (APNPs).[56]

It is important for all nurses to understand their scope of practice as outlined in the Nurse Practice Act (NPA) and Wisconsin Board of Nursing Administrative Rules. Each nurse is accountable for the quality of care he or she provides and is expected to practice at the level of education, knowledge, and skill ordinarily expected of one who has completed an approved nursing program. Furthermore, all nurses are expected to recognize the limits of their knowledge and experience and to appropriately address situations that are beyond their competency. Nurses are responsible to be knowledgeable regarding all laws and rules that relate to their nursing practice.

⌕ Wisconsin Board of Nursing[57]

Wisconsin Practice Act: Standards of Practice

The Wisconsin Nurse Practice Act outlines the standards of care provided by a registered nurse (RN), also known as the **Nursing Process**. An RN utilizes the nursing process in the execution of general nursing procedures in the maintenance of health, prevention of illness, or care of the ill. This standard is met through steps of the nursing process, including:

- **Assessment:** The systematic and continual collection and analysis of data about the health status of a patient culminating in the formulation of a nursing diagnosis.

- **Planning:** Development of a nursing plan of care for a patient, which includes goals and priorities derived from the nursing diagnosis.

- **Intervention:** The nursing action to implement the plan of care by directly administering care or by directing and supervising nursing acts delegated to LPNs or less skilled assistants.

- **Evaluation:** The determination of a patient's progress or lack of progress toward goal achievement, which may lead to modification of the nursing diagnosis.[58]

---

55   Wisconsin Department of Safety and Professional Services. (n.d.). *Wisconsin nurse practice act (NPA) course.* https://dsps.wi.gov/Documents/BoardCouncils/NUR/20190110NURAdditionalMaterials.pdf.

56   Wisconsin Department of Safety and Professional Services. (n.d.). *Wisconsin nurse practice act (NPA) course.* https://dsps.wi.gov/Documents/BoardCouncils/NUR/20190110NURAdditionalMaterials.pdf.

57   Wisconsin Department of Safety and Professional Services. (n.d.). *Board of nursing Wisconsin Administrative Code.* https://dsps.wi.gov/Pages/RulesStatutes/Nursing.aspx.

58   Wisconsin Department of Safety and Professional Services. (n.d.). *Wisconsin nurse practice act (NPA) course.* https://dsps.wi.gov/Documents/BoardCouncils/NUR/20190110NURAdditionalMaterials.pdf.

Wisconsin Practice Act: Rules of Conduct

The Wisconsin Nurse Practice Act also outlines Rules of Conduct expected of nurses. Nurses can receive disciplinary action from the Board of Nursing ranging from a reprimand to revocation of their license if they do not follow the Rules of Conduct. It is important for nurses to protect their licenses to maintain current knowledge about expected rules of conduct in each state where they practice nursing. Details regarding rules and conduct and grounds for denying or taking disciplinary action by the Wisconsin Board of Nursing can be found in Chapter N7, "Rules of Conduct."[59, 60]

Chapter N7, "Rules of Conduct," of the Wisconsin Nurse Practice Act.

Common reasons related to medication administration for the Board of Nursing to take disciplinary action against a nursing license include, but are not limited to:

- Noncompliance with federal, jurisdictional, or reporting requirements, including:
  - Practicing beyond the scope of practice.
- Confidentiality, patient privacy, consent, or disclosure violations.
- Fraud, deception or misrepresentation, including:
  - Falsification of patient documentation.
- Unsafe practice or substandard care, including:
  - Failing to perform nursing with reasonable skill and safety.
  - Departing from or failing to conform to the minimal standards of acceptable nursing practice that may create unnecessary risk or danger to a patient's life, health, or safety. Actual injury to a patient need not be established.
  - Failing to report to or leaving a nursing assignment without properly notifying appropriate supervisory personnel and ensuring the safety and welfare of the patient or client.
  - Practicing nursing while under the influence of alcohol, illicit drugs, or while impaired by the use of legitimately prescribed pharmacological agents or medications.
  - Inability to practice safely due to alcohol or other substance use, psychological or physical illness or impairment.
  - Executing an order which the licensee knew or should have known could harm a patient.
- Improper supervision or allowing unlicensed practice.
- Improper prescribing, dispensing, or administering medication or drug-related offenses.[61]

---

59 Wisconsin Department of Safety and Professional Services. (n.d.). *Wisconsin nurse practice act (NPA) course*. https://dsps. wi.gov/Documents/BoardCouncils/NUR/20190110NURAdditionalMaterials.pd.

60 Wisconsin State Legislature. (2016, August). *Chapter N 7 rules of conduct*.https://docs.legis.wisconsin.gov/ code/admin_code/n/7.pdf.

61 Wisconsin Department of Safety and Professional Services. (n.d.). *Wisconsin nurse practice act (NPA) course*. https://dsps. wi.gov/Documents/BoardCouncils/NUR/20190110NURAdditionalMaterials.pdf.

Wisconsin Statutes, Chapter 961: Uniform Controlled Substances Act

The Wisconsin Statutes are a compilation of the general laws of the state of Wisconsin and include chapters related to the regulation of nursing, as well as the Uniform Controlled Substances Act.

✐ Wisconsin Statutes

Chapter 441 defines the Board of Nursing and relates to the Regulation and Licensure of Nursing. Chapter 961 is the Uniform Controlled Substances Act. The Wisconsin legislature finds that the abuse of controlled substances constitutes a serious problem for society. As a partial solution, laws regulating controlled substances have been enacted with penalties. Chapter 961 does not apply to the nondrug use of peyote and mescaline in the bona fide religious ceremonies of the Native American Church. See the link below for more information about the regulations related to Schedule I through V drugs in the State of Wisconsin.[62]

✐ Chapter 961: Uniform Controlled Substances Act

Wisconsin's Enhanced Prescription Drug Monitoring Program (ePDMP)

The ePDMP is a new tool to help combat the ongoing prescription drug abuse epidemic in Wisconsin. By providing valuable information about controlled substance prescriptions that are dispensed in the state, it aids healthcare professionals in their prescribing and dispensing decisions. The ePDMP also fosters the ability of pharmacies, healthcare professionals, law enforcement agencies, and public health officials to work together to reduce the misuse, abuse, and diversion of prescribed controlled substance medications. See the link below to read more information about Wisconsin's ePDMP.[63]

✐ Wisconsin's Enhanced Prescription Drug Monitoring Program (ePDMP)

Wisconsin Department of Safety and Professional Services: Professional Assistance Procedure (PAP)

The Professional Assistance Procedure (PAP) is a voluntary non-disciplinary program to provide support for credentialed professionals with substance abuse disorder who are committed to their own recovery. The goal is to protect the public by promoting early identification of chemically dependent professionals and encouraging rehabilitation. It provides an opportunity for qualified participants to continue practicing, without public discipline, while being monitored and supported in their recovery.

✐ Wisconsin's Professional Assistance Procedure[64]

---

62 Wisconsin State Legislature. (n.d.). *Chapter 961 uniform uncontrolled substances act.* https://docs.legis.wisconsin.gov/statutes/statutes/961.

63 Wisconsin ePDMP. (2019). https://pdmp.wi.gov/.

64 Wisconsin Department of Safety and Professional Services. (n.d.). *Wisconsin nurse practice act (NPA) course.* https://dsps.wi.gov/Documents/BoardCouncils/NUR/20190110NURAdditionalMaterials.pdf.

Critical Thinking Activity 2.3d

A nurse is disciplined by the Wisconsin Board of Nursing for an incident reported by her employer that she arrived at her shift intoxicated. The nurse shares with a nursing colleague, "I love taking care of patients. I worked so hard to obtain my nursing license – I don't want to lose it. I know my drinking has gotten out of control, but I don't know where to turn."

What is the best advice by the nursing colleague for this nurse with a drinking problem?

Note: Answers to the Critical Thinking activities can be found in the "Answer Key" sections at the end of the book.

2.4   CULTURAL AND SOCIAL DETERMINANTS RELATED TO MEDICATION ADMINISTRATION

Critical Thinking Activity

A nurse is providing patient education to a mother regarding a liquid antibiotic prescribed for her child to take at home. The prescription states amoxicillin 250 mg 1 teaspoon (5 ml) every 8 hours for 7 days. After talking with the mother, the nurse realizes the family does not have measuring spoons in their home.

What is the nurse's best response?

Note: Answers to the Critical Thinking activities can be found in the "Answer Key" sections at the end of the book.

In additional to the legal and ethical considerations affecting the safe administration of medication, there are also cultural and social influences that the nurse must consider. The United States has become increasingly diverse in the last century. According to the 2010 U.S. Census, approximately 36 percent of the population belongs to a racial or ethnic minority group. Though health indicators such as life expectancy and infant mortality have improved for most Americans, some minorities experience a disproportionate burden of preventable disease, death, and disability compared with non- minorities.[65]

The American Nurses Association Scope and Standards of Practice states that the need for health care is universal and transcends differences with respect to the culture; values; and preferences of the individual, family, group, community, and population. Diversity characterizes today's healthcare environment, and nursing is responsive to the changing needs of society. To effectively promote meaningful patient outcomes that maximize quality of life across the life span, the ANA states that nurses must embrace diversity and engage in culturally congruent practice. **Culturally congruent practice** is the application of evidence-based nursing that is in agreement with the preferred cultural values, beliefs, worldview, and practices of the healthcare consumer and other stakeholders. **Cultural competence** represents the process by which nurses demonstrate culturally congruent practice.[66]

In addition to cultural beliefs, conditions in the places where people live, learn, work, and play affect a wide range of health risks and outcomes. These conditions are known as social determinants of health (SDOH). Differences in health are striking in communities with poor SDOH such as unstable housing, low income, unsafe neighborhoods, or substandard education. By applying what we know about SDOH, nurses can not only improve an individual's health, but also improve health equity for communities and the population as a whole. Healthy People is a government agency that provides science-based, ten-year national objectives for improving the health of all

---

65   Centers for Disease Control and Prevention. (2018, July 17). *Health equity.* https://www.cdc.gov/minorityhealth/index. html.

66   American Nurses Association. (2015). *Nursing: Scope and Standards of Practice* (3rd edition). Available for all Chippewa Valley Technical College students and employees through OneSearch.

Americans. Healthy People 2020 highlights the importance of addressing SDOH with a goal to "create social and physical environments that promote good health for all" as one of the four overarching goals for the decade.[67, 68]

The U.S. Department of Health and Human Services has also set national standards for Culturally and Linguistically Appropriate Services (CLAS) in health and healthcare. The national CLAS standards are intended to advance health equity, improve quality, and help eliminate health care disparities by "providing effective, equitable, understandable, and respectful quality care and services that are responsive to diverse cultural health beliefs and practices, preferred languages, health literacy, and other communication needs."[69]

The U.S. Department of Health and Human Services (HHS) defines **health literacy** as "the degree to which individuals have the capacity to obtain, process, and understand basic health information needed to make appropriate health decisions. Adequate health literacy may include being able to read and comprehend essential health-related materials such as information on a prescription bottle. A nurse that values health literacy makes it a priority to implement systems and interventions such as visual aids and counseling that increase understanding and thereby advance patient safety.[70]

National CLAS Standards

Examples of Culturally Congruent Practice Related to Medication Therapy

There are several instances when a nurse must assess and accommodate a patient's culture or social determinants of health when administering or teaching about medications. One example was provided above when a nurse should assist a patient to read a prescription bottle and its instructions to advocate for patient safety.

Another example of culturally congruent practice is when a nurse must consider cultural or religious beliefs, such as fasting, when administering medications. For example, a Muslim patient may participate in the Ramadan, which requires 12-hour fasting. A nurse can advocate for the patient and assist in altering the scheduling of medication to accommodate the patient's belief and avoid the risk of treatment failure.

Drug Intake During Ramadan[71]

A third example of culturally congruent practice is considering when a patient's ethnic background may affect their ability to respond to medications. For example, African Americans often require combination therapy to treat hypertension, whereas Asian and Hispanic patients often respond better to lower doses of antidepressants.

---

67   Social Determinants of Health: Know What Affects Health by Centers for Disease Control and Prevention is available in the public domain.

68   Social Determinants of Health by Healthypeople.gov is available in the public domain.

69   U.S. Department of Health and Human Services, Offce of Minority Health. (n.d.). *National standards for culturally and linguistically appropriate services (CLAS) in health and health care.* https://thinkculturalhealth.hhs.gov/assets/pdfs/Enhanced-NationalCLASStandards.pdf.

70   Health Literacy by Healthypeople.gov is available in the public domain.

71   Aadil, N., Houti, I. E., and Moussamih, S. (2004). Drug intake during Ramadan. *BMJ (Clinical research ed.), 329,* 778–782. https://doi.org/10.1136/bmj.329.7469.778.

You can read more about these cultural accommodations at the following article links:

🔗 **Treatment of Hypertension Among African Americans: The Jackson Heart Study**

🔗 **Prescribing Medication for Asians with Mental Disorders**[72, 73]

The US Department of Health and Human Services has created a free module for nurses to learn more about cultural competency.

🔗 **Culturally Competent Nursing Care: A Cornerstone of Caring**

---

72   Harman, J., Walker, E. R., Charbonneau, V., Akylbekova, E. L., Nelson, C., and Wyatt, S. B. (2013). Treatment of hypertension among African Americans: the Jackson heart study. *Journal of Clinical Hypertension, 15*(6), 367–374. https://www.ncbi.nlm.nih.gov/pubmed/23730984.

73   Chen, J. P., Barron, C., Lin, K. M., and Chung, H. (2002). Prescribing medication for Asians with mental disorders. *The Western Journal of Medicine, 176*(4), 271–275.

2.5 PREVENTING MEDICATION ERRORS

When a nurse administers medication, the ultimate goal is to provide patient safety and to prevent harm from medications. However, medical errors and adverse effects of medication therapy continue to be a significant problem in the United States. This section will discuss initiatives established by the Institute of Medicine (IOM), the World Health Organization (WHO), the Institute for Safe Medication Practices (ISMP), and Quality and Safe Education for Nurses (QSEN).

Institute of Medication (IOM)

IOM Report: To Err is Human

The national focus on reducing medical errors has been in place for almost two decades. The Institute of Medicine (IOM) released an initial report in 1999 titled *To Err is Human: Building a Safer Health System*. The report stated that at that time, errors caused between 44,000 and 98,000 deaths every year in American hospitals and over one million injuries. Health care appeared to be far behind other high-risk industries in ensuring basic safety. The IOM report called for a 50% reduction in medical errors over five years. Its goal was to break the cycle of inaction regarding medical errors by advocating a comprehensive approach to improving patient safety. The IOM 1999 report changed the nature of the patient safety conversation from focusing on dispensing blame to improving systems.[74]

IOM: Preventing Medication Errors

Despite the progress made in patient safety since the *To Err is Human* report, medication errors remain extremely common, and the national health care system continues to implement initiatives to prevent error. In 2007, the IOM published a follow-up report titled *Preventing Medication Errors*, reporting that more than 1.5 million Americans are injured every year in American hospitals, and the average hospitalized patient experiences at least one medication error each day. This report emphasized actions that health care systems, providers, funders, and regulators could take to improve medication safety. These recommendations included actions such as having all U.S. prescriptions written and dispensed electronically, promoting widespread use of medication reconciliation, and performing additional research on drug errors and their prevention. The report also emphasized actions that patients can take to prevent medication errors, such as maintaining active medication lists and bringing their medications to appointments for review.[75]

The *Preventing Medication Errors* report included specific actions for nurses to improve medication safety. Figure 2.2 lists these key actions.

---

74 Institute of Medicine. (2000). *To Err Is Human: Building a Safer Health System.* The National Academies Press. https://doi.org/10.17226/9728 footnote]Stelfox, H. T., Palmisani, S., Scurlock, C., Orav, E. J., and Bates, D. W. (2006). The "To Err is Human" report and the patient safety literature. *Quality and Safety in Health Care, 15*(3), 174–178. doi: 10.1136/qshc.2006.017947.

75 Institute of Medicine. (2007). *Preventing medication errors.* The National Academies Press. https://doi.org/ 10.17226/11623.

Figure 2.2: Improving Medication Safety: Actions By Nurses

- Establish safe work environments for medication preparation, administration, and documentation; for instance, reduce distractions and provide appropriate lighting.

- Maintain a culture of rigorous commitment to principles of safety in medication administration (for instance, the five rights of medication safety and cross-checks with colleagues, where appropriate).

- Remove barriers and facilitate the involvement of patient surrogates in checking the administration and monitoring the medication effects.

- Foster a commitment to patients' rights as co-consumers of their care.

- Develop aids for patients or their surrogates to support self-management of medications.

- Enhance communication skills and team training to be prepared and confident in questioning medication orders and evaluating patient responses to drugs.

- Actively advocate for the development, testing, and safe implementation of electronic health records.

- Work to improve systems that address "near misses" in the work environment.

- Realize they are part of a system and do their part to evaluate the efficacy of new safety systems and technology.

- Contribute to the development and implementation of error reporting systems, and support a culture that values accurate reporting of medication errors.

WHO Global Patient Safety Challenge: Medication Without Harm

Unsafe medication practices and medication errors are a leading cause of injury and avoidable harm in health care systems in America and across the world. Globally, the cost associated with medication errors has been estimated at $42 billion USD annually. Errors can occur at different stages of the medication use process. Multiple interventions to address the frequency and impact of medication errors have already been developed, yet their implementation is varied. In 2019, the World Health Organization (WHO) identified "Medication Without Harm" as the theme for the third Global Patient Safety Challenge with the goal of reducing severe, avoidable medication-related harm by 50% over the next five years. As part of the *Global Patient Safety Challenge: Medication Without Harm,* WHO has prioritized three areas to protect patients from harm while maximizing the benefit from medication:

- Medication safety in high-risk situations

- Medication safety in **polypharmacy**

- Medication safety in transitions of care[76]

ᘓ The World's Health Organization's Patient Safety Page

A summary of these three areas and the strategies to reduce harm is provided below. View the patient video explaining how to avoid harm from medications, or click on the "Real Life Stories" link to read patient stories about harm caused by medications.

---

76 World Health Organization. (2019). *Medication safety in key action areas.* https://www.who.int/patientsafety/medication-safety/technical-reports/en/.

Medication Without Harm

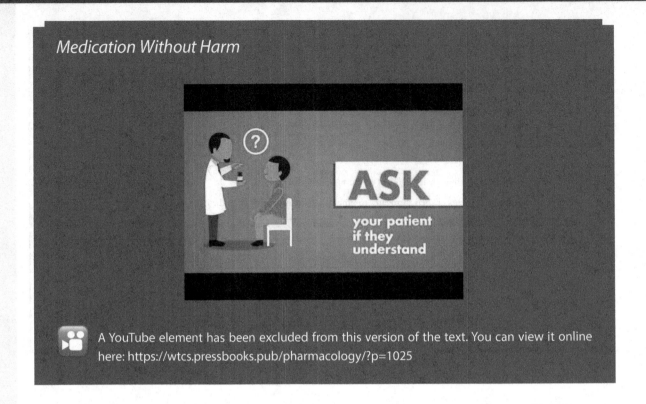

A YouTube element has been excluded from this version of the text. You can view it online here: https://wtcs.pressbooks.pub/pharmacology/?p=1025

Real Life Stories

Figure 2.3[77] describes the key steps for ensuring medication safety.

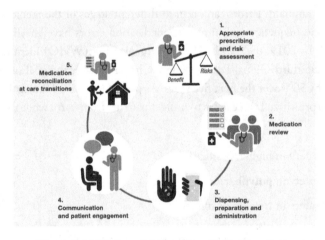

Figure 2.3 Key Steps for Ensuring Medication Safety

Medication Safety in High-Risk Situations

Medication safety in high-risk situations include high-risk medications, provider-patient relations, and systems factors.

---

77   This image is a derivative of *Medication Safety in High Risk Situations* by World Health Organization, https://apps.who.int/iris/handle/10665/325131 page 7, licensed under CC BY-NC-SA 3.0.

High-Risk (High-Alert) Medications

High-risk medications are drugs that bear a heightened risk of causing significant patient harm when they are used in error. Although mistakes may or may not be more common with these medications, the consequences of an error are more devastating to patients. High-risk medication can be remembered using the mnemonic "A PINCH." Figure 2.4 describes these medications included with the "A PINCH" mnemonic.

Figure 2.4: Demonstrating "A Pinch"

High-Risk Medicine Group	Examples of Medicines
A: Anti-infective	Amphotericin Aminoglycosides
P: Potassium and Other Electrolytes	Injections of potassium, magnesium, calcium, hypertonic sodium chloride
I: Insulin	All insulins
N: Narcotics and Other Sedatives	Hydromorphone, oxycodone, morphine Fentanyl Benozdiazepines
C: Chemotherapeutic Agents	Methotrexate, Vincristine
H: Heparin and Anticoagulants	Warfarin, Enoxaparin

Note: Based on research, the Institute of Safe Medication Practices (ISMP) has expanded this list. The list can be viewed at:

✐ ISMP List of High-Alert Medications in Acute Care Settings

Provider-Patient Relations

In addition to high-risk medications, a second component of medication safety in high-risk situations includes provider and patient factors. This component relates to either the health care professional providing care or the patient being treated. Even the most dedicated health care professional is fallible and can make errors. The act of prescribing, dispensing, and administering a medicine is complex and involves several health care professionals.

The patient should be the center of what should be a "prescribing partnership."[78] See Figure 2.5.[79]

---

78   This work is a derivative of *Medication Safety in High Risk Situations* by World Health Organization and is licensed under CC BY-NC-SA 3.0.

79   This image is a derivative of (2019) *Medication Safety in High Risk Situations* by World Health Organization, https://apps.who.int/iris/handle/10665/325131 page 24, licensed under CC BY-NC-SA 3.0.

Patients also can present risk factors. For example, it is well-known that adverse drug events occur most often at the extremes of life (in the very young and in older people). In the older population, frail patients are likely to be receiving several medications concurrently, which adds to the risk of adverse drug events. In addition, the harm of some of these medication combinations may sometimes be synergistic and be greater than the sum of the risks of harm of the individual agents. In neonates (particularly premature neonates), elimination routes through the kidney or liver may not be fully developed. The very young and those of old age are also less likely to tolerate adverse drug reactions, either because their homeostatic mechanisms are not yet fully developed or may have deteriorated. Medication errors in children, where doses may have to be calculated in relation to body weight or age, are also a source of major concern. Additionally, certain medical conditions predispose patients to an increased risk of adverse drug reactions, particularly renal or hepatic dysfunction and cardiac failure. Interprofessional strategies to address these potential harms are based on a systems approach with a "prescribing partnership" between the patient, the prescriber, the pharmacist, and the nurse, as outlined in Figure 2.5.

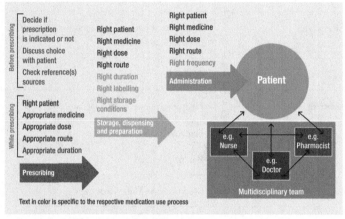

Source: Adapted, with the permission of the publisher, from Routledge *(94)*.

Figure 2.5 Prescribing partnership

Systems Factors

In addition to high-risk medications and provider-patient relations, systems factors also contribute to medication safety in high-risk situations. Systems factors, also called the environment in hospitals, can contribute to error-provoking conditions for several reasons. The unit may be busy or understaffed, which can contribute to inadequate supervision or failure to remember to check important information. Interruptions during critical processes (e.g., administration of medicines) can also occur, which can have significant implications for patient safety. Tiredness and the need to multitask when busy or flustered can also contribute to error and can be compounded by poor electronic medical record design. Preparing and administering intravenous medications is also particularly error prone. Strategies for reducing errors include checking at each step of the medication administration process; preventing interruptions; electronic provider order entry; and utilizing prescribing assessment tools, such as the Beers Criteria for 9 potentially inappropriate medication use in older adults.[80]

80   This work is a derivative of *Medication Safety in High Risk Situations* by World Health Organization and is licensed under CC BY-NC-SA 3.0.

Medication Safety in Polypharmacy

A second area of the WHO *Medications Without Harm* initiative relates to medication safety in polypharmacy. Polypharmacy is the concurrent use of multiple medications. Although there is no standard definition, polypharmacy is often defined as the routine use of five or more medications. This includes over-the-counter, prescription and/or traditional, and complementary medicines used by a patient. As the population ages, more people are likely to suffer from multiple long-term illnesses and take multiple medications. It is therefore essential to take a person-centered approach to ensure that medications are appropriate for the individual to gain the most benefits without harm and to ensure that patients are integral to the decision making process. Appropriate polypharmacy is present when all medicines are prescribed for the purpose of achieving specific therapeutic objectives that have been agreed with the patient; therapeutic objectives are actually being achieved or there is a reasonable chance they will be achieved in the future; medication therapy has been optimized to minimize the risk of adverse drug reactions; and the patient is motivated and able to take all medicines as intended. **Inappropriate polypharmacy** is present when one or more medicines are prescribed that are not or no longer needed, either because there is no evidence-based indication, the indication has expired or the dose is unnecessarily high; one or more medicines fail to achieve the therapeutic objectives they are intended to achieve; one or the combination of several medicines put the patient at a high risk of adverse drug reactions; or because the patient is not willing or able to take one or more medicines as intended. When patients move across care settings, medication review is important to prevent harm caused by inappropriate polypharmacy. Figure 2.6 includes the questions that should be addressed during a medication review with a multidisciplinary approach that includes the nurse.

Step-By-Step Approach to Conducting a Patient-Centered Medication Review

Figure 2.6: Step-by-Step Approach to Conducting a Patient-Centered Medication Review		
Aims	1. What matters to the patient?	**Review diagnoses and identity therapeutic objectives with respect to:** ■ Understanding goals of medication therapy ■ Management of existing health problems ■ Prevention of future health problems
Need	2. What are the essential medications?	**Identify essential medications (not to be stopped without specialist advice) such as:** ■ Medications that have essential replacement functions (e.g., thyroxine) ■ Medications to prevent rapid symptomatic decline (e.g., medications for Parkinson's disease)
	3. Does the patient take unnecessary medications?	**Identify and review the (continued) need for medications:** ■ With temporary indications ■ With higher-than-usual maintenance doses ■ With limited benefit in general for the indication they are used for ■ With limited benefit for the particular patient under review
Effectiveness	4. Are therapeutic objectives being achieved?	**Identify the effect of adding/intensifying medication therapy to achieve therapeutic objectives:** ■ To achieve symptom control ■ To achieve biochemical/ clinical targets ■ To prevent disease progression/ exacerbation

Safety	5. Does the patient have/ is at risk of adverse drug reactions?	**Identify patient safety risks by checking for:** ■ Drug-disease interactions ■ Drug-to-drug interactions ■ Robustness of monitoring mechanisms for high-risk medications ■ Risk of accidental overdosing
	6. Does the patient know what to do if they are ill?	**Identify adverse drug effects by checking for:** ■ Specific symptoms/ laboratory markers (e.g., hypokalaemia) ■ Cumulative adverse drug effects ■ Medications that may be used to treat adverse drug reactions caused by other medications
Costs	7. Is therapy cost-effective?	**Identify unnecessarily costly medication by:** ■ Considering more cost-effective alternative (but balance against effectiveness, safety, convenience)
Patient-centeredness	8. Is the patient willing and able to take medication as intended?	**Evaluate the patient understanding of the outcomes:** ■ Does the patient understand the rationale for taking their medications? ■ Consider teach-back technique to ensure full understanding **Ensure medication changes are tailored to patient preferences:** ■ Is the medication route appropriate for this patient? ■ Is the dosing schedule convenient for this patient? ■ Consider what assistance the patient might have and when this is available ■ Consider the patient's ability to take the medicines as intended.
		Agree and communicate plan: ■ Discuss with the patient therapeutic objectives and treatment priorities ■ Collaborate with the patient to determine which medicines are sufficiently effective to continue or consider discontinuation ■ Inform relevant health care and social care change in treatments across care transitions

Medication Safety in Transitions of Care

A third area of the WHO *Medications Without Harm* initiative relates to medication safety during transitions of care. View the interactive activity below to see how medications are reconciled during transitions of care from admission to discharge in a hospital setting.

> ## Interactive Activity
>
> An interactive or media element has been excluded from this version of the text. You can view it online here: https://wtcs.pressbooks.pub/pharmacology/?p=1025

Medication errors can occur during these changes in settings. Figure 2.7[81] is an image from the World Health Organization showing ranges of percentage of errors that occur during common transitions of care.

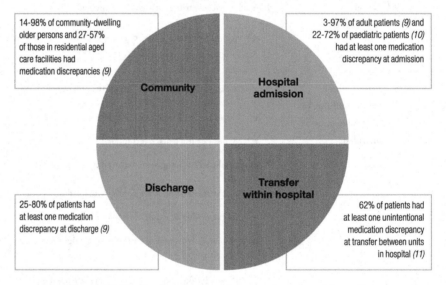

Figure 2.7 Medication discrepancies at various transitions of care

Key strategies for improving medication safety during transitions of care include:

- Implementing formal structured processes for medication reconciliation at all transition points of care. Steps of effective medication reconciliation are to build the best possible medication history by interviewing the patient and verifying with at least one reliable information source, reconciling and updating the medication list, and communicating with the patient and future health care providers about changes in their medications.

- Partnering with patients, families, caregivers, and health care professionals to agree on treatment plans, ensuring patients are equipped to manage their medications safely, and ensuring patients have an up-to-date medication list.

---

81 This work is a derivative of (2019) *Medication Safety in Transition of Care* by World Health Organization, https://apps.who. int/iris/bitstream/handle/10665/325453/WHO-UHC-SDS-2019.9-eng.pdf?ua=1 page 15, licensed under CC BY-NC-SA 3.0.

■ Where necessary, prioritizing patients at high risk of medication-related harm for enhanced support such as post-discharge contact by a nurse. [82]

Critical Thinking Activity

A nurse is performing medication reconciliation for an elderly patient admitted from home. The patient does not have a medication list and cannot report the names, dosages, and frequencies of the medication taken at home.

What other sources can the nurse use to obtain medication information?

Note: Answers to the Critical Thinking activities can be found in the "Answer Key" sections at the end of the book.

Institute for Safe Medication Practices (ISMP)

The Institute for Safe Medication Practices (ISMP) is respected as the gold standard for medication safety information. It is a nonprofit organization devoted entirely to preventing medication errors. ISMP collects and analyzes thousands of medication error and adverse event reports each year through its voluntary reporting program and then issues alerts regarding errors happening across the nation. The ISMP has established several prevention strategies for safe medication administration, including lists of high-alert medications, error-prone abbreviations to not use, Do Not Crush medications, look alike-sound alike drugs, and error-prone conditions that lead to error by student nurses. Each of these initiatives is further described below. [83]

℘ ISMP website

High-Alert Medications

High-alert medications are drugs that bear a heightened risk of causing significant patient harm when they are used in error. Although mistakes may or may not be more common with these drugs, the consequences of an error are clearly more devastating to patients. As discussed earlier in the "WHO" section of this chapter, an acronym that can be used to remember the basic list of high-alert medication is "A PINCH." The ISMP list contains additional medication to the mnemonic "A PINCH."

Strategies for safe administration of high-alert medication include:

■ Standardizing the ordering, storage, preparation, and administration of these products

■ Improving access to information about these drugs

■ Employing clinical decision support and automated alerts

■ Using redundancies such as automated or independent double checks when necessary

---

82   This image is a derivative of *Medication Safety in Transition of Care* by World Health Organization licensed under CC BY-NC-SA 3.0.

83   Institute for Safe Medication Practices. (2007, October 18). *Error-prone conditions that lead to student nurse- related errors.* https://www.ismp.org/resources/error-prone-conditions-lead-student-nurse-related-errors.

🔗 ISMP List of High-Alert Medications in Acute Care Settings

Error-Prone Abbreviations

ISMP's List of Error-Prone Abbreviations, Symbols, and Dose Designations contains abbreviations, symbols, and dose designations that have been reported through the ISMP National Medication Errors Reporting Program as being frequently misinterpreted and involved in harmful medication errors. These abbreviations, symbols, and dose designations should never be used when communicating medical information. Note that this list has additional abbreviations than those contained in the Joint Commission's Do Not Use List of Abbreviations. Click on the link below for the ISMP list of error-prone abbreviations to avoid. Some examples of abbreviations that were commonly used that should now be avoided are qd, qod, qhs, BID, QID, D/C, subq, and APAP.[84]

Strategies to avoid mistakes related to error-prone abbreviations include not using these abbreviations in medical documentation. Furthermore, if a nurse receives a prescription containing an error-prone abbreviation, it should be clarified with the provider and the order rewritten without the abbreviation.

🔗 ISMP List of Error-Prone Abbreviations to Avoid

Do Not Crush List

The IMSP maintains a list of oral dosage medication that should not be crushed, commonly referred to as the "Do Not Crush" list. These medications are typically extended-release formulations. The list can be accessed by using the link below.[85]

Strategies for preventing harm related to oral medication that should not be crushed include requesting an order for a liquid form or a different route if the patient cannot safely swallow the pill form.

🔗 ISMP Do Not Crush List

Look-Alike and Sound-Alike (LASA) Drugs

ISMP maintains a list of drug names containing look-alike and sound-alike name pairs such as Adderall and Inderal. These medications require special safeguards to reduce the risk of errors and minimize harm.

Safeguards may include:

- Using both the brand and generic names on prescriptions and labels
- Including the purpose of the medication on prescriptions
- Changing the appearance of look-alike product names to draw attention to their dissimilarities
- Configuring computer selection screens to prevent look-alike names from appearing consecutively[86]

---

84 Institute for Safe Medication Practices. (2017, October 2). *List of error-prone abbreviations.* https://www.ismp.org/recommendations/error-prone-abbreviations-list.

85 Institute for Safe Medication Practices. (2020, February 21). *Oral dosage forms that should not be crushed.* https://www.ismp.org/recommendations/do-not-crush.

86 Institute for Safe Medication Practices. (2019, February 28). *List of confused drug names.* https://www.ismp.org/recommendations/confused-drug-names-list.

⊘ ISMP Look Alike-Sound Alike List of Medications

Error Prone Conditions That Lead to Student Nurse Related Error

When analyzing errors involving student nurses reported to the USP-ISMP Medication Errors Reporting Program and the PA Patient Safety Reporting System, it appears that many errors arise from a distinct set of error-prone conditions or medications. Some student-related errors are similar in origin to those that seasoned licensed healthcare professionals make, such as misinterpreting an abbreviation, misidentifying drugs due to look-alike labels and packages, misprogramming a pump due to a pump design flaw, or simply making a mental slip when distracted. Other errors stem from system problems and practice issues that are rather unique to environments where students and hospital staff are caring together for patients. See the link to the list of these error prone conditions that should be avoided.

⊘ Error Prone Conditions That Lead to Student Nurse Related Error

Critical Thinking Activity 2.5b

A nurse is preparing to administer insulin to a patient. The nurse is aware that insulin is a medication on the ISMP list of high-alert medications.

What strategies should the nurse implement to ensure safe administration of this medication to the patient?

Note: Answers to the Critical Thinking activities can be found in the "Answer Key" sections at the end of the book.

Quality and Safety Education for Nurses (QSEN)

The Quality and Safety Education for Nurses (QSEN) project's vision is to "inspire health care professionals to put quality and safety as core values to guide their work." QSEN began in 2005 and is funded by the Robert Wood Johnson Foundation. Based on the Institute of Medicine (2003) competencies for nursing, QSEN further defined these quality and safety competencies for educating nursing students:

- Patient-Centered Care
- Teamwork & Collaboration
- Evidence-Based Practice
- Quality Improvement
- Safety
- Informatics[87]

Learn activities that teach nursing students how to provide safe, quality care to their patients.

⊘ QSEN website

---

87   QSEN Institute. (n.d.). *Project overview.* http://qsen.org/about-qsen/project-overview/.

My Notes

Below are supplementary learning resources related to patient safety and preventing error during medication administration.

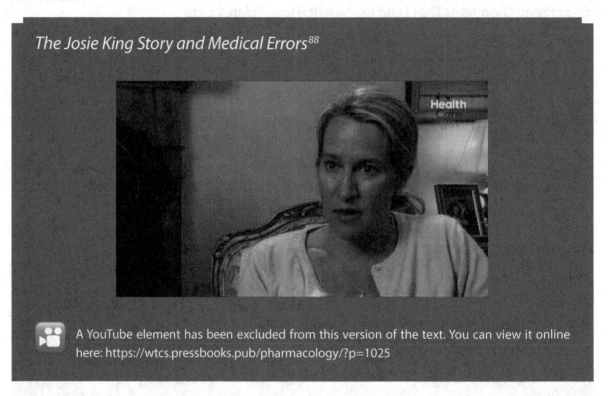

The Josie King Story and Medical Errors[88]

A YouTube element has been excluded from this version of the text. You can view it online here: https://wtcs.pressbooks.pub/pharmacology/?p=1025

As a student, when you prepare to administer medications to your patients during clinical, your instructor will ask you questions to ensure safe medication administration.

See an example of the typical questions that a clinical instructor might ask.

⚲ Enhancing Medication Safety in Clinical: A Video for Students and Nursing Faculty

Watch a QSEN PowerPoint presentation related to the revision of hospital policies to reduce error prone conditions for student nurses when administering medication.

⚲ QSEN PowerPoint

Summary of Nursing Considerations for Safe and Effective Medication Administration

Medication administration by nurses is not just a task on a daily task list; it is a system-wide process in collaboration with the healthcare team to ensure safe and effective treatment. As part of the medication administration process, the nurse must consider ethics, laws, national guidelines, and cultural/social determinants before administering medication to a patient. The nurse is the vital "last stop" for preventing errors and potential harm from

---

88   Healthcare.gov. (2011, May 25). Introducing the Partnerships for Patients with Sorrel King [Video]. YouTube. https://youtu.be/ak_5X66V5Ms.

medications before they reach the patient. A list of nursing considerations whenever administering medications are outlined below.

Nursing Considerations for Safe and Effective Medication Administration

BEFORE Administering Medication

Ethics

- Will this medication do more good than harm for this patient at this point in time?

- Has the patient (or the patient's decision maker) had a voice in the decision making process regarding use of this medication? Have they been informed about this medication and the potential risks/benefits to consider?

- If there are any ethical concerns, advocate for patient rights and autonomy and contact the provider and/or pursue the proper chain of command.

Legal and National Guidelines

- Be sure the prescription/order contains the proper information according to CMS guidelines.

- Are there any FDA Black Box Warnings for this drug? If so, is the patient aware of the risks and what to do if they occur? This discussion should be documented.

- Is this a controlled substance? If so, follow guidelines for controlled substances in terms of counting, wasting, and disposal. For prescriptions for outpatient use, advocate that Prescription Drug Monitoring Program guidelines are followed.

- Be aware of signs of drug diversion in other healthcare team members and follow up appropriately in the chain of command. You can also directly submit an online tip to the DEA at Rx Abuse Online Reporting.

- Follow the Joint Commission "SPEAK UP" guidelines if you have any concerns about the safe use of this medication, including, but not limited to:
  - Unclear or "do not use" abbreviations
  - Strategies for look alike-sound alike medications
  - Any other concerns for error

- Follow your state's practice act regarding Scope of Practice and Rules of Conduct. Is administering this medication appropriate for your scope of practice and for this patient? If not, protect your patient from harm and your nursing license by notifying the appropriate contacts within your agency.

- Is this medication administration occuring during a transition of care from unit to unit, home to agency, or in preparation for discharge? If so, be sure proper medication reconciliation has been completed.

DURING Administration

- Use the Nursing Process as you ASSESS if this drug is appropriate to administer at this time and PLAN continued monitoring. Consider life span and disease process implications. If you NOTICE any findings that this medication may not be appropriate at this time for this patient, withhold the medication and contact the provider.

- Assess if there are any cultural or social determinants that will impact the patient's ability to use these medications safely and effectively. IMPLEMENT appropriate accommodations as needed and notify the provider.

- Follow National Patient Safety Goals as you correctly identify the patient and follow guidelines to use medicines safely.

- If this is a "high-alert" medication, follow recommendations for safe administration (such as adding a second RN check, etc.).

- Reduce distractions in your environment as you prepare and administer medications.

- Do not crush medications unless safe to do so.

- Follow JC and CMS standards:

    - Check 5 rights before administering to patient

    - Educate the patient about their medication

    - Dispose of waste controlled substances appropriately

    - Document appropriately

AFTER Administration

- Continue to EVALUATE the patient for potential side effects/adverse effects, as well as therapeutic effects of the medications.

- Document and verbally share your findings during handoff reports for safe continuity of care.

- If an error occurs, file an incident report and participate in root cause analysis to determine how to prevent it from happening again.

Supplementary Resources

For more information related to medication safety, go to these supplementary resources.

- **Culturally Competent Nursing Care: A Cornerstone of Caring. Free Educational Program.**

- **FDA (2018) Safe Use Initiative – Current Projects**

- **Institute for Safe Medication Practices. The Five Rights: A Destination Without a Map.**

- **Improvement Stories: Beyond the Five Rights.**

- **ISMP. 2018-2019 Targeted Medication Safety Best Practices for Hospitals.**

- **Koharchik, L., and Flavin, P. M. (2017). Teaching students to administer medications safely. American Journal of Nursing, (1), 62. Retrieved from OneSearch.**

🔗 **Lippincott Procedures (2018). Safe medication administration practices, general. Accessed August 16, 2019.**

🔗 **WHO (2014). The High 5s Project: Implementation guide. Assuring medication accuracy at transitions in care: medication reconciliation**

2.6 MODULE LEARNING ACTIVITIES

> *Interactive Activity*
>
> An interactive or media element has been excluded from this version of the text. You can view it online here: https://wtcs.pressbooks.pub/pharmacology/?p=1165

Glossary

American Nurses Association (ANA): The professional organization that represents the interests of the nation's 4 million registered nurses.

Beneficence: To "do good."

Black Box Warnings: The strongest warnings issued by the Federal Drug Association (FDA) that signify a drug carries a significant risk of serious or life-threatening adverse effects.

Code of Ethics for Nurses: Developed by the American Nurses Association as a guide for carrying out nursing responsibilities in a manner consistent with quality in nursing care and the ethical obligations of the profession.

Cultural Competence: The process by which nurses demonstrate culturally congruent practice.

Culturally Congruent Practice: The application of evidence-based nursing that is in agreement with the preferred cultural values, beliefs, worldview, and practices of the healthcare consumer and other stakeholders.

Do Not Crush List: A list of medications that should not be crushed, often due to a sustained-release formulation.

Drug Diversion: The transfer of any legally prescribed controlled substance from the individual for whom it was prescribed to another person for any illicit use.

Error-Prone Abbreviations: Abbreviations, symbols, and dose designations that are frequently misinterpreted and involved in harmful medication errors.

Five Rights of Medication Administration: Standards of practice that require the following information is confirmed prior to each administration of medication: right patient, right drug, right dose, right time, and right route.

Health Literacy: The degree to which individuals have the capacity to obtain, process, and understand basic health information needed to make appropriate health decisions.

High-Risk Medications: Drugs that bear a heightened risk of causing significant patient harm when they are used in error.

Inappropriate Polypharmacy: Present when one or more medicines are prescribed that are not or no longer needed.

Joint Commission: A national organization that accredits and certifies health care organizations in the United States.

Look-Alike and Sound-Alike (LASA) Drugs: Medications that require special safeguards to reduce the risk of errors and minimize harm.

Maleficence: Causing harm to patients.

National Patient Safety Goals (NPSGs): Goals established by the Joint Commission to help accredited organizations address specific areas of concern related to patient safety.

Nursing: The protection, promotion, and optimization of health and abilities, prevention of illness and injury, facilitation of healing, alleviation of suffering through the diagnosis and treatment of human response, and advocacy in the care of individuals, families, groups, communities, and populations, as defined by the American Nurses Association.

Nursing Process: Standards of Practice that include Assessment; Diagnosis; Outcome Identification; Planning; Implementation; and Evaluation components of providing patient care.

Nursing Scope and Standards of Practice: A document created by the American Nurses Association that outlines professional nursing performance according to national standards.

Polypharmacy: The concurrent use of multiple medications.

Prescription Drug Monitoring Programs (PDMP): A statewide electronic database that collects designated data on substances dispensed in a state to address prescription drug abuse, addiction, and diversion.

Professional Assistance Procedure: A voluntary non-disciplinary program to provide support for credentialed professionals in Wisconsin with substance abuse disorder who are committed to their own recovery.

Registered Nurse (RN): An individual who is educationally prepared and licensed by a state to practice as a registered nurse.

Root Cause Analysis: An analysis after an error occurs to help identify not only what and how an event occurred, but also why it happened. When investigators are able to determine why an event or failure occurred, they can create workable corrective measures that prevent future errors from occurring.

Safety Culture: The culture of a health care agency that empowers staff to speak up about risks to patients and to report errors and near misses, all of which drive improvement in patient care and reduce the incident of patient harm.

Scheduled Medications: The Controlled Substances Act (CSA) places all substances that are regulated under existing federal law into one of five schedules, ranging from Schedule I drugs with a high potential for abuse and the potential to create severe psychological and/or physical dependence, to Schedule V drugs with the least potential for abuse.

Social Determinants of Health: Poverty, education, safe medication, and other healthcare disparities that affect a patient's health.

Standards of Practice: Authoritative statements of duties by the American Nursing Association that all registered nurses, regardless of role, population, or specialty, are expected to perform competently. Standards of Practice include Assessment, Diagnosis, Outcome Identification, Planning, Implementation, and Evaluation components of providing patient care.

Standards of Professional Performance: Describe a competent level of behavior in the professional role, including activities related to ethics, culturally congruent practice, communication, collaboration, leadership, education, evidence-based practice, and quality of practice as defined by the American Nursing Association.

State Nurse Practice Act: Laws enacted by state legislatures setting professional standards of nursing care to which nurses are held accountable by the State Board of Nursing.

State Board of Nursing: A group of officials who enforce the State Nurse Practice Act.

Substance Use Disorder: A pattern of behaviors that ranges from misuse to dependency or addiction, whether it is alcohol, legal drugs, or illegal drugs. Addiction is a complex disease with serious physical, emotional, financial, and legal consequences.

Chapter III

Antimicrobials

3.1   ANTIMICROBIALS INTRODUCTION

Learning Objectives

- Identify the classifcations and actions of antimicrobial medications
- Give examples of when, how, and to whom antimicrobial drugs may be administered
- Identify the side effects and special considerations associated with antimicrobial therapy
- Include considerations and implications of using antimicrobial medications across the life span
- Include evidence-based concepts when using the nursing process
- Identify and interpret related laboratory tests

Have you ever been prescribed an antibiotic for an infection and asked, "Why do I have to fnish taking all these pills when I already feel better"? Or, perhaps you wondered why the healthcare provider chose a certain medication over another or why the pharmacist told you to avoid certain foods when taking a certain antibiotic.

You may have had these questions in your own healthcare experiences. It is important to remember that if you have these questions, many of your patients will as well. Learning about the various types of antimicrobials and how they work will help you provide better health education to your patients.

Did you know that the use of antimicrobial agents dates back to ancient times?

Although the discovery of antimicrobials and their subsequent widespread use is commonly associated with modern medicine, there is evidence that humans have been exposed to antimicrobial compounds for millennia. Chemical analyses of the skeletal remains of people from between 350 and 550 AD of people living near the Nile River have shown residue of the antimicrobial agent tetracycline in high enough quantities to suggest the purposeful fermentation of tetracycline-producing Streptomyces during the beer-making process. The resulting beer, which was thick and gruel-like, was used to treat a variety of ailments in both adults and children, including gum disease and wounds.

Additionally, the antimicrobial properties of plants and honey have been recognized by various cultures around the world, including Indian and Chinese herbalists who have long used plants for a wide variety of medical purposes. Healers of many cultures understood the antimicrobial properties of fungi, and their use of moldy bread or other mold-containing products to treat wounds have been well documented for centuries.[1]

---

1   This work is a derivative of *Microbiology* by OpenStax and is licensed under CC BY 4.0.

3.2   ANTIMICROBIAL BASICS

Basic Concepts Related to Antimicrobial Therapy

Before we learn about medications that are used to treat infections in our patients, we must frst understand the basics of microbiology. Let's begin with a review of bacteria. Bacteria are found in nearly every habitat on earth, including within and on humans. Most bacteria are harmless or considered helpful, but some are pathogens. A **pathogen** is defned as an organism causing disease to its host. Pathogens, when overgrown, can cause signifcant health problems or even death for your patients.

Bacteria may be identifed when a patient has an infection by using a culture and sensitivity test or a gram stain test. Antimicrobials may be classifed as broad-spectrum or narrow-spectrum, based on the variety of bacteria they effectively treat. Additionally, antibiotics may be bacteriostatic or bactericidal in terms of how it targets the bacteria. Finally, the mechanism of action is also considered in the selection of an antibiotic.

In addition to antibiotics, antimicrobials also include medications used to treat viruses and fungi. Each of these topics will be discussed in more detail below, along with the issue of drug resistance.

Culture and Sensitivity

When a patient presents signs or symptoms of an infection, healthcare providers will begin the detective work needed to identify the source of the infection. A **culture** is a test performed to examine different body substances for the presence of bacteria or fungus.[2] These culture samples are commonly collected from a patient's blood, urine, sputum, wound bed, etc. Nurses are commonly responsible for the collection of culture samples and must be conscientious to collect the sample prior to the administration of antibiotics. Antibiotic administration prior to a culture can result in a delayed identifcation of the organism and complicate the patient's recovery. Once culture samples are collected, they are then incubated in a solution that promotes bacterial or fungal growth and spread onto a special culture plate.[3] Clinical microbiologists subsequently monitor the culture for signs of organism growth to aid in the diagnosis of the infectious pathogen. A **sensitivity analysis** is often performed to select an effective antibiotic to treat the microorganism. If the organism shows **resistance** to the antibiotics used in the test, those antibiotics will not provide effective treatment for the patient's infection. Sometimes a patient may begin antibiotic treatment for an infection, but will be switched to a different, more effective antibiotic based on the culture and sensitivity results.[4]

Gram Positive versus Gram Negative

A **gram stain** is another type of test that is used to assist in classifcation of pathogens. Gram stains are useful for quickly identifying if bacteria are "gram positive" or "gram negative," based on the staining patterns of their cellular walls. Utilizing gram stain allows microbiologists to look for characteristic violet (Gram +) or red/pink (Gram -)

---

2   This work is a derivative of *Microbiology* by OpenStax licensed under CC BY 4.0. Access for free at https://openstax.org/books/microbiology/pages/1-introduction.

3   Kristof, K. and Pongracz, J. (2016). Interpretation of blood microbiology results - function of the clinical microbiologist. *The Journal of the International Federation of Clinical Chemistry and Laboratory Medicine, 27*(2), 147–155. https://www.ncbi.nlm.nih.gov/pmc/articles/PMC4975230/.

4   Vorvick, L. (Ed.). (2019, February 7). *Sensitivity analysis.* https://medlineplus.gov/ency/ article/003741.htm.

staining patterns when they examine the organisms under a microscope.[5] Identifcation of bacteria as gram positive or gram negative assists the healthcare provider in quickly selecting an appropriate antibiotic to treat the infection.

Sample Gram Positive Infections

Streptococcus the name which comes from the Greek word for twisted chain, is responsible for many types of infectious diseases in humans. Streptococcus is an example of a **Gram + infection** and is identifed by its ability to lyse, or breakdown, red blood cells when grown on blood agar.

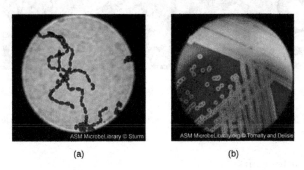

(a)   (b)

Figure 3.1 Gram Stain Specimen Streptococcus

S. pyogenes is a type of ß-hemolytic *Streptococcus*. This species is considered a pyogenic pathogen because of the associated pus production observed with infections it causes (see Figure 3.1[6] for an image of Streptococcus undergoing gram staining). *S. pyogenes* is the most common cause of bacterial pharyngitis (strep throat); it is also a common cause of various skin infections that can be relatively mild (e.g., impetigo) or life threatening (e.g., necrotizing fasciitis, also known as flesh-eating disease).[7]

Staphylococcus is a second example of a Gram + bacteria. The bacteria Staphylococcus comes from a Greek word for bunches of grapes, which describes their microscopic appearance in culture. Strains of S. aureus cause a wide variety of infections in humans, including skin infections that produce boils, carbuncles, cellulitis, or impetigo. Many strains of S. aureus have developed resistance to antibiotics. Some antibiotic-resistant strains are designated as **methicillin-resistant S. aureus (MRSA)** and **vancomycin-resistant S. aureus (VRSA)**. These strains are some of the most difficult to treat because they exhibit resistance to nearly all available antibiotics, not just methicillin and vancomycin. Because they are difficult to treat with antibiotics, infections can be lethal. MRSA and VRSA are also contagious, posing a serious threat in hospitals, nursing homes, dialysis facilities, and other places where there are large populations of elderly, bedridden, and/or immunocompromised patients.[8] See Figure 3.2[9] for an image of Staphylococcus bacteria microscopically.

---

5   This work is a derivative of *Microbiology* by OpenStax licensed under CC BY 4.0. Access for free at https://openstax.org/books/microbiology/pages/1-introduction.

6   "OSC Microbio 04 04 Strep.jpg" by CNX OpenStax is licensed under CC BY 4.0 Access for free at https://openstax.org/books/microbiology/pages/4-4-gram-positive-bacteria.

7   This work is a derivative of *Microbiology* by OpenStax licensed under CC BY 4.0. Access for free at https://openstax.org/books/microbiology/pages/1-introduction.

8   This work is a derivative of *Microbiology* by OpenStax licensed under CC BY 4.0. Access for free at https://openstax.org/books/microbiology/pages/1-introduction.

9   This work is a derivative of "CDC-10046-MRSA.jpg" by Janice Haney Carr, Centers for Disease Control and Prevention is licensed under CC0.

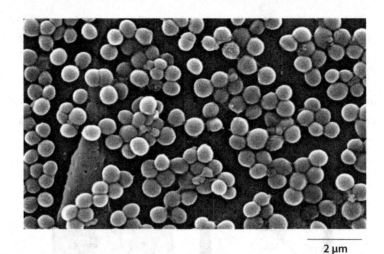

Figure 3.2 Staphylococcus aureus illustrates the typical "grape-like" clustering of cells

Sample Gram Negative Infections

Gram Negative bacteria often grow between aerobic and anaerobic areas (such as in the intestines). Some gram negative bacteria cause severe, sometimes life-threatening disease. The genus *Neisseria*, for example, includes the bacteria *N. gonorrhoeae*, the causative agent of the sexually transmitted infection gonorrhea, and *N. meningitides*, the causative agent of bacterial meningitis. See Figure 3.3[10] for an image of Neisseria meningitides. Another common gram negative infection that is seen in hospitalized patients is *Escherichia coli* (E. Coli). This is a frequent culprit for urinary tract infections due to its presence in the GI tract.

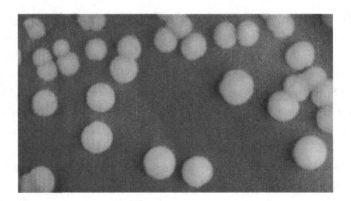

Figure 3.3 Neisseria meningitidis growing in colonies on a chocolate agar plate

Broad-Spectrum versus Narrow-Spectrum Antimicrobials

Spectrum of activity is one of the factors that providers use when selecting antibiotics to treat a patient's infection. A **narrow-spectrum antimicrobial** targets only specifc subsets of bacterial pathogens.[11] For example, some

---

10 "OSC Microbio 04 02 Neisseria.jpg" by CNX OpenStax is licensed under CC BY 4.0 Access for free at https://openstax.org/books/microbiology/pages/4-2-proteobacteria.

11 This work is a derivative of *Microbiology* by OpenStax licensed under CC BY 4.0. Access for free at https://openstax.org/books/microbiology/pages/1-introduction.

narrow-spectrum drugs only target gram positive bacteria, but others target only gram negative bacteria. If the pathogen causing infection has been identifed in a culture and sensitivity test, it is best to use a narrow-spectrum antimicrobial and minimize collateral damage to the normal microbacteria.

A **broad-spectrum antimicrobial** targets a wide variety of bacterial pathogens, including both gram positive and gram negative species, and is frequently used to cover a wide range of potential pathogens while waiting on the laboratory identifcation of the infecting pathogen. Broad-spectrum antimicrobials are also used for polymicrobial infections (a mixed infection with multiple bacterial species) or as prophylactic prevention of infections with surgery/invasive procedures. Finally, broad-spectrum antimicrobials may be selected to treat an infection when a narrow-spectrum drug fails because of development of drug resistance by the target pathogen.[12]

One risk associated with using broad-spectrum antimicrobials is that they will also target a broad spectrum of the normal microbacteria that can cause diarrhea. They also increase the risk of a **superinfection**, a secondary infection in a patient having a preexisting infection. A superinfection develops when the antibacterial intended for the preexisting infection kills the protective microbiota, allowing another pathogen resistant to the antibacterial to proliferate and cause a secondary infection. Common examples of superinfections that develop as a result of antimicrobial use include yeast infections (candidiasis) and pseudomembranous colitis caused by **Clostridium diffcile (C-diff)**, which can be fatal.[13] Probiotics, such as lactobacillus, are commonly used for individuals with C-diff to introduce normal bacteria into the gastrointestinal system and improve bowel function. See Figure 3.4[14] for an image of C-diff microscopically.

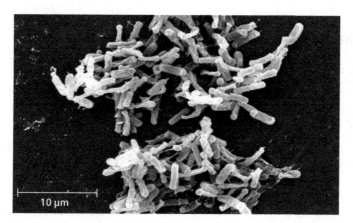

Figure 3.4 Clostridium diffcile, a gram-positive, rod-shaped bacterium, causes severe colitis and diarrhea, often after the normal gut microbiota is eradicated by antibiotics

Let's recap . . .

- A broad-spectrum antibiotic will treat gram positive **and** gram negative bacteria.
- A narrow-spectrum antibiotic will treat **either** gram positive **or** gram negative bacteria.

---

12   This work is a derivative of *Microbiology* by OpenStax licensed under CC BY 4.0. Access for free at https://openstax.org/books/microbiology/pages/1-introduction.

13   This work is a derivative of *Microbiology* by OpenStax licensed under CC BY 4.0. Access for free at https://openstax.org/books/microbiology/pages/1-introduction.

14   This work is a derivative of "Clostridium diffcile 01.jpg" by Lois D Wiggs at Centers of Disease Control and Prevention is licensed under CC0.

If a patient is started on an antibiotic that is gram + and the culture identifes a gram–organism, the medication will not improve the patient's status. The selection of an incorrect antibiotic can lead to adverse reactions and increase bacterial resistance.

At times, a broad spectrum antibiotic may be administered prior to receiving the culture report due to the severity of the illness of the patient. Once the culture is reported, the antibiotic therapy is tailored to the patient. It is the nurse's responsibility to review culture results and ensure that the results have been communicated to the prescribing provider.

Antibacterials Actions — Bacteriostatic versus Bactericidal

When a provider selects an antibacterial drug, it is important to consider how and where the drug will ultimately target the bacteria. Antibacterial drugs can be either bacteriostatic or bactericidal in their interactions with the offending bacteria. **Bacteriostatic** drugs cause bacteria to stop reproducing; however, they may not ultimately kill the bacteria. In contrast, **bactericidal** drugs kill their target bacteria.

The decision about whether to use a bacteriostatic or bactericidal drug often depends on the type of infection and the overall immune status of the patient. In a healthy patient with strong immune defenses, both bacteriostatic and bactericidal drugs can be effective in achieving clinical cure. However, when a patient is immunocompromised, a bactericidal drug is essential for the successful treatment of infections. Regardless of the immune status of the patient, life-threatening infections such as acute endocarditis require the use of a bactericidal drug to eliminate all offending bacteria.[15]

Mechanism of Action

Another consideration in the selection of an antibacterial drug is the drug's mechanism of action. Each class of antibacterial drugs has a unique **mechanism of action**, the way in which a drug affects microbes at the cellular level. For example, cephalosporins act on the integrity of the cell wall. In contrast, aminoglycosides impact ribosome function and inhibit protein synthesis, which stops the proliferation of cells.[16] See Figure 3.5[17] for a summary of how various antibiotics affect the cell wall, the plasma membrane, the ribosomes, the metabolic pathways, or DNA synthesis of bacteria.

15   This work is a derivative of *Microbiology* by OpenStax licensed under CC BY 4.0. Access for free at https://openstax.org/books/microbiology/pages/1-introduction.

16   This work is a derivative of *Microbiology* by OpenStax licensed under CC BY 4.0. Access for free at https://openstax.org/books/microbiology/pages/1-introduction.

17   "OSC Microbio 14 02 Modes.jpg" by CNX Openstax is licensed under CC BY 4.0 Access for free at https://openstax.org/books/microbiology/pages/14-3-mechanisms-of-antibacterial-drugs.

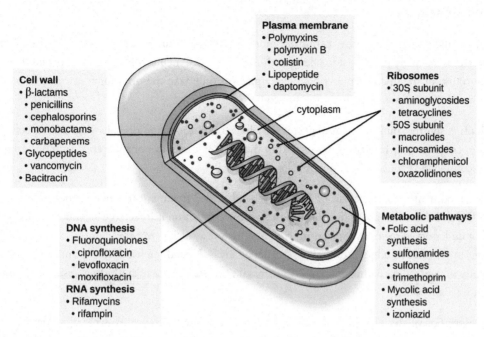

Figure 3.5 Various mechanisms of actions of antimicrobial medication

Antiviral

Similar to antibacterial medications, **antiviral** drugs directly impact interaction and reproduction of the offending microorganism. Antibacterial medications are required for treating bacterial infections; antivirals treat specifc viral infections. For example, oseltamivir (Tamifu) is commonly prescribed to treat infuenza. Unlike antimicrobials, antiviral medications do not kill the offending virus, but they work to reduce replication and development of the virus.[18]

Antifungal

Antifungal, or antimycotic agents, are medications that are used to treat fungal infections. These medications work by killing the cells of the fungus or inhibiting the reproduction of the cells. Unlike antibacterial and antiviral medications, many antifungals are applied topically to the affected area. Fungal infections commonly affect surface areas of the body, including the toes, nails, mouth, groin, etc. For example, *Candida albicans* is a type of fungi that when overgrown in the mouth produces oral thrush. Patients experiencing thrush may be prescribed oral antifungal swish and spit medication such as nystatin.

Drug Resistance

Although there is a wide availability of medications that are useful for treating infection, greater limitations in effectiveness are being seen. According to the Centers for Disease Control (2019), each year in the United States, at least 2 million people are infected with an antibiotic-resistant infection, and more than 23,000 die.[19]

---

18   This work is a derivative of *Microbiology* by OpenStax licensed under CC BY 4.0. Access for free at https://openstax.org/ books/microbiology/pages/1-introduction.

19   Centers for Disease Control and Prevention. (2019). *About antimicrobial resistance*. https://www.cdc.gov/drugresistance/ about.html.

Prevention Strategies

In the United States and many other countries, most antimicrobial drugs are self-administered by patients at home. Unfortunately, many patients stop taking antimicrobials once their symptoms dissipate and they feel better. If a 10-day course of treatment is prescribed, many patients only take the drug for 5 or 6 days, unaware of the negative consequences of not completing the full course of treatment.

The Problem: A shorter course of treatment not only fails to kill the target organisms to the expected levels but also assists in creating drug-resistant variants within the body. A patient's nonadherence amplifes drug resistance when the recommended course of treatment is long.

For example, treatment for tuberculosis (TB) has a recommended treatment regimen lasting from 6 months to a year. The CDC estimates that about one third of the world's population is infected with TB, most living in under-developed or underserved regions where antimicrobial drugs are available over the counter. In such countries, there may be even lower rates of adherence than in developed areas. Nonadherence leads to antibiotic resistance and more diffculty in controlling pathogens. As a direct result, the emergence of multidrug-resistant strains of TB is becoming a huge problem.

The over prescription of antimicrobials also contributes to antibiotic resistance. Patients often demand antibiotics for diseases that do not require them, like viral colds and ear infections. Pharmaceutical companies aggressively market drugs to physicians and clinics, making it easy for them to give free samples to patients, and some pharmacies even offer certain antibiotics free to low-income patients with a prescription.

In recent years, various initiatives have aimed to educate parents and clinicians about the judicious use of antibiotics. However, previous studies have shown the parental expectations for antimicrobial prescriptions for children actually increased.

One possible solution that is being explored is a regimen called directly observed therapy (DOT), which involves the supervised administration of medications to patients. Patients are either required to visit a health-care facility to receive their medications, or health-care professionals must administer medication in patients' homes or another designated location. DOT has been implemented in many cases for the treatment of TB and has been shown to be effective; indeed, DOT is an integral part of WHO's global strategy for eradicating TB.

But is this a practical strategy for all antibiotics? Would patients taking penicillin, for example, be more or less likely to adhere to the full course of treatment if they had to travel to a health-care facility to receive each dose? Who would pay for the increased cost associated with DOT? When it comes to overprescription, should providers or drug companies be policed when it comes to over prescribing antibiotics to enforce best practices? What group should assume this responsibility, and what penalties would be effective in discouraging overprescription?

This is a complex issue with no clear, easy solution. However, what is clear is that all patients need extensive education regarding the judicious and complete use of medications to increase adherence and decrease the opportunity for antimicrobial resistance.[20]

---

20   This work is a derivative of *Microbiology* by OpenStax licensed under CC BY 4.0. Access for free at https://openstax.org/books/microbiology/pages/1-introduction.

Critical Thinking Activity 3.2a

Refecting on current healthcare challenges regarding the ongoing emergence of antimicrobial resistant organisms, what actions could you take within your nursing practice to help prevent drug resistance?

Note: Answers to the Critical Thinking activities can be found in the "Answer Key" sections at the end of the book.

Interactive Activity

 An interactive or media element has been excluded from this version of the text. You can view it online here: https://wtcs.pressbooks.pub/pharmacology/?p=256

3.3   ADMINISTRATION CONSIDERATIONS

The administration of antimicrobial drug therapy involves special considerations to ensure that the therapeutic drug effect is achieved while maintaining patient safety and minimizing complications.

Let's consider some of the variables that may impact antimicrobial administration:

Half-Life

Many antimicrobial medications are administered to ensure a certain therapeutic level of medication remains in the bloodstream and may require interval or repeated dosing throughout the day. For example, the **half-life**, or rate at which 50% of a drug is eliminated from the plasma, can vary signifcantly between drugs. Some drugs have a short half-life of only 1 hour and must be given multiple times a day, but other drugs have half-lives exceeding 12 hours and can be given as a single dose every 24 hours. Although a longer half-life can be considered an advantage for an antibacterial when it comes to convenient dosing intervals, the longer half-life can also be a concern for a drug with serious side effects. Medications that have longer half-life and more concerning side effects will exert these side effects over a longer period of time.

See Figure 3.6[21] for an illustration of half-lives and the time it takes for a medication to be eliminated from the bloodstream.

Concentration vs. number of half-life periods

Figure 3.6 Medication concentration over time demonstrates half-life

Life Span Considerations

A majority of medications are calculated specifcally based on the patient's size, weight, and renal function. Patient age and size are especially vital in pediatric patients. A child's stage of development and the size of their internal organs will greatly impact how the body absorbs, digests, metabolizes, and eliminates medications.

---

21   "Concentration_vs_number_of_half-life_periodes.png" by OPPSD is licensed under CC BY-SA 3.0.

Liver and Renal Function

Additionally, there are many antimicrobial medications that will require tailored dosing based on individual patient response and the potential impact of the medication on the patient's liver and renal function. For more information about the effects of liver and renal function on medications, refer to Chapter 1 regarding metabolism and excretion. Often times, pharmacists and providers will collect drug peak and trough drug blood levels to determine how an individual patient's body is responding to an antimicrobial. Follow-up interval dosing is then prescribed based on these blood levels. This is especially important for older adults or those with known liver/renal impairment. Individuals with diminished liver and renal function are more prone to drug toxicity because of the reduced ability of the body to metabolize or clear medications from the body. For more information about peak and trough levels, refer to Chapter 1 regarding medication safety.[22]

Dose Dependency/Time Dependency

The goal of antimicrobial therapy is to select an optimal dosage that will result in clinical cure, while reducing the patient complications or signifcant side effects. Many medications may be **dose dependent**. This means that there is a more signifcant killing of the bacterial with increasing levels of the antibiotic. For example, furoquinolones are dose-dependent medications with the treatment goal to optimize the amount of the drug. Other medications are **time dependent**. Time-dependent medications have optimal bacterial killing effect at lower doses over a longer period of time. Time-dependent antimicrobials exert the greatest effect by binding to the microorganism for an extensive length of time. Penicillin is an example of a time-dependent medication where the goal is to optimize the duration of exposure.[23]

Route

It is also important to consider the route of drug administration within the patient's body. Many of us may have been prescribed oral antibiotics and have simply filled our prescription and completed the drug regimen within the comfort of our own homes. However, there are many types of infections or disease processes that do not respond well to the use of oral antimicrobial therapy. For these diseases, patients may require intravenous or intramuscular injections. Patients requiring intravenous or intramuscular injections may need to be hospitalized, have home health nursing arranged, or travel to the hospital/clinic for their therapy. Concerns with treatment compliance exists with all routes of administration. For more information about considerations regarding routes of adminis-tration, refer to Chapter 1 on absorption. See Figure 3.7[24] for an illustration of three common routes of medication within the body.

---

22   This work is a derivative of *Microbiology* by OpenStax licensed under CC BY 4.0. Access for free at https://openstax.org/books/microbiology/pages/1-introduction.

23   This work is a derivative of *Microbiology* by OpenStax licensed under CC BY 4.0. Access for free at https:// openstax.org/books/microbiology/pages/1-introduction.

24   A drug's life in the body (with labels)" by National Institute of General Medical Sciences Image and Video Gallery is licensed under CC NC-SA 3.0.

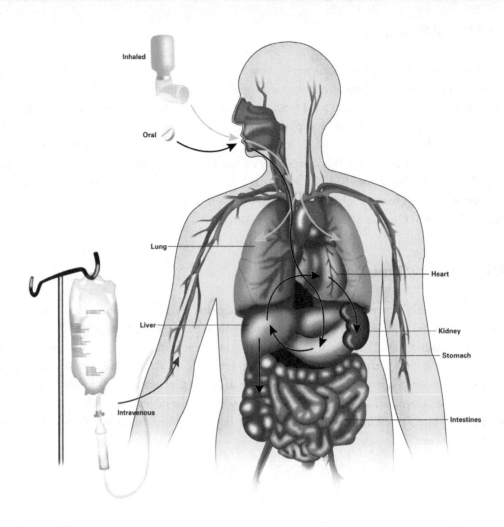

Figure 3.7 Common routes of medication administration include oral, inhalation, and IV

Drug Interactions

For the optimum treatment of select infections, two antibacterial drugs may be administered together. Concurrent drug administration produces a **synergistic interaction** that is better than the effcacy of either drug alone. In this case, TWO is truly better than ONE! A classic example of synergistic drug combinations is trimethoprim and sulfamethoxazole (Bactrim). Individually, these two drugs provide only bacteriostatic inhibition of bacterial growth, but combined, the drugs are bactericidal.[25]

Although synergistic drug interactions provide a benefit to the patient, **antagonistic interactions** produce harmful effects. Antagonism can occur between two antimicrobials or between antimicrobials and non-antimicrobials being used to treat other conditions. The effects vary depending on the drugs involved, but antagonistic

---

25   This pwork is a derivative of *Microbiology* by OpenStax licensed under CC BY 4.0. Access for free at https://openstax.org/books/microbiology/pages/1-introduction.

interactions cause diminished drug activity, decreased therapeutic levels due to elevated metabolism and elimination, or increased potential for toxicity due to decreased metabolism and elimination.

Let's consider an example of these antagonistic interactions.

Many antibacterials are absorbed most effectively from the acidic environment within the stomach. However, if a patient takes antacids, the antacids increase the pH of the stomach and negatively impact the absorption of the antibacterial, thus decreasing their effectiveness in treating an infection.

Interactive Activity

 An interactive or media element has been excluded from this version of the text. You can view it online here: https://wtcs.pressbooks.pub/pharmacology/?p=258

3.4   NURSING PROCESS

Now that we have reviewed antimicrobial basics and administration considerations, we will take a closer look at specifc antimicrobial classes and administration considerations, therapeutic effects, adverse effects, and specifc teaching needed for each class of antimicrobials. But before we do that, let's reexamine the importance of the nursing process in guiding the nurse who administers antimicrobial medications. The nursing process consists of assessment, diagnosis, outcome identifcation, planning, implementation of interventions, and evaluation. For more information about the nursing process, refer to the Chapter 2 sub-module on "Ethical and Professional Foundations of Safe Medication Administration by Nurses." Because diagnosis, outcome identifcation, and planning are specifcally tailored to the individual patient, we will broadly discuss considerations related to assessment, implementation of interventions, and evaluation when administering antimicrobials.

Nursing Process: Assessment

Although there are numerous details to consider when administering medications, it is important to always frst think more broadly about what you are giving and why. As a nurse who is administering an antimicrobial, you must remember some important broad considerations.

First, Let's think of the why?

Antimicrobials are given to prevent or treat infection. If a patient is prescribed an antimicrobial, an important piece of the nursing assessment should be to look for signs and symptoms of infection. The nurse should always know WHY the patient is receiving an antimicrobial to evaluate if the patient is improving or deteriorating. Remember, the nurse must assess how this medication is working, and having pre-administration assessment information is an important part of this process. Typical data that a nurse collects at the start of a shift include a baseline temperature, heart rate, blood pressure, and white blood cell count. Focused assessments are then made based on the type of infection. For example, if it is a wound infection, the wound should be assessed. If it is a respiratory infection, the nurse should assess the patient's lung sounds. If a patient has a urinary tract infection (UTI), the urine and symptoms related to a UTI should be assessed. Additionally, whenever a patient has an infection, it is important to continually monitor for the development of sepsis, a life-threatening condition caused by severe infection. Early signs of sepsis include new onset confusion, elevated heart rate, decreased blood pressure, increased respiratory rate, and elevated fever.

Additional baseline information to collect prior to the administration of any new medication order includes a patient history, current medication use including herbals or other supplements, and history of allergy or previous adverse response. Many patients with an allergy to one type of antimicrobial agent may experience cross-reactivity to other classes. This information should be appropriately communicated to the prescribing provider prior to the administration of any antimicrobial medication.

Nursing Process: Implementation of Interventions

With administration of the antimicrobial medication, it is important for the nurse to anticipate any additional interventions associated with the medications. For example, antimicrobials often cause gastrointestinal upset (GI) such as nausea, diarrhea, etc. The patient should be educated about these potential side effects, and proper interventions should be taken to minimize these occurrences. For example, the nurse may instruct the patient to take certain antimicrobials with food to diminish the chance of GI upset, whereas other medications should be taken on an empty stomach for optimal absorption.

Hypersensitivity/allergic reactions are always a potential adverse reaction, especially when administering the first dose of a new antibiotic, and the nurse should monitor for these symptoms closely and respond appropriately by immediately notifying the prescriber. Hypersensitivity reactions are immune responses that are exaggerated or inappropriate to an antigen and can range from itching to anaphylaxis. Anaphylaxis is a medical emergency that can cause life-threatening respiratory failure. Early signs of anaphylaxis include, but are not limited to, hives and itching, the feeling of a swollen tongue or throat, shortness of breath, dizziness, and low blood pressure.

Nursing Process: Evaluation

Finally, it is important to always evaluate the patient's response to a medication. With antimicrobial medications, the nurse should assess for absence of or decreasing signs of infection, indicating the patient is improving. It is important to document these findings to reflect the patient's trended response.

Additionally, it is also important for the nurse to promptly identify and communicate signs of worsening infection to the provider. For example, increasing white blood cell count, temperature, heart rate, and respiratory rate may indicate that the patient's body is experiencing a life-threatening response to the infection. These signs of worsening clinical assessment require prompt intervention to prevent further clinical deterioration. Additionally, patients receiving antibiotics should be closely monitored for developing a complication called "C-diff," resulting in frequent, foul-smelling stools. C-diff requires the implementation of modified contact precautions, including the use of soap and water, not hand sanitizer, as well as antibiotic therapy.[26]

---

26   Kelly, C.P., Lamon, J.T., and Bakken, J.S. (2019). Clostridioides (formerly Clostridium) diffcile infection in adults: Treatment and prevention. *UpToDate*. Retrieved on July 8, 2019, from https://www.uptodate.com/contents/ clostridioides-formerly-clostridium-diffcile-infection-in-adults-treatment-and-prevention?search=Clostridioides%20(formerly%20Clostridium)%20diffcile%20infection%20in%20adults&source=search_result&selectedTitle=1~150&usage_type=default&display_rank=1.

3.5   PENICILLINS

Now that we have reviewed antimicrobial basics, administration considerations, and the nursing process when administering antimicrobials, we will take a closer look at specifc antimicrobial classes and administration considerations, therapeutic effects, adverse effects, and specifc teaching needed for each class of antimicrobials. Each of the following sections of this chapter is based on a class or subclass of anti-infective medications. Each section discusses the mechanism of action, specifc administration considerations, and common patient teaching for this class/subclass of medication. Each section is then followed by a medication table with a common generic medication and its specifc administration considerations, therapeutic effects, and side effects/adverse effects for this medication.

Penicillins

Penicillin was the first antibiotic discovered and its detection came as a bit of an accident. In 1928, Alexander Fleming, a professor of bacteriology at St. Mary's Hospital in London, discovered penicillin accidentally growing in a petri dish in his lab. The penicillin was the result of mold juice that had grown there inadvertently. Fleming noted that this "mold juice" inhibited the growth of Staphylococcus bacteria that was previously growing in the petri dish. Subsequently, the first antibiotic discovery was made.[27]

Indications

Penicillins are prescribed to treat a variety of infectious processes such as Streptococcal infections, Pneumococcal infections, and Staphylococcal infections. Penicillins may be administered orally, IV, or intramuscularly.

Mechanism of Action

Penicillins are bactericidal and kill bacteria by interfering with the synthesis of proteins needed in their cellular walls.[28] When the bacterial cell wall is impaired, the cell is rapidly broken down and destroyed.

Specifc Administration Considerations

In addition to general antimicrobial administration considerations, it is important to monitor patients who receive penicillins for signs of superinfections such as C-diff or yeast infections. There is also a cross-sensitivity for patients allergic to cephalosporins. It is important to remember that patients who are prescribed high doses of penicillin may experience signifcant coagulation abnormalities. [29]Other notable drug interactions include the use of diuretic therapy with penicillin. Penicillin contains a signifcant amount of potassium. Patients receiving potassium-sparing diuretics or supplementation should be monitored for signs of hyperkalemia. Penicillin is best absorbed on an empty stomach; however, many patients may experience GI upset and subsequently take the medication with food.

Patient Teaching and Education

---

27   American Chemical Society International Historic Chemical Landmarks. *Discovery and development of penicillin*. http://www.acs.org/content/acs/en/education/whatischemistry/landmarks/flemingpenicillin.html.

28   This work is a derivative of *Principles of Pharmacology* by LibreTexts licensed under CC BY-NC-SA 4.0.

29   *Pharmacology Notes: Nursing Implications for Clinical Practice* by Gloria Velarde is licensed under CC BY-NA- SA 4.0.

The patient should notify the health care provider (HCP) if fever or diarrhea develops, especially if the stool contains blood, pus, or mucus. Advise the patient not to treat diarrhea without advice from HCP. If GI upset occurs, the patient may take the medication with meals but should avoid taking with citrus-based products, which can impede absorption. Additionally, patients should be instructed to chew oral chewable tablets thoroughly before swallowing. The patient should report a rash or any signs of superinfection (black, furry overgrowth on tongue; vaginal itching or discharge; loose or foul-smelling stool).

Patients should be instructed to take medication around the clock and to finish the drug completely as directed. Doses should be spaced evenly to achieve the desired therapeutic effect. Additionally, patients should receive instruction to not share medication and that any sharing of medications may be dangerous. Patients with a history of rheumatic heart disease or valve replacement should receive instruction regarding the importance of using antimicrobial prophylaxis before invasive medical or dental procedures. Female patients taking oral contraceptives should use an alternative form of contraception during therapy with amoxicillin and until next period. Patients should notify their HCP if symptoms do not improve.[30]

Now let's take a closer look at the penicillin medication grid in Table 3.5.[31] Medication grids are intended to assist students to learn key points about each medication. Basic information related to a common generic medication in this class is outlined, including administration considerations, therapeutic effects, and side effects/adverse effects. **Prototype**/generic medications listed in the medication grid are also hyperlinked directly to a free resource from the United States National Library of Medicine called *Daily Med*. Because information about medication is constantly changing, nurses should always consult evidence-based resources to review current recommendations before administering specific medication. On the home page of *Daily Med*, enter the drug name in the search bar to read more about the medication.

Table 3.5: Penicillin Medication Grid

Class/ Subclass	Prototype-Generic	Administration Considerations	Therapeutic Effects	Side/Adverse Effects
Penicillin	penicillin V (PO) penicillin G (IV) ■ amoxicillin ■ piperacillin/ tazobactam (combination product)	Check for allergies to penicillin or cephalosporins Obtain culture, if ordered, before first dose Take with full glass of water; no acidic juice Best absorbed orally on empty stomach; give with food if stomach upset If high doses; monitor INR, platelets, PT	Monitor for systemic signs of infection: ■ WBCs ■ Temp ■ Culture results Monitor actual site of infection for improvement	Common: nausea, vomiting, epigastric distress, diarrhea, and black hairy tongue Monitor for C-diff, candidiasis, and hyperkalemia Hypersensitivity: Rash (maculopapular to exfoliative dermatitis), urticaria, laryngeal edema, and anaphylaxis SAFETY: If an allergic reaction occurs, penicillin should be discontinued and appropriate therapy instituted. Serious anaphylactic reactions require emergency treatment with epinephrine and airway management

---

30   uCentral from Unbound Medicine. https://www.unboundmedicine.com/ucentral.

31   *Pharmacology Notes: Nursing Implications for Clinical Practice* by Gloria Velarde is licensed under CC BY-NA- SA 4.0.

My Notes

Critical Thinking Activity 3.5a

Using the above grid information, consider the following clinical scenario question:

Mr. Jones was admitted to the medical surgical foor with a Pneumococcal respiratory infection and prescribed penicillin V 500 mg PO every 6 hours. You bring the patient his 0800 medications, which include his penicillin. The patient has just finished his breakfast that included orange juice. Would you proceed with the penicillin administration at this time? Why or why not?

Note: Answers to the Critical Thinking activities can be found in the "Answer Key" sections at the end of the book.

3.6   CEPHALOSPORINS

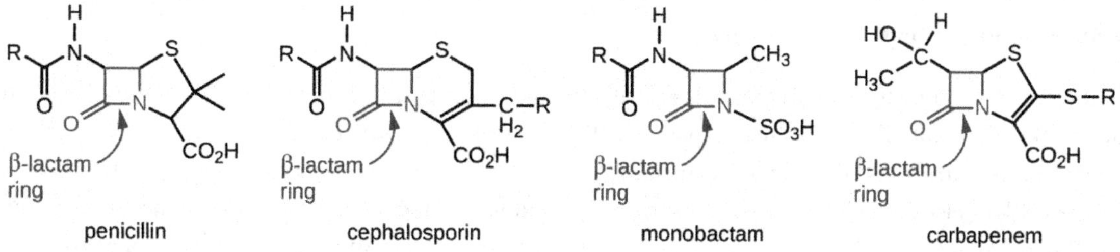

β-lactam ring
penicillin

β-lactam ring
cephalosporin

β-lactam ring
monobactam

β-lactam ring
carbapenem

R group	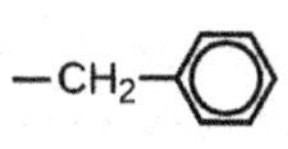 $-CH_2-$⬡	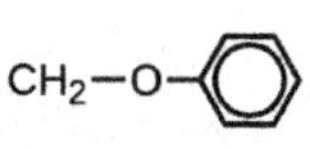 CH_2-O-⬡	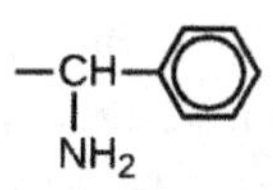 $-CH-$⬡ $\vert$ NH_2	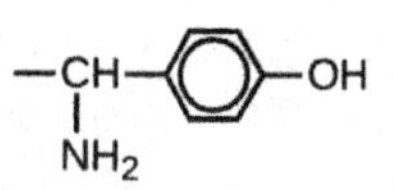 $-CH-$⬡$-OH$ $\vert$ NH_2	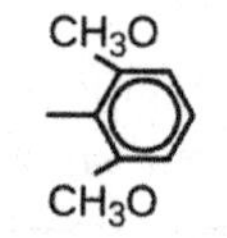 CH_3O ⬡ CH_3O
Drug name	penicillin G	penicillin V	ampicillin	amoxicillin	methicillin
Spectrum of activity	G+ and a few G−	similar to penicillin G	G+ and more G− than penicillin	similar to ampicillin	G+ only, including β-lactamase producers
Route of administration	parenteral	oral	parenteral and oral	oral (better than ampicillin)	parenteral

Figure 3.8 Comparison of beta-lactam ring structure across different classes of medications, spectrum of activity and routes of administration[footnote]"OSC Microbio 14 02 BetaLactam.jpg" by CNX Openstax is licensed under CC BY 4.0 Access for free at https://openstax.org/books/microbiology/ pages/14–3-mechanisms-of-antibacterial-drugs[/footnote]

Cephalosporins are a slightly modifed chemical "twin" to penicillins due to their beta lactam chemical structure. (See Figure 3.8 for a comparison of the beta-lactam ring structure, spectrum of activity, and route of administration across different classes of medications.) Because of these similarities, some patients who have allergies to penicillins may experience cross-sensitivity to cephalosporins.

Indications

Cephalosporins are used to treat skin and skin-structure infections, bone infections, genitourinary infections, otitis media, and community-acquired respiratory tract infections.

Mechanism of Action

Cephalosporins are typically bactericidal and are similar to penicillin in their action within the cell wall. Cephalosporins are sometimes grouped into "generations" by their antimicrobial properties. The 1st-generation drugs are effective mainly against gram-positive organisms. Higher generations generally have expanded spectra against

My Notes

aerobic gram-negative bacilli. The 5th-generation cephalosporins are active against methicillin-resistant Staphylococcus aureus (MRSA) or other complicated infections.[32]

Specifc Administration Considerations

Patients who are allergic to pencillins may also be allergic to cephalosporins. Patients who consume cephalosporins while drinking alcoholic beverages may experience disulfram-like reactions including severe headache, flushing, nausea, vomiting, etc.[33] Additionally, like penicillins, cephalosporins may interfere with coagulability and increase a patient's risk of bleeding. Cephalosporin dosing may require adjustment for patients experiencing renal impairment. Blood urea nitrogen (BUN) and creatinine should be monitored carefully to identify signs of nephrotoxicity.

Patient Teaching and Education

Patients who are prescribed cephalosporins should be specifcally cautioned about a disulfram reaction, which can occur when alcohol is ingested while taking the medication. Additionally, individuals should be instructed to monitor for rash and signs of superinfection (such as black, furry overgrowth on tongue; vaginal itching or discharge; loose or foul-smelling stool) and report to the prescribing provider.

It is also important to note that cephalosporin can enter breastmilk and may alter bowel fora of the infant. Thus, use during breastfeeding is often discouraged.[34]

Now let's take a closer look at the cephalosporin medication grid in Table 3.6.[35]

---

32   Werth, B.J. (2018, August). *Cephalosporins.* Merck Manual Professional Version. https://www.merckmanuals.com/professional/infectious-diseases/bacteria-and-antibacterial-drugs/ cephalosporins.

33   Ren, S., Cao, Y., Zhang, X., Jiao, S., Qian, S., and Liu, P. (2014). Cephalosporin induced disulfram-like reaction: a retrospective review of 78 cases. *International Surgery, 99*(2), 142–146. https://www.internationalsurgery.org/ doi/full/10.9738/INTSURG-D-13-00086.1.

34   uCentral from Unbound Medicine. https://www.unboundmedicine.com/ucentral.

35   *Daily Med*, https://dailymed.nlm.nih.gov/dailymed/index.cfm, used for hyperlinked medications in this module. Retrieved June 27, 2019.

Table 3.6: Cephalosporin Medication Grid

Class/ Subclass	Prototype/Generics	Administration Considerations	Therapeutic Effects	Side/ Adverse Effects
Cephalosporins	1st generation: cephalexin Cefazolin 2nd generation: cefprozil 3rd generation: ceftriaxone 4th generation: cefepime 5th generation: ceftolozane	Check for allergies, including if allergic to penicillin Dosage adjustment if renal impairment Use with caution with seizure disorder PO: Administer without regard to food; if GI distress, give with food IV: Reconstitute drug with sterile water or normal saline; shake well until dissolved. Inject into large vein or free-fowing IV solution over 3–5 minutes Drug interaction: anticoagulants	Monitor for systemic signs of infection: ■ WBCs ■ Fever Monitor actual site of infection Monitor culture results, if obtained	Common side effects: ■ Nausea ■ Vomiting ■ Epigastric distress ■ Diarrhea Monitor for: ■ Rash ■ C-diff ■ Nephrotoxicity if pre-existing renal disease ■ Elevated INR and bleeding risk ■ Development of hemolytic anemia

Critical Thinking Activity 3.6a

Using the above grid information, consider the following clinical scenario question:

Mrs. Jenkins is an 89-year-old patient admitted to the medical surgical foor for treatment of a skin infection. The admitting provider prescribes Cefazolin 1 gram every 8 hours IV.

Mrs. Jenkins' admission laboratory tests include renal laboratory studies refecting:

Creatinine: 1.3 mg/dL (Normal range: 1.2 mg/dL [36]

Blood urea nitrogen (BUN): 25 mg/dL (Normal: 8-20 mg/dL)

Glomerular Filtration Rate: 55 ml/min (Normal: 90-120 ml/min)

On Day 3 Mrs. Jenkins has renal laboratory studies performed again. The results are:

Creatinine: 1.6 mg/dL

Blood urea nitrogen (BUN): 57 mg/dL

Glomerular Filtration Rate: 20 ml/min [37]

Are Day 3 fndings expected or not? What course of action should the nurse take?

Note: Answers to the Critical Thinking activities can be found in the "Answer Key" sections at the end of the book.

---

36   U.S. National Library of Medicine, Medline Plus. (2020, February 13). *Basic metabolic panel.* https://medlineplus.gov/ency/article/003462.htm.

37   U.S. National Library of Medicine, Medline Plus. (2020, February 13). *Glomerular filtration rate.* https://medlineplus.gov/ency/article/007305.htm.

3.7   CARBAPENEMS

Carbapenems are a beta- lactam "cousin" to penicillins and cephalosporins.

Indications

Carbapenems are useful for treating life-threatening, multidrug-resistant infections due to their broad spectrum of activity.[38] These antibiotics are effective in treating gram-positive and gram-negative infections. Because of their broad spectrum of activity, these medications can be especially useful for treating complex hospital-acquired infections or for patients who are immunocompromised.

Mechanism of Action

Carbapenems are typically bactericidal and work by inhibiting the synthesis of the bacterial cell wall.

Specifc Administration Considerations

Carbapenems are similar to cephalosporins. Cross sensitivity may occur in patients allergic to pencillin or cephalosporins.

Patient Teaching and Education

Patients should monitor for signs of superinfection and report any occurrence to the provider. If a patient experiences fever and bloody diarrhea, they should contact the provider immediately. The patient should also be advised that side effects can occur even weeks after the medication is discontinued.[39]

Now let's take a closer look at the medication grid for imipenem in Table 3.7.[40]

Table 3.7: Carbapenem Medication Grid

Class/Subclass	Prototype/ Generic	Administration Considerations	Therapeutic Effects	Side/Adverse Effects
Carbapenems	imipenem	Route: IV Check for allergies, including penicillin and cephalosporins Dosage adjustment if renal impairment Use with caution with seizure disorder or renal dysfunction	Monitor for systemic signs of infection: ■ WBCs ■ Fever Monitor actual site of infection Monitor culture results, if obtained	Similar to cephalosporins

38   Papp-Wallace, K. M., Endimiani, A., Taracila, M. A., and Bonomo, R. A. (2011). Carbapenems: past, present, and future. *Antimicrobial agents and chemotherapy, 55*(11), 4943–4960. https://www.ncbi.nlm.nih.gov/pmc/articles/PMC3195018/.

39   uCentral from Unbound Medicine. https://www.unboundmedicine.com/ucentral.

40   *Daily Med*, https://dailymed.nlm.nih.gov/dailymed/index.cfm, used for hyperlinked medications in this module. Retrieved June 27, 2019.

My Notes

Critical Thinking Activity 3.7a

Using the above grid information, consider the following clinical scenario question:

John Smith was admitted to the hospital with a serious abdominal infection. The nurse notices that this patient is allergic to penicillin as he prepares to administer the first dose of imipenem medication. What is the nurse's next best action?

Note: Answers to the Critical Thinking activities can be found in the "Answer Key" sections at the end of the book.

3.8   MONOBACTAMS

Like penicillins, cephalosporins, and carbapenems, monobactams also have a beta-lactam ring structure.

Indications

Monobactams are narrow-spectrum antibacterial medications that are used primarily to treat gram-negative bacteria such as Pseudomonas aeruginosa.

Mechanism of Action

Monobactams are bactericidal and work to inhibit bacterial cell wall synthesis.[41]

Specifc Administration Considerations

Patients taking monobactams may experience adverse effects similar to other beta-lactam medications, so nurses should monitor for GI symptoms, skin sensitivities, and coagulation abnormalities.

Patient Teaching and Education

Patients should monitor for signs of superinfection and report any occurrence to the provider. If the patient experiences fever and bloody diarrhea, they should contact the provider immediately. The patient should also be advised to notify the provider immediately if symptoms progress or if any sign of allergic response occurs.[42]

Now let's take a closer look at the medication grid for aztreonam in Table 3.8.[43]

Table 3.8: Monobactam Medication Grid

Class/Subclass	Prototype/ Generic	Administration Considerations	Therapeutic Effects	Side/Adverse Effects
Monobactams	aztreonam	Check for allergies to any beta lactams—penicillin, cephalosporins, or carbapenems Can be administered IM, IV, or via inhalation	Monitor for systemic signs of infection: ■ WBCs ■ Fever Monitor actual site of infection Monitor culture results, if obtained	Similar to cephalosporins

---

41   This work is a derivative of *Microbiology* by OpenStax licensed under CC BY 4.0. Access for free at https://openstax.org/books/microbiology/pages/1-introduction.

42   uCentral from Unbound Medicine. https://www.unboundmedicine.com/ucentral.

43   *Daily Med*, https://dailymed.nlm.nih.gov/dailymed/index.cfm, used for hyperlinked medications in this module. Retrieved June 27, 2019.

My Notes

Critical Thinking Activity 3.8a

Using the above grid information, consider the following clinical scenario question:

A patient with cystic fbrosis is diagnosed with ventilator-associated pneumonia and is prescribed Aztreonam 1 gm IV daily for a suspected Pseudomonas aeruginosa infection. The nurse reviews the culture results that just arrived and notices that the results indicate the infection is caused by Methicillin-resistant Staphylococcus aureus. Will this medication be effective against this bacteria? What is the nurse's next best response?

Note: Answers to the Critical Thinking activities can be found in the "Answer Key" sections at the end of the book.

3.9   SULFONAMIDES

Sulfonamides are one of the oldest broad-spectrum antimicrobial agents that work by competitively inhibiting bacterial metabolic enzymes needed for bacterial function.

Indications

Sulfonamides are used to treat urinary tract infections, otitis media, acute exacerbations of chronic bronchitis, and travelers' diarrhea.

Mechanism of Action

This mechanism of action provides bacteriostatic inhibition of growth against a wide spectrum of gram-positive and gram-negative pathogens.

Specifc Administration Considerations

Allergic reactions to sulfonamide medications are common and, therefore, patients should be monitored carefully for adverse effects including delayed hypersensitivity reactions. Sulfonamide medications increase the risk of crystalluria that can cause kidney stones or decreased kidney function; therefore, patients should increase their water intake while taking these medications.[44]

Patient Teaching and Education

The patient should receive education to complete the full prescribed dose of medications and take measures to not skip doses. If a dose is missed, the patient should take the missed dose as soon as possible unless it is near the next dosing time. The medication can cause increased photosensitivity, and patients should be educated to use sunscreen and protective clothing with sun exposure. The patient should also report any rash, sore throat, fever, or mouth sores that might occur. Unusual bleeding or bruising should also be reported to the provider. If patients are receiving prolonged therapy, they may require platelet count monitoring.[45]

Now let's take a closer look at the medication grid for trimethoprim-sulfamethoxazole in Table 3.9.[46]

---

44   This work is a derivative of *Microbiology* by OpenStax licensed under CC BY 4.0. Access for free at https://openstax.org/books/microbiology/pages/1-introduction.

45   uCentral from Unbound Medicine. https://www.unboundmedicine.com/ucentral.

46   *Daily Med*, https://dailymed.nlm.nih.gov/dailymed/index.cfm, used for hyperlinked medications in this module. Retrieved June 27, 2019.

Table 3.9: Sulfonamides Medication Grid

Class/Subclass	Prototype/Generic	Administration Considerations	Therapeutic Effects	Side/Adverse Effects
Sulfonamides	trimethoprim-sulfamethoxazole	Check for allergies Dose adjustment for renal impairment Administer PO with 8 oz of water Monitor urine output and for cloudiness or crystals Do not administer IM Use cautiously with cardiac antidysrhythmics Use cautiously with oral antidiabetics; may increase hypoglycemic effects. Monitor glucose level carefully Use cautiously with anticoagulant medications such as warfarin; may increase risk of bleeding. Monitor INR and patient for signs of bleeding	Monitor for systemic signs of infection: ■ WBCs ■ Fever Monitor actual site of infection Monitor culture results, if obtained	SAFETY: Sulfonamides, including sulfonamide-containing products such as sulfamethoxaole/trimethoprim, should be discontinued at the first appearance of skin rash of any sign of adverse reaction

Critical Thinking Activity 3.9a

Using the above grid information, consider the following clinical scenario question:

A nurse is caring for an elderly diabetic patient who has been prescribed trimethoprim-sulfamethoxazole for a urinary tract infection. What nursing interventions will be implemented prior to medication administration?

Note: Answers to the Critical Thinking activities can be found in the "Answer Key" sections at the end of the book.

3.10 FLUOROQUINOLONES

Indications

Fluoroquinolones may be used to treat pneumonia or complicated skin or urinary tract infections.

Mechanism of Action

Fluoroquinolones are a synthetic antibacterial medication that work by inhibiting the bacterial DNA replication. They are bacteriocidal due to the action they take against the DNA of the bacterial cell wall. Many fuoroquinolones are broad spectrum and effective against a wide variety of both gram-positive and gram-negative bacteria.

Specifc Administration Considerations

Patients taking oral fuoroquinolones should avoid the use of antacid medication as antacids signifcantly impede absorption. Patients should also be instructed to take oral fuoroquinolones with a full glass of water two hours before or after meals to enhance absorption and prevent crystalluria. Fluoroquinolone therapy is contraindicated in children except for complicated UTIs, pyelonephritis, plague, or post Anthrax exposure and should be used cautiously in pregnancy.[47]

Black Box Warning

Black Box Warnings are the strongest warnings issued by the Federal Drug Association (FDA) and signify that the medical studies have indicated that the drug carries a signifcant risk of serious or life- threatening adverse effects.

Fluoroquinolones, including levofoxacin, have been associated with disabling and potentially irreversible serious adverse reactions, including:

- Tendinitis and tendon rupture
- Peripheral neuropathy
- Central nervous system effects
- Exacerbation of muscle weakness in patients with myasthenia gravis

In patients who experience any of these serious adverse reactions, discontinue the medication immediately, and avoid the useof fuoroquinolones.

Patient Teaching and Education

All patients on fuoroquinolone therapy should be instructed to avoid direct and indirect sunlight due to the photosensitivity that can be experienced while on these medications. The patient should take measures to ensure that dosages are spaced evenly throughout the day and that fluid balance is maintained. It is important to maintain an intake of 1500mL–2000mL per day while taking the medication. The patient should be advised that medications containing calcium, aluminum, iron, or zinc may impair absorption and should be avoided. Other side effects of fuoroquinolones increase drowsiness. Additionally, the patient should be cautioned to monitor for episodes of fainting or decreased heart rate and report any history of prolonged QT syndrome. If a patient notices

---

47   This work is a derivative of *Microbiology* by OpenStax licensed under CC BY 4.0. Access for free at https://openstax.org/ books/microbiology/pages/1-introduction.

My Notes

peripheral neuropathy occurring, this should be reported to the healthcare provider. Additional side effects to monitor include increased tendon pain, jaundice, rash, or mood changes.[48]

Now let's take a closer look at the medication grid for levofoxacin in Table 3.10.[49]

Table 3.10: Fluoroquinolone Medication Grid

Class/ Subclass	Prototype/ Generic	Administration Considerations	Therapeutic Effects	Side/Adverse Effects
Fluoroquinolones	levofloxacin	Check for allergies Give with plenty of fuids Oral: Administer 2 hours before or after meals, antacid, or iron IV: Infuse 500 mg or less over 60 minutes and doses of 750 mg over 90 minutes Dosage adjustment if renal or hepatic impairment Use cautiously if history of seizures	Monitor for systemic signs of infection: ■ WBCs ■ Fever Monitor actual site of infection Monitor culture results, if obtained	Discontinue immediately if tendonitis, tendon rupture, peripheral neuropathy, CNS effects, or muscle weakness in patients with Myasthenia Gravis Monitor for: ■ GI upset ■ Hypersensitivity ■ Photosensitivity ■ Hypoglycemia ■ C-diff

Critical Thinking Activity 3.10a

Utilizing the above grid information, consider the following clinical scenario question:

A nurse is administering levofoxacin to a patient diagnosed with pneumonia. The patient reports that he has pain "above his heel" today. The nurse assesses and discovers the pain is over the Achilles tendon. What is the nurse's next best response?

Note: Answers to the Critical Thinking activities can be found in the "Answer Key" sections at the end of the book.

---

48   uCentral from Unbound Medicine. https://www.unboundmedicine.com/ucentral.

49   *Daily Med*, https://dailymed.nlm.nih.gov/dailymed/index.cfm, used for hyperlinked medications in this module. Retrieved June 27, 2019.

3.11   MACROLIDES

Macrolides are complex antibacterial broad-spectrum medications that are effective against both gram-positive and gram-negative bacteria.

Mechanism of Action

Macrolides inhibit RNA protein synthesis and suppress reproduction of the bacteria. Macrolides are bacteriostatic as they do not actually kill bacteria, but inhibit additional growth and allow the body's immune system to kill the offending bacteria.[50]

Indications

Macrolides are often used for respiratory infections, otitis media, pelvic infammatory infections, and Chlamydia.

Specifc Administration Considerations

Macrolides can have signifcant impact on liver function and should be used cautiously in patients with liver disease or impairment.

Patient Teaching and Education

GI upset is common and patients can be advised to take medication with food. Patients should also be advised to avoid excessive sunlight and to wear protective clothing and use sunscreen when outside, as well as to report any adverse reactions immediately. Advise patients to report symptoms of chest pain, palpitations, or yellowing of eyes or skin. Additionally, patients should be advised that these medications can cause drowsiness.[51]

Now let's take a closer look at the medication grid for erythromycin and azithromycin in Table 3.11.[52]

50   This work is a derivative of *Microbiology* by OpenStax licensed under CC BY 4.0. Access for free at https://openstax.org/books/microbiology/pages/1-introduction.

51   uCentral from Unbound Medicine. https://www.unboundmedicine.com/ucentral.

52   *Daily Med*, https://dailymed.nlm.nih.gov/dailymed/index.cfm, used for hyperlinked medications in this module. Retrieved June 28, 2019.

Table 3.11: Macrolides Medication Grid

Class/Subclass	Prototype/ Generic	Administration Considerations	Therapeutic Effects	Side/Adverse Effects
Macrolides	erythromycin azithromycin	Check for allergies PO: Reconstitute suspension with water. Can be given with or without food. Take with food if GI upset occurs IV: Reconstitute and shake until well dissolved. Dilute as instructed. Infuse a 500-mg dose of azithromycin IV over 1 hour or longer. Never give as a bolus or IM injection May prolong QT interval segment. Monitor for dysrhythmias	Monitor for systemic signs of infection: ■ WBCs ■ Fever Monitor actual site of infection	GI upset Hypersensitivity Photosensitivity Discontinue immediately if: ■ QT prolongation or dysrhythmias ■ Signs of liver damage or jaundice ■ Onset or worsening of myasthenia gravis

Critical Thinking Activity 3.11a

Using the above grid information, consider the following clinical scenario question:

A nurse is administering azithromycin to a patient with an acute bacterial worsening of COPD. Today the patient's sclera appear yellow, which is a new finding. What is the nurse's next best response?

Note: Answers to the Critical Thinking activities can be found in the "Answer Key" sections at the end of the book.

3.12 AMINOGLYCOSIDES

Aminoglycosides are a potent broad spectrum of antibiotics that are useful for treating severe infections. Many aminoglycosides are poorly absorbed in the GI tract; therefore, the majority are given IV or IM. Aminoglycosides are potentially nephrotoxic and neurotoxic. They should be administered cautiously. Blood peak and trough levels should be performed to titrate a safe dose for each patient.

Indications

Streptomycin is used for streptococcal endocarditis and a second line treatment for tuberculosis. Neomycin is used in the treatment of hepatic encephalopathy as adjunct therapy to lower ammonia levels and is also used as a bowel prep for colon procedures.

Mechanism of Action

Aminoglycosides are bactericidal and bind with the area of the ribosome known as the 30S subunit, inhibiting protein synthesis in the cell wall and resulting in bacterial death (see Figure 3.9).[53] Aminoglycosides may be given with beta-lactam medications to facilitate transport of aminoglycoside across the cellular membrane, resulting in a synergistic effect and increasing drug effectiveness.

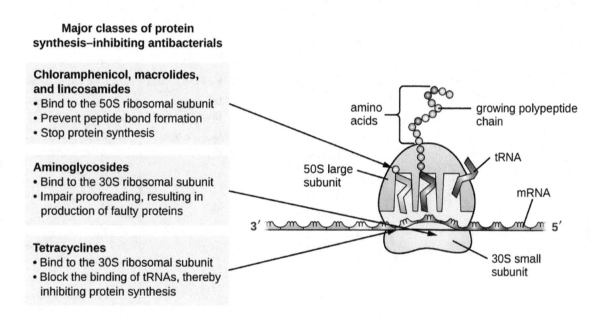

Figure 3.9 Medications that inhibit protein synthesis

Special Administration Considerations

Aminoglycosides can result in many adverse effects for the patient and, therefore, the nurse should monitor the patient carefully for signs of emerging concerns. Peak and trough levels are used to titrate this medication to a safe dose. Aminoglycosides can be nephrotoxic (damaging to kidney), neurotoxic (damaging to the nervous system), and ototoxic (damaging to the ear). Nurses should monitor the patient receiving aminoglycosides for signs

---

53   This work is a derivative of *Microbiology* by OpenStax licensed under CC BY 4.0. Access for free at https://openstax.org/ books/microbiology/pages/1-introduction.

of decreased renal function such as declining urine output and increasing blood urea nitrogen (BUN), creatinine, and declining glomerular filtration rate (GFR). Indications of damage to the neurological system may be assessed as increasing peripheral numbness or tingling in the extremities. Additionally, the patient should be carefully assessed for hearing loss or hearing changes throughout the course of drug administration.

Patient Teaching and Education

Patients receiving aminoglycosides should be advised to monitor for signs of hypersensitivity and auditory changes. This may include tinnitus and hearing loss. Patients may also experience accompanying vertigo while on the medication. Patients should be advised to drink plenty of fluids while taking the medication. Female patients should notify their provider if pregnancy is planned or if they are actively breastfeeding.[54]

Now let's take a closer look at the medication grid for streptomycin and gentamycin in Table 3.12.[55]

Table 3.12: Streptomycin and Gentamycin Medication Grid

Class/Subclass	Prototype/ Generic	Administration Considerations	Therapeutic Effects	Side/Adverse Effects
Aminoglycosides	streptomycin gentamicin	Check for allergies Obtain culture before administering IM: Blood sample for peak level should be obtained 1 to 2 hours after IM injection; obtain blood for trough level just before next dose Inject in a large muscle Handle carefully; use gloves to prepare Monitor peak and trough levels	Monitor for systemic signs of infection: ■ WBCs ■ Fever Monitor actual site of infection Monitor culture results	GI upset Rash Report diarrhea immediately SAFETY: Nephrotoxicity: monitor renal function closely Risk for severe neurotoxic reactions, especially with renal impairment. Can result in respiratory paralysis if given soon after anesthesia or muscle relaxant Risk for ototoxicity, especially if administered with a loop diuretic Can cause harm to fetus and breastfed infants

---

54   uCentral from Unbound Medicine. https://www.unboundmedicine.com/ucentral.

55   *Daily Med*, https://dailymed.nlm.nih.gov/dailymed/index.cfm, used for hyperlinked medications in this module. Retrieved June 27, 2019.

Critical Thinking Activity 3.12a

Using the above grid information, consider the following clinical scenario question:

A patient is admitted with streptococcal endocarditis and the nurse is preparing the morning dose of streptomycin. The lab has not yet arrived to obtain the trough level, and the drug is now overdue to be given. What is the nurse's next best response?

Note: Answers to the Critical Thinking activities can be found in the "Answer Key" sections at the end of the book.

3.13 TETRACYCLINES

Tetracyclines are broad-spectrum antibiotics that are bacteriostatic, subsequently inhibiting bacterial growth.

Indications

Tetracycline medications are useful for the treatment of many gram-positive and gram-negative infectious processes, yet are limited due to the signifcance of side effects experienced by many patients.

Mechanism of Action

Tetracyclines work by penetrating the bacterial cell wall and binding to the 30S ribosome, inhibiting the protein synthesis required to make the cellular wall.[56]

Special Administration Considerations

Signifcant side effects of tetracycline drug therapy include photosensitivity, discoloration of developing teeth and enamel hypoplasia, and renal and liver impairment.[57] Tetracyclines are contraindicated in pregnancy and for children ages 8 and under. Small amounts may be excreted in breast milk.

Patient Teaching and Education

Patients should be instructed to avoid direct sunlight exposure and wear sunscreen to prevent skin sensitivities.

Additionally, it is important for patients to be educated regarding potential impaired absorption of tetracycline with the use of dairy products. Patients who are on oral contraceptives should be educated that tetracyclines may impede the effectiveness of the oral contraceptive and an alternative measure of birth control should be utilized while on the antibiotic. Female patients must be aware to immediately stop tetracycline if they become pregnant. Expired tetracycline should be immediately disposed of as it can become toxic.[58]

Now let's take a closer look at the medication grid for tetracycline in Table 3.13.[59]

---

56   This work is a derivative of *Microbiology* by OpenStax licensed under CC BY 4.0. Access for free at https://openstax.org/books/microbiology/pages/1-introduction.

57   This work is a derivative of *Microbiology* by OpenStax licensed under CC BY 4.0. Access for free at https://openstax.org/books/microbiology/pages/1-introduction.

58   uCentral from Unbound Medicine. https://www.unboundmedicine.com/ucentral.

59   *Daily Med*, https://dailymed.nlm.nih.gov/dailymed/index.cfm, used for hyperlinked medications in this module. Retrieved June 27, 2019.

Table 3.13: Tetracycline Medication Grid

Class/ Subclass	Prototype/ Generic	Administration Considerations	Therapeutic Effects	Side/Adverse Effects
Tetracyclines	tetracycline	Check allergies Alert: Check expiration date. Using outdated or deteriorated drug has been linked to severe reversible nephrotoxicity (Fanconi syndrome) Effectiveness is reduced when drug is given with milk or other dairy products, antacids, or iron products For best drug absorption, give drug with a full glass of water on an empty stomach at least 1 hour before or 2 hours after meals Give drug at least 1 hour before bedtime to prevent esophageal irritation or ulceration Use caution with renal or hepatic impairment Avoid using in children younger than age 8 because drug may cause permanent discoloration of teeth, enamel defects, and bone growth retardation Avoid in pregnancy due to toxic effects on the developing fetus (often related to retardation of skeletal development and teeth)	Monitor for systemic signs of infection: ■ WBCs ■ Fever Monitor actual site of infection	Gastrointestinal symptoms C-diff Photosensitivity Oral candidiasis Permanent teeth discoloration if given to patients < 8 y.o. Intracranial hypertension: Monitor for headache, blurred vision, diplopia, and vision loss Decreased effectiveness of oral contraceptives

Critical Thinking Activity 3.13a

Using the above grid information, consider the following clinical scenario question:

The nurse is providing medication teaching to a parent of a six-year-old child with strep throat in a clinic setting. Due to multiple drug allergies, tetracycline was prescribed by a doctor who is new to the clinic. What is the nurse's best response and why?

Note: Answers to the Critical Thinking activities can be found in the "Answer Key" sections at the end of the book.

3.14 ANTIVIRALS

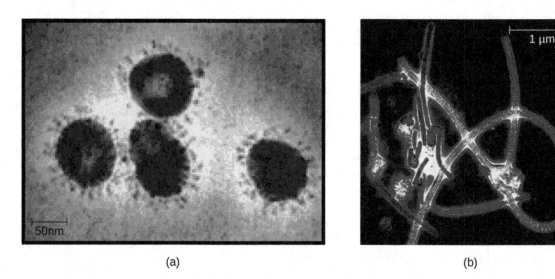

(a)   (b)

Figure 3.10 Images of viruses (a) Members of the Coronavirus family can cause respiratory infections like the common cold, severe acute respiratory syndrome (SARS), and Middle East respiratory syndrome (MERS). Here they are viewed under a transmission electron microscope (TEM). (b) Ebolavirus, a member of the Filovirus family. (credit a: modifcation of work by Centers for Disease Control and Prevention; credit b: modifcation of work by Thomas W. Geisbert)

Unlike the complex structure of fungi or protozoa, viral structure is simple. There are several subclasses of antiviral medications: antiherpes, antiinfuenza, anti-hepatitis, and antiretrovirals. Each subclass will be discussed in more detail below. See Figure 3.10[60] for images of viruses.

Subclass: Antiherpes

Indications

Acyclovir (Zovirax) and its derivatives are frequently used for the treatment of herpes and varicella virus infections, including genital herpes, chickenpox, shingles, Epstein-Barr virus infections, and cytomegalovirus infections.

Mechanism of Action

Acyclovir causes termination of the DNA chain during the viral replication process. Acyclovir can be administered either topically or systemically, depending on the infection.[61]

Special Administration Considerations

Acyclovir use may result in nephrotoxicity.

---

60 "Unknown" by CNX OpenStax is licensed under CC BY 4.0 Access for free at https://openstax.org/books/microbiology/pages/1-3-types-of-microorganisms.

61 This work is a derivative of *Microbiology* by OpenStax licensed under CC BY 4.0. Access for free at https://openstax.org/books/microbiology/pages/1-introduction.

Patient Teaching and Education

Patients who are being treated with antiviral therapy should be instructed about the importance of medication compliance. They may also experience signifcant fatigue, so periods of rest should be encouraged.[62]

Subclass: AntiInfluenza

Indications

Tamifu (oseltamivir) is used to target the influenza virus by blocking the release of the virus from the infected cells.

Mechanism of Action

Tamifu prevents the release of virus from infected cells.

Special Administration Considerations

This medication does not cure influenza, but can decrease flu symptoms and shorten the duration of illness if taken in a timely manner. Patients are prescribed the medication for prophylaxis against infection, known exposure, or to lesson the course of the illness. If patients experience fu-like symptoms, it is critical that they start treatment within 48 hours of symptom onset.

Patient Teaching and Education

Patients who are being treated with antiviral therapy should be instructed about the importance of medication compliance. They may also experience signifcant fatigue, so periods of rest should be encouraged.[63]

The influenza virus is one of the few RNA viruses that replicates in the nucleus of cells. Antivirals block the release stage. See Figure 3.11.[64]

---

62   uCentral from Unbound Medicine. https://www.unboundmedicine.com/ucentral.

63   uCentral from Unbound Medicine. https://www.unboundmedicine.com/ucentral.

64   "Unknown" by CNX OpenStax is licensed under CC BY 4.0 Access for free at https://openstax.org/ books/microbiology/ pages/6-2-the-viral-life-cycle.

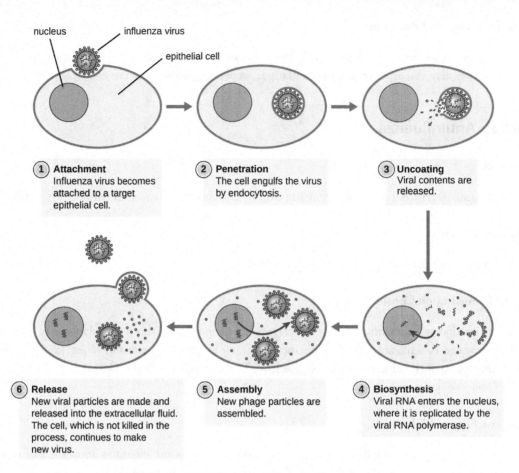

Figure 3.11 Influenza virus replication stages

Subclass: Antiretrovirals

Viruses with complex life cycles, such as HIV, can be more difficult to treat. These types of viruses require the use of antiretroviral medications that block viral replication. (See Figure 3.12 to view the viral replication process of HIV.)[65] Additionally, antiretrovirals fall under the class of antiviral medications.

---

65   This work is a derivative of "HIV Virus Replication Cycle" by NIAID is licensed under CC BY 2.0.

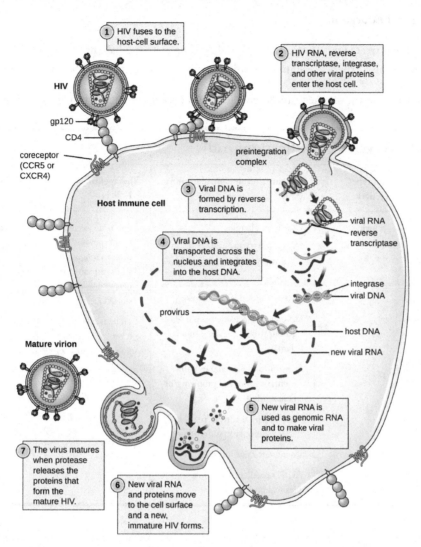

Figure 3.12 HIV attaches to a cell surface receptor of an immune cell and fuses with the cell membrane. Viral contents are released into the cell, where viral enzymes convert the single-stranded RNA genome into DNA and incorporate it into the host genome

Indications

Antiretrovirals are used for the treatment of illnesses like HIV.

Mechanism of Action

Antiretrovirals impede virus replication.

Special Administration Considerations

Many antiretrovirals may impact renal function; therefore, the patient's urine output and renal labs should be monitored carefully for signs of decreased function.

Patient Teaching and Education

Patients who are being treated with antiviral therapy should be instructed about the importance of antiretroviral compliance. They may also experience signifcant fatigue, so periods of rest should be encouraged.[66]

Now let's take a closer look at the medication grids for the subclasses of antivirals in Table 3.14a-d.[67]

Tables 3.14a: Acyclovir MedicationGrid				
Class/Subclass	**Prototype/ Generic**	**Administration Considerations**	**Therapeutic Effects**	**Side/Adverse Effects**
Antivirals: Antiherpes	acyclovir	Check for allergies Route: PO, IV, or topical; do not give IM or subcutaneously (subq) Give with food if GI distress IV: Give IV infusion over at least 1 hour to prevent renal tubular damage Use cautiously if renal impairment, neurological problems, or dehydration Start therapy as early as possible after signs or symptoms occur Encourage fluid intake Avoid sexual contact while lesions present	Drug is not a cure for herpes but improves signs and symptoms of herpes lesions if started early Can be used long term for prevention of outbreaks	GI distress Monitor renal function in long-term use, especially if renal impairment Lowers seizure threshold

---

66   uCentral from Unbound Medicine. https://www.unboundmedicine.com/ucentral.

67   *Daily Med*, https://dailymed.nlm.nih.gov/dailymed/index.cfm, used for hyperlinked medications in this module. Retrieved June 27, 2019.

Tables 3.14b: Oseltamivir Medication Grid

Class/Subclass	Prototype/ Generic	Administration Considerations	Therapeutic Effects	Side/Adverse Effects
Antivirals: AntiInfuenza Agents	oseltamivir	Check for allergies Route: PO Must be given within 48 hours of onset of symptoms Administer with food to avoid GI distress Does not replace need for annual influenza vaccination	Reduce duration of flu symptoms	GI distress Serious skin/hyper-sensitivity reactions; discontinue immediately Monitor for neuropsychiatric symptoms Use cautiously in patients with renal failure, chronic cardiac or respiratory diseases, or any medical condition that may require imminent hospitalization

Tables 3.14c: Adefovir Medication Grid

Class/Subclass	Prototype/ Generic	Administration Considerations	Therapeutic Effects	Side/Adverse Effects
Antivirals: Anti-Hepatitis Agents	adefovir	Route: PO Prolonged therapy (>1 year or indefinitely) based on patient status Offer HIV testing; may promote resistance to antiretrovirals in patients with chronic HBV infection who also have unrecognized or untreated HIV infection Do not stop taking medication unless directed Monitor hepatic function several months after stopping therapy	Maintain or improve liver function when active disease is present	Severe acute exacerbations of Hepatitis B Nephrotoxicity - Lactic acidosis - Severe hepatomegally

My Notes

Tables 3.14d: Lamuvadine-Zidovudine Medication Grid

Class/Subclass	Prototype/ Generic	Administration Considerations	Therapeutic Effects	Side/Adverse Effects
Antivirals: Antiretrovirals ■ Nucleoside– nucleotide Reverse transcriptase inhibitors	lamivudine– zidovudine	Check for allergies Lamivudine used to treat HIV-1 infection contains a higher dose of the active ingredient than the lamivudine used to treat chronic HBV infection. Patients with HIV-1 infection should receive only dosing forms appropriate for HIV-1 treatment Use cautiously in patients with renal impairment Inform patient that drug doesn't cure HIV infection, that opportunistic infections and other complications of HIV infection may still occur, and that transmission of HIV to others through sexual contact or blood contamination is still possible. Taking these medications, along with practicing safer sex and making other lifestyle changes, may decrease the risk of transmitting (spreading) the HIV or hepatitis B virus to other people Teach symptoms of pancreatitis	Decreases chance of developing acquired immunodeficiency syndrome (AIDS) and HIV-related illnesses such as serious infections or cancer	Lactic acidosis Severe hepatomegaly Stop treatment immediately if pancreatititis

Critical Thinking Activity 3.14a

Using the above grid information, consider the following clinical scenario question:

A patient is prescribed oseltamivir (Tamifu) for infuenza symptoms. The patient states to the nurse, "I hope this medication works quickly! I have felt lousy for the past 5 days!" What is the nurse's next best response?

Note: Answers to the Critical Thinking activities can be found in the "Answer Key" sections at the end of the book.

3.15 ANTIFUNGALS

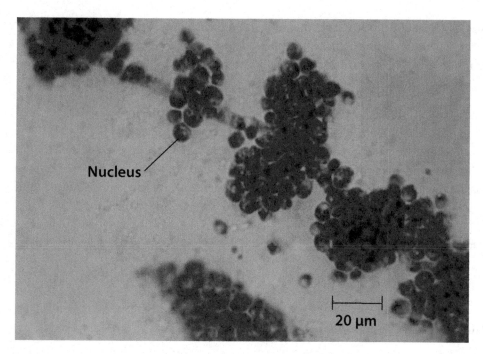

Figure 3.13 Candida albicans is a unicellular fungus, or yeast. It is the causative agent of vaginal yeast infections as well as oral thrush, a yeast infection of the mouth that commonly affects infants.[68]

Fungi are important to humans in a variety of ways. Both microscopic and macroscopic fungi have medical relevance, but some pathogenic species that can cause **mycoses** (illnesses caused by fungi). See Figure 3.13 for a microscopic image of candida albicans that is the causative agent of yeast infections. Some pathogenic fungi are opportunistic, meaning that they mainly cause infections when the host's immune defenses are compromised and do not normally cause illness in healthy individuals. Fungi are important in other ways. They act as decomposers in the environment, and they are critical for the production of certain foods such as cheeses. Fungi are also major sources of antibiotics, such as penicillin from the fungus *Penicillium*.[69]

Indications

Imidazoles are synthetic fungicides commonly used in medical applications and also in agriculture to keep seeds and harvested crops from molding. Examples include miconazole, ketoconazole, and clotrimazole, which are used to treat fungal skin infections such as ringworm, specifcally tinea pedis (athlete's foot), tinea cruris (jock itch), and tinea corporis.

Triazole drugs, including fuconazole, can be administered orally or intravenously for the treatment of several types of systemic yeast infections, including oral thrush and cryptococcal meningitis, both of which are prevalent

---

68   This image is a derivative of "Candida albicans" by Dr. Gordon Roberstad, Centers of Disease Control and Prevention. https://cnx.org/contents/y54zcuVm@1/Characteristics-of-Fungi, licensed under CC0.

69   This work is a derivative of *Microbiology* by OpenStax licensed under CC BY 4.0. Access for free at https://openstax.org/books/microbiology/pages/1-introduction.

in patients with AIDS. Triazoles also exhibit more selective toxicity, compared with the imidazoles, and are associated with fewer side effects.[70]

Allylamines, a structurally different class of synthetic antifungal drugs, are most commonly used topically for the treatment of dermatophytic skin infections like athlete's foot, ringworm, and jock itch. Oral treatment with terbinafne is also used for fngernail and toenail fungus, but it can be associated with the rare side effect of hepatotoxicity.[71]

Polyenes are a class of antifungal agents naturally produced by certain actinomycete soil bacteria and are structurally related to macrolides. Common examples include nystatin and amphotericin B. Nystatin is typically used as a topical treatment for yeast infections of the skin, mouth, and vagina, but may also be used for intestinal fungal infections. The drug amphotericin B is used for systemic fungal infections like aspergillosis, cryptococcal meningitis, histoplasmosis, blastomycosis, and candidiasis. Amphotericin B was the only antifungal drug available for several decades, but its use has associated serious side effects, including nephrotoxicity.[72]

Mechanism of Action

Antifungals disrupt ergosterol biosyntheses of the cell membrane increasing cellular permeability and causing cell death.

Special Administration Considerations

Administration guidelines will vary depending on the type of fungal infection being treated. It is important to monitor response of the affected area and examine class specifc administration considerations to monitor patient response.

Patient Teaching and Education

The patient should be advised to follow dosage instructions carefully and fnish the drug completely, even if they feel their symptoms have resolved. The patient should report any skin rash, abdominal pain, fever, or diarrhea to the provider. The patient should monitor carefully for unexplained bruising or bleeding, which may be a sign of liver dysfunction.[73]

Now let's take a closer look at the medication grid for various antifungals in Table 3.15.[74]

70   This work is a derivative of *Microbiology* by OpenStax licensed under CC BY 4.0. Access for free at https://openstax.org/books/microbiology/pages/1-introduction.

71   This work is a derivative of *Microbiology* by OpenStax licensed under CC BY 4.0. Access for free at https://openstax.org/books/microbiology/pages/1-introduction.

72   This work is a derivative of *Microbiology* by OpenStax licensed under CC BY 4.0. Access for free at https://openstax.org/books/microbiology/pages/1-introduction.

73   uCentral from Unbound Medicine. https://www.unboundmedicine.com/ucentral.

74   *Daily Med*, https://dailymed.nlm.nih.gov/dailymed/index.cfm, used for hyperlinked medications in this module. Retrieved June 27, 2019.

Table 3.15: Antifungal Medication Grid

Class/Subclass	Prototype/ Generic	Administration Considerations	Therapeutic Effects	Side/Adverse Effects
Antifungals	clotrimazole	Check for allergies Topical cream: apply liberally twice daily to affected area	Improve symptoms of athlete's foot (tinea pedis), jock itch (tinea cruris), or ringworm	Topical-skin irritation, rash
	fluconazole	Check for allergies Route: PO/IV ■ Single or multiple doses ■ Caution if liver dysfunction ■ Potential for fetal harm	Improve symptoms of yeast infection	Hepatotoxicity
	terbinafne	Cream or aerosol Wash affected area with soap and water and allow to dry completely before applying	Improve symptoms of athlete's foot (tinea pedis), jock itch (tinea cruris), or ringworm	External use only
	nystatin	PO: If order is "swish and swallow," instruct patient to hold medication in mouth for several minutes before swallowing Topical cream/powder: apply liberally twice daily	Improve symptoms of yeast infection of skin	External use only

	amphotericin B	Check for allergies	Improvement of systemic fungal infection such as aspergillis	Monitor fluid intake and output; report change in urine appearance or volume
		Route: IV		Monitor BUN and creatinine levels two or three times weekly. Kidney damage may be reversible if drug is stopped at first sign of renal dysfunction
		Reconstitute and dilute as directed on packaging		
		Administer slowly over several hours initially and monitor VS every 30 minutes; may require premedication		
		Therapy may take several months		Hydrate patient before infusion to reduce risk of nephrotoxicity
		Alert: Different amphotericin B preparations aren't interchangeable		Obtain liver function tests once or twice weekly
		Caution if renal impairment		Monitor CBC weekly
		Black Box Warning		Monitor potassium level closely and report signs of hypokalemia
		Don't use to treat noninvasive forms of fungal disease in patients with normal neutrophil counts		Check calcium and magnesium levels twice weekly
				Drug may be ototoxic. Report evidence of hearing loss, tinnitus, vertigo, or unsteady gait

Critical Thinking Activity 3.15a

Using the above grid information, consider the following clinical scenario question:

A patient in a skilled nursing facility has been receiving nystatin applied to groin folds twice daily for several weeks, but there is no sign of improvement. What is the nurse's best response?

Note: Answers to the Critical Thinking activities can be found in the "Answer Key" sections at the end of the book.

3.16   ANTIMALARIALS

Malaria is a prevalent protozoal disease impacting individuals across the world. According to the Centers for Disease Control, approximately 1,700 cases of malaria are diagnosed in the United States each year.[75]

Indications

Antimalarials are used for the prevention or treatment of malaria.

Mechanism of Action

Antimalarial agents work by targeting specifc intracellular processes that impact cell development.[76]

Special Administration Considerations

Antimalarial medications may impact hearing and vision so patients should be monitored carefully for adverse effects. Additionally, antimalarial medications may cause GI upset, so patients should be instructed to take these medications with food.

Patient Teaching and Education

Patients should receive instruction to take medication as prescribed and adhere to the full prescription regimen. Patients should minimize additional exposure to mosquitoes using preventative means such as repellents, protective clothing, netting, etc. Patients on chloroquine therapy should also avoid alcohol. Chloroquine can be extremely toxic to children and should be safely stored and out of reach. Patients receiving antimalarial therapy may have increased sensitivity to light and should be counseled to wear protective glasses to prevent ocular damage. Treatment often requires sustained regimens of six months or greater so patients should be monitored carefully for adherence and compliance.[77]

Now let's take a closer look at the medication grid on chloroquine in Table 3.16.[78]

75   Centers for Disease Control and Prevention. (2018, November 15). *Choosing a drug to prevent malaria.* https://www.cdc.gov/malaria/travelers/drugs.html.

76   Achieng, A., Rawat, M., Ogutu, B., Guyah, B., Ong'echa, J.M., Perkins, D., and Kempaiah, P. (2017). Antimalarials: Molecular drug targets and mechanism of action. *Current Topics in Medicinal Chemistry, 17,* 1–15.

77   uCentral from Unbound Medicine. https://www.unboundmedicine.com/ucentral.

78   *Daily Med,* https://dailymed.nlm.nih.gov/dailymed/index.cfm, used for hyperlinked medications in this module. Retrieved June 27, 2019.

Table 3.16: Chloroquine Medication Grid

Subclass	Prototype/ Generic	Administration Considerations	Therapeutic Effects	Side/Adverse Effects
Antimalarials	chloroquine	Check for allergies Contraindicated in patients hypersensitive to drug and in those with retinal or visual feld changes Use cautiously in patients with severe GI, neurologic, or blood disorders; hepatic disease or alcoholism; or G6PD defciency or psoriasis Take with food to prevent GI upset In severe or resistant cases, artesunate IV may be prescribed	Prevention of malaria or improvement of an acute attack of malaria For malaria prevention, the CDC recommends that patients take drug for 4 weeks after leaving the area	Changes in vision Changes in hearing Monitor renal function closely Monitor patient for overdose, which can quickly lead to toxic symptoms: headache, drowsiness, visual disturbances, nausea and vomiting, cardiovascular collapse, shock, and convulsions

Critical Thinking Activity 3.16a

Using the above grid information, consider the following clinical scenario question:

A nurse is providing medication teaching to a patient who is planning on visiting a country with high rates of malaria to do mission work. The patient states, "I'm glad I only have to take this medication for a week. The side effects sound horrific!" What is the nurse's best response regarding the length of therapy?

Note: Answers to the Critical Thinking activities can be found in the "Answer Key" sections at the end of the book.

3.17   ANTIPROTOZOALS

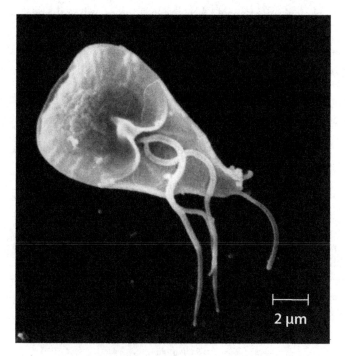

Figure 3.14 Giardia lamblia

Antiprotozoal drugs target infectious protozoans such as Giardia, an intestinal protozoan parasite that infects humans and other mammals, causing severe diarrhea (see Figure 3.14 for a microscopic image of Giardia).[79]

Indications

Metronidazole is an example of an antiprotozoal antibacterial medication gel that is commonly used to treat acne rosacea, bacterial vaginosis, or trichomonas. Metronidazole IV is used to treat Giardia and also serious anaerobic bacterial infections such as Clostridium diffcile (C-diff).

Mechanism of Action

Many antiprotozoal agents work to inhibit protozoan folic acid synthesis, subsequently impairing the protozoal cell.[80]

Special Administration Considerations

It can be administered PO, parenterally, or topically. Orally is the preferred route for GI infections. The nurse should monitor the patient carefully for side effects such as seizures, peripheral neuropathies, and dizziness. Psychotic reactions have been reported with alcoholic patients taking disulfram.

---

79   "Giardia lamblia SEM 8698 lores.jpg" by CDC/ Janice Haney Carr is licensed under CC0.

80   This work is a derivative of *Microbiology* by OpenStax licensed under CC BY 4.0. Access for free at https://openstax.org/books/microbiology/pages/1-introduction.

My Notes

Patient Teaching and Education

Patients taking antiprotozoal medications should receive education regarding the need for medication compliance and prevention of reinfection. They should be advised that the medication may cause dizziness and dry mouth. Additionally, the medication may cause darkening of the urine. They should also avoid alcoholic beverages during medication therapy to prevent a disulfram-like reaction.

If patients are being treated for protozoal infections such as trichomoniasis, they should be advised that sexual partners might be sources of reinfection even if asymptomatic. Partners should also receive treatment.[81]

Patients teaching should include the avoidance of alcohol during therapy. Now let's take a closer look at the medication grid in Table 3.17.[82]

Table 3.17: Metronidazole Medication Grid

Class/Subclass	Prototype/ Generic	Administration Considerations	Therapeutic Effects	Side/Adverse Effects
Antiprotozoal-antibacterial	metrogel metronidazole IV	Check for allergies Topical, vaginal, PO, or IV Don't give by IV push. Infuse over 30 to 60 minutes Contraindications: pregnancy, hypersensitivity, use of alcohol or disulfram during therapy Use cautiously with hepatic impairment, blood dyscrasias, or CNS diseases	Improvement of symptoms	Seizures Peripheral neuropathy Psychotic reactions Hepatotoxicity

Critical Thinking Activity 3.17a

Using the above grid information, consider the following clinical scenario question:

A patient develops C-diff after taking multiple antibiotics for a non-healing wound. What medication is commonly used to treat C-diff, and what route is used?

Note: Answers to the Critical Thinking activities can be found in the "Answer Key" sections at the end of the book.

---

81   uCentral from Unbound Medicine. https://www.unboundmedicine.com/ucentral.

82   *Daily Med*, https://dailymed.nlm.nih.gov/dailymed/index.cfm, used for hyperlinked medications in this module. Retrieved June 27, 2019.

3.18 ANTIHELMINTIC

There are two major groups of parasitic helminths in the human body: the roundworms (Nematoda) and fatworms (Platyhelminthes). See Figure 3.15 for images of a tapeworm and a guinea worm.[83] Of the many species that exist in these groups, about half are parasitic and some are important human pathogens.

Indications

Anthelmintic medications target parasitic helminths.[84]

Mechanism of Action

Because helminths are multicellular eukaryotes like humans, developing drugs with selective toxicity against them is extremely challenging. Despite this, several effective classes have been developed. Many anthelmintic medications work by preventing microtubule formation within the parasitic cell, compromising glucose uptake. Others work by blocking neuronal transmission within the parasite, subsequently causing starvation, paralysis, and death of the worms. Additionally, many antihelminths inhibit ATP formation and impair calcium uptake inducing paralysis and death.[85]

Special Administration Considerations

Prolonged therapy using antihelmintic medication can result in liver damage and bone marrow suppression.

Patient Teaching and Education

Patients on antihelmintic drug therapy should receive special instruction to ensure rigorous hygienic precautions to minimize the risk of reinfection. They should also wash all bedding, linens, towels, and clothing following treatment to minimize reinfection risk.[86]

---

83   This work is a derivative of "Taenia saginata adult 5260 lores.jpg" and "Dracunculus medinensis.jpg" by Centers for Disease Control and Prevention is licensed under CC0.

84   This work is a derivative of *Microbiology* by OpenStax licensed under CC BY 4.0. Access for free at https://openstax.org/books/microbiology/pages/1-introduction.

85   This work is a derivative of *Microbiology* by OpenStax licensed under CC BY 4.0. Access for free at https://openstax.org/books/microbiology/pages/1-introduction.

86   uCentral from Unbound Medicine. https://www.unboundmedicine.com/ucentral.

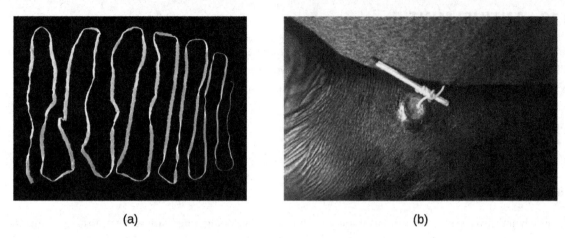

(a)   (b)

Figure 3.15 A. The tapeworm Taenia saginata, that infects both cattle and humans. Eggs are microscopic, but the adult tapeworm like the one show here can reach 4–10 meters, taking up residence in the digestive system B. An adult guinea worm, Dracunculus medinensis, is removed through a lesion in the patient's skin by winding it around a matchstick

Now let's take a closer look at the medication grid on mebendazole in Table 3.18.[87]

Table 3.18: Mebendazole Medication Grid

Class/Subclass	Prototype/ Generic	Administration Considerations	Therapeutic Effects	Side/Adverse Effects
Antihelmintic	mebendazole	Contraindicated during pregnancy; may cause fetal harm To help prevent reinfection: ■ Wash hands and fingernails with soap often during the day, especially before eating and after using the toilet ■ Wash all fruits and vegetables thoroughly or cook them well ■ Wear shoes	Elimination of worms	In prolonged treatment: ■ Hepatic effects ■ Bone marrow suppression

87   *Daily Med*, https://dailymed.nlm.nih.gov/dailymed/index.cfm, used for hyperlinked medications in this module. Retrieved June 27, 2019.

Critical Thinking Activity 3.18a

Using the above grid information, consider the following clinical scenario question:

A mother reports that her four-year-old son had a worm in his stool this morning. They live on a dairy farm. She reports that her son enjoys being in the barn during chore time, and it is common for the live-stock to develop "worms." Mebendazole was prescribed. What patient teaching should the nurse provide to the child and the mother?

Note: Answers to the Critical Thinking activities can be found in the "Answer Key" sections at the end of the book.

3.19 ANTITUBERCULARS

M. tuberculosis is the causative agent of tuberculosis (TB), a disease that primarily impacts the lungs but can infect other parts of the body as well. It has been estimated that one third of the world's population has been infected with M. tuberculosis and millions of new infections occur each year. Treatment of M. tuberculosis is challenging and requires patients to take a combination of drugs for an extended time. Complicating treatment even further is the development and spread of multidrug-resistant strains of this pathogen.[88]

Indications

Antitubercular medications are selective for mycobacteria work by inhibiting growth or selectively destroying mycobacteria.[89]

Mechanism of Action

They work impacting the synthesis or transcription of mycobacteria RNA or inhibiting the synthesis of mycolic acids in the cellular wall. Mycobacteria can develop resistance to antitubercular medications; therefore, strict compliance to drug regimen must be emphasized.

Special Administration Considerations

Antitubicular medications require at least six months of treatment. Many antitubercular medications may impact liver function, and liver enzymes should be monitored carefully. Other side effects to medication administration include GI symptoms, peripheral neuropathy, and vision changes.[90]

Patient Teaching and Education

Advise patients that medications must be taken as directed. It is important that patients understand the significance of continuing drug therapy even after symptoms have resolved to prevent the spread of disease. Drug therapy may be continued for six months to two years. If a patient notices any change in visual acuity or eye discomfort, it should be reported immediately to the healthcare provider.

Patients should also be advised to avoid alcohol during antitubercular therapy because of the increased risk of liver toxicity. Foods containing tyramine such as tuna and Swiss cheese should be avoided.[91]

---

88   This work is a derivative of *Microbiology* by OpenStax licensed under CC BY 4.0. Access for free at https://openstax.org/books/microbiology/pages/1-introduction.

89   This work is a derivative of *Microbiology* by OpenStax licensed under CC BY 4.0. Access for free at https://openstax.org/books/microbiology/pages/1-introduction.

90   This work is a derivative of *Microbiology* by OpenStax licensed under CC BY 4.0. Access for free at https://openstax.org/books/microbiology/pages/1-introduction.

91   uCentral from Unbound Medicine. https://www.unboundmedicine.com/ucentral.

Now let's take a closer look at the medication grid on isoniazid in Table 3.19.[92, 93]

Table 3.19: Isoniazid Medication Grid

Class/Subclass	Prototype/ Generic	Administration Considerations	Therapeutic Effects	Side/Adverse Effects
Antitubercular (also known as antimycobacterials)	isoniazid	Direct observed therapy (DOT) may be initiated to ensure compliance with long-term therapeutic regimen Multiple-drug resistant tuberculosis (i.e., resistance to at least isoniazid and rifampin) presents diffcult treatment problems. Treatment must be individualized and based on susceptibility studies May decrease effectiveness of oral contraceptives. Patients should be counseled to use alternate form of oral contraception Vitamin B6 supplementation is necessary in some patients for prevention of peripheral neuropathy	Negative sputum smears Prevention or elimination of TB symptoms: (productive cough, fever, night sweats)	GI upset Hepatotoxicity May decrease effectiveness of oral contraceptives

92 *Daily Med*, https://dailymed.nlm.nih.gov/dailymed/index.cfm, used for hyperlinked medications in this module. Retrieved June 27, 2019.

93 Allen, R.H. (2019). Combined estrogen-progestin oral contraceptives: Patient selection, counseling, and use. UpTo-Date. Retrieved on July 8, 2019 from https://www.uptodate.com/contents/combined-estrogen-progestin-oral-contra ceptives-patient-selection-counseling-and-use?search=Combined%20estrogen-progestin%20oral%20contraceptives:& source=search_result&selectedTitle=1~150&usage_type=default&display_ rank=1.

Critical Thinking Activity 3.19a

Using the above grid information, consider the following clinical scenario question:

A patient has been prescribed isoniazid as part of a multi-drug regimen for resistant TB. Direct observed therapy (DOT) has been initiated. The patient asks the nurse, "What does 'direct observed therapy' mean?" What is the nurse's best response?

Note: Answers to the Critical Thinking activities can be found in the "Answer Key" sections at the end of the book.

3.20 MISCELLANEOUS ANTIBACTERIALS: GLYCOPEPTIDES

Vancomycin is a glycopeptide commonly used to treat MRSA.

Indications

Vancomycin is a popular glycopeptide that is active against gram-positive bacteria. Vancomycin is commonly used to treat serious or severe infections when other antibiotics are ineffective or contraindicated, including those caused by MRSA.

Mechanism of Action

Glycopeptides are a class of medications that inhibit bacterial cell wall synthesis.

Special Administration Considerations

It is poorly absorbed from the GI tract, so it must be given by IV to treat a systemic infection. Oral vancomycin, on the other hand, is used to treat antibiotic-associated clostridium diffcile (C-diff). Vancomycin poses a signifcant risk to kidney function and hearing; therefore, patients' trough levels must be monitored carefully for effective IV dosing to avoid complications. Patients receiving IV vancomycin may also experience a complication known as "red man syndrome" in which they experience a flushing of the skin and a reddish rash on the upper body when the infusion is administered too rapidly.

Patient Teaching and Education

Patients should be counseled to take medications as directed for the full course of antibacterial therapy. They should monitor for side effects such as hypersensitivity, tinnitus, hearing loss, and vertigo. Patients should promptly follow-up with their healthcare provider if no improvement in symptoms is identifed.[94]

Now let's take a closer look at the medication grid on vancomycin in Table 3.20.[95]

---

94   uCentral from Unbound Medicine. https://www.unboundmedicine.com/ucentral.

95   *Daily Med*, https://dailymed.nlm.nih.gov/dailymed/index.cfm, used for hyperlinked medications in this module. Retrieved June 27, 2019.

Table 3.20: Vancomycin Medication Grid

Class/Subclass	Prototype/ Generic	Administration Considerations	Therapeutic Effects	Side/Adverse Effects
Miscellaneous Antibacterials: Glycopeptides	vancomycin	Check for allergies Route: IV but PO for C-diff Obtain culture prior to administering frst dose Dosage adjustment is required for renal impairment Monitor trough levels IV should be administered in a diluted solution over a period of 60 minutes or more to avoid rapid-infusion-related reactions	Monitor for systemic signs of infection: ■ WBCs ■ Fever Monitor actual site of infection for improvement Monitor and report trough levels for targeted dosing	Nephrotoxicity Ototoxicity C-diff can occur up to 2 months after therapy ends Red-man syndrome can occur if drug is infused too rapidly. Signs and symptoms include maculopapular rash on face, neck, trunk, and limbs and pruritus and hypotension caused by histamine release. Stop infusion and contact provider. Prepare to administer diphenhydramine 50mg IV or PO. Monitor BP closely; IV fuids and/or vasopressors may be required if hypotensive. Infusion may be restarted at a slower rate after rash and itching resolve

Critical Thinking Activity 3.20a

Using the above grid information, consider the following clinical scenario question:

A nurse is caring for a patient who was prescribed vancomycin IV for a MRSA infection. The dose of medication is due now, but a trough level is not yet available in the chart. What is the nurse's next best response?

Note: Answers to the Critical Thinking activities can be found in the "Answer Key" sections at the end of the book.

3.21 MODULE LEARNING ACTIVITIES

Now that you've learned all about antimicrobials, practice applying your knowledge with the following activities.

Interactive Activities

 An interactive or media element has been excluded from this version of the text. You can view it online here: https://wtcs.pressbooks.pub/pharmacology/?p=334

Glossary

Antagonistic Interactions: Concurrent administration of two drugs causes harmful effects such as a decrease of drug activity, decreased therapeutic levels due to increased metabolism and elimination, or increased potential for toxicity due to decreased metabolism and elimination. An example of an antagonistic interaction is taking antacids with antibiotics, causing decreased absorption of the antibiotic.

Antifungal: Medications that are used to treat fungal infections. For example, nystatin is used to treat Candida Albicans, a fungal infection.

Antiviral: Medications used to treat viral infections. For example, Tamifu is used to treat infuenza.

Bactericidal: Antimicrobial drugs that kill their target bacteria.

Bacteriostatic: Antimicrobial drugs that cause bacteria to stop reproducing but may not ultimately kill the bacteria.

Black Box Warnings: The strongest warnings issued by the Federal Drug Administration (FDA) that signify the drug carries a signifcant risk of serious or life-threatening adverse effects.

Broad-Spectrum Antimicrobial: An antibiotic that targets a wide variety of bacterial pathogens, including both gram-positive and gram-negative species.

Clostridium Diffcile (C-diff): Clostridium diffcile causes pseudomembranous colitis, a superinfection that can be caused by broad spectrum antibiotic therapy.

Culture: A test performed on various body substances for the presence of bacteria or fungus.

Dose Dependent: A more signifcant response occurs in the body when the medication is administered in large doses to provide a large amount of medication to the site of infection for a short period of time.

Gram-Positive: Gram-positive bacteria are classifed by the color they turn after a chemical called Gram stain is applied to them. Infections caused by Streptococcus and Staphylococcus bacteria are examples of gram-positive infections.

Gram-Negative: Gram-negative bacteria are classifed by the color they turn after a chemical called Gram stain is applied to them. Escherichia Coli (also known as E. Coli) is an example of a gram-negative infection.

Gram Stain: A test used to quickly diagnose types of bacterial infection. Gram-positive and gram-negative bacteria stain differently because their cell walls are different. Identifcation of bacteria as gram positive or gram negative assists the healthcare provider in selecting an appropriate antibiotic to treat the infection.

Half-Life: The rate at which 50% of a drug is eliminated from the bloodstream.

Indications

The use of a drug for treating a particular condition or disease. The FDA determines if there is enough evidence for a labeled indication of a drug. Providers may also prescribe medications for off-label indications if there is reasonable scientifc evidence that the drug is effective, but these uses have not been approved by the FDA.

Mechanism of Action

The way in which a drug affects microbes at the cellular level.

Methicillin-Resistant S. Aureus (MRSA): An infection caused by Methicillin-resistant Staphylococcus aureus that is diffcult to treat because it exhibits resistance to nearly all available antibiotics.

Narrow-Spectrum Antimicrobial: An antibiotic that targets only specifc subsets of bacterial pathogens.

Pathogen: An organism causing disease to its host.

Prototype: A common individual drug that represents a drug class or group of medications having similar chemical structures, mechanism of actions, and modes of action.

Resistance: A characteristic of bacteria when sensitivity analysis is performed demonstrating lack of effective treatment by a particular antibiotic.

Sensitivity Analysis: A test performed in addition to a culture to select an effective antibiotic to treat a microorganism.

Superinfection: A secondary infection in a patient having a preexisting infection. C-diff and yeast infections as a result of antibiotic therapy are examples of superinfections.

Synergistic Interaction: Concurrent drug administration producing a synergistic interaction that is better than the effcacy of either drug alone. An example of synergistic drug combinations is trimethoprim and sulfamethoxazole (Bactrim).

Time Dependent: Time dependency occurs when greater therapeutic effects are seen with lower blood levels over a longer period of time.

Vancomycin-Resistant S. Aureus (VRSA): An infection caused by Vancomycin-resistant Staphylococcus aureus that is diffcult to treat because it exhibits resistance to nearly all available antibiotics.

Chapter IV

Autonomic Nervous System

4.1   AUTONOMIC NERVOUS SYSTEM INTRODUCTION

Learning Objectives

- Identify the classifications and actions of autonomic nervous system drugs

- Give examples of when, how, and to whom autonomic nervous system drugs may be administered

- Identify the side effects and special considerations associated with autonomic nervous system drugs

- Include considerations and implications of using autonomic nervous system drugs across the life span

- Include evidence-based concepts when using the nursing process related to medications that affect the autonomic nervous system

- Identify and interpret related laboratory tests

Have you ever wondered what causes your heart to beat or your lungs to breathe? These are examples of **involuntary responses** the brain controls without the need for conscious thought. The autonomic nervous system (ANS) works using a balance of the sympathetic and parasympathetic nervous systems that regulate the body's involuntary functions, including heart rate, respiratory rate, digestion, and sweating. Many medications are used to control various cardiovascular, respiratory, and gastrointestinal conditions by acting on ANS receptors. Beta blockers and anticholinergic medications are the most commonly prescribed medications in this category.

My Notes

4.2   AUTONOMIC NERVOUS SYSTEM BASICS

This section will review key anatomy concepts in the autonomic nervous system (ANS) related to the mechanism of action of medications. For more detailed information regarding the concepts reviewed, use the links provided to review detailed autonomic nervous system content in the Open Stax *Anatomy and Physiology* book:[1]

🔗 **Review the basic structure and function of the nervous system**

🔗 **Review the anatomy of sensory perception.**

🔗 **Review the anatomy of motor responses.**

🔗 **Review the divisions of the autonomic nervous system.**

🔗 **Review autonomic reflexes and homeostasis.**

🔗 **Review information on a few drugs that affect the autonomic nervous system.**

Components and Functions of the Nervous System

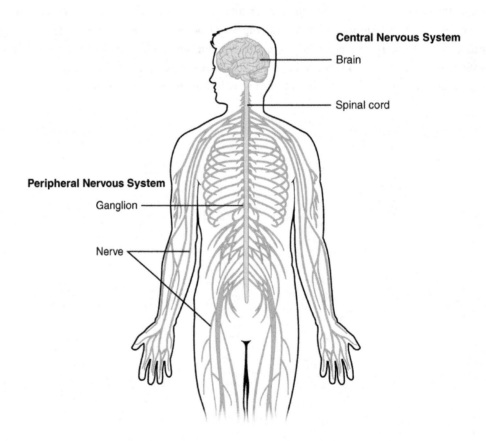

Figure 4.1 Central and Peripheral Nervous System

---

1   Content can be found at https://openstax.org/books/anatomy-and-physiology/pages/12-1-basic-structure-and-function -of-the-nervous-system.

The nervous system has two major components: the central nervous system (CNS) and the peripheral nervous system. See Figure 4.1.[2] The **central nervous system (CNS)** is composed of the brain and the spinal cord. The **peripheral nervous system** includes nerves outside the brain and spinal cord and consists of sensory neurons and motor neurons. **Sensory neurons** sense the environment and conduct signals to the brain that become a conscious perception of that stimulus. This conscious perception may lead to a motor response that is conducted from the brain to the peripheral nervous system via motor neurons to cause a movement. **Motor neurons** consist of the **somatic nervous system** that stimulates voluntary movement of muscles and the **autonomic nervous system**[3] that controls involuntary responses. This chapter will focus on the autonomic nervous system.

The two divisions[4] of the autonomic nervous system are the **sympathetic division (SNS)** and the **parasympathetic division (PNS)**. The SNS contains alpha and beta receptors, and the PNS contains nicotinic and muscarinic receptors. Each type of receptor has a specific action when stimulated (see Figure 4.2 for an image of the divisions of the nervous system and the receptors in the ANS).

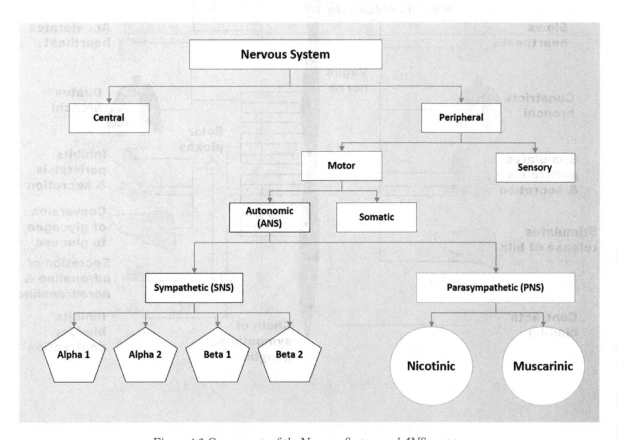

Figure 4.2 Components of the Nervous System and ANS receptors

2   "1201 Overview of Nervous System.jpg" by CNX OpenStax. is licensed under CC BY 4.0 Access for free at https://openstax.org/books/anatomy-and-physiology/pages/12-1-basic-structure-and-function-of-the-nervous- system.

3   "Component of the Nervous System" by Blaire Babbit at Chippewa Valley Technical College is licensed under CC BY 4.0.

4   "Component of the Nervous System" by Blaire Babbit at Chippewa Valley Technical College is licensed under CC BY 4.0.

SNS and PNS Functions and Homeostasis

The sympathetic system is associated with the **"fight-or-flight"** response, and parasympathetic activity is often referred to as "rest and digest." See Figure 4.3[5] to compare the effects on PNS and SNS stimulation on target organs. The autonomic nervous system regulates many of the internal organs through a balance of these two divisions and is instrumental in homeostatic mechanisms in the body.[6]

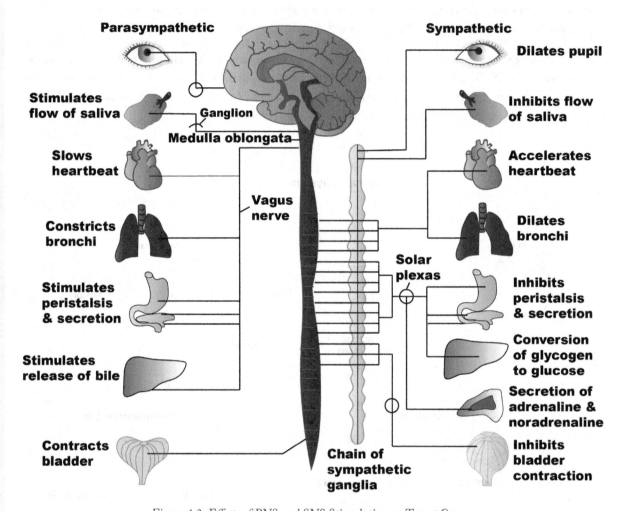

Figure 4.3. Effects of PNS and SNS Stimulation on Target Organs

Stimulation of SNS primarily produces increased heart rate, increased blood pressure via the constriction of blood vessels, and bronchial dilation. In comparison, stimulation of the PNS causes slowing of the heart, lowering of blood pressure due to vasodilation, bronchial constriction, and focuses on stimulating intestinal motility, salivation, and relaxation of the bladder.

---

5 "a7 autonomic nervous system" by unknown is licensed under CC BY-NC-SA 3.0 Access for free at https://blog.coturnix .org/2010/08/24/bio101-physiology-regulation-and-control/.

6 This work is a derivative of *Anatomy and Physiology* by OpenStax licensed under CC BY 4.0. Access for free at Access for free at https://openstax.org/books/anatomy-and-physiology/pages/1-introduction.

Homeostasis is the balance between the two systems. At each target organ, dual innervation determines activity. For example, the heart receives connections from both the sympathetic and parasympathetic divisions. SNS stimulation causes the heart rate to increase, whereas PNS stimulation causes the heart rate to decrease.

To respond to a threat—to "fight or flight"—the sympathetic system stimulates many different target organs to achieve this purpose. For example, if a person sees a grizzly bear in the wilderness, the individual has the choice to stand and fight the bear or to run away. For either choice, several things must occur for additional oxygen and glucose to be delivered to skeletal muscle to fight or run. The respiratory, cardiovascular, and musculoskeletal systems are all activated to breathe rapidly, cause bronchodilation in the lungs to inhale more oxygen, stimulate the heart to pump more blood, and increase blood pressure to deliver it to the muscles.[7] The liver creates more glucose for energy for the muscles to use. The pupils dilate to see the threat (or the escape route) more clearly. Sweating prevents the body from overheating from excess muscle contraction. Since the digestive system is not needed during this time of threat, the body shunts oxygen-rich blood to the skeletal muscles. To coordinate all these targeted responses, catecholamines such as epinephrine and norepinephrine are released in the sympathetic system and disperse to the many neuroreceptors on the target organs simultaneously.[8]

Chemical Signaling in the Autonomic Nervous System

Neurons conduct impulses to the synapse of a target organ. The **synapse** is a connection between the neuron and its target cell. See Figures 4.4[9] and 4.5[10] for images of synapse connections.

Preganglionic Neurons

The synapse is composed of a preganglionic (presynaptic) neuron and a postganglionic (postsynaptic) neuron. **Preganglionic neurons** release **acetylcholine (ACh)** onto nicotinic receptors on the postganglionic neuron. Nicotine, found in tobacco products, also binds to and activates nicotinic receptors, mimicking the effects of ACh. This is worth noting, because if medications were developed to impact the nicotinic receptors, then it would impact both the SNS and PNS systems at the preganglionic level. Instead, most medications target the **postganglionic neurons**, because each type of postganglionic neuron has different neurotransmitters and different target receptors.

---

7   This work is a derivative of *Anatomy and Physiology* by OpenStax licensed under CC BY 4.0. Access for free at https://openstax.org/books/anatomy-and-physiology/pages/1-introduction.

8   This work is a derivative of *Anatomy and Physiology* by OpenStax licensed under CC BY 4.0. Access for free at Access for free at https://openstax.org/books/anatomy-and-physiology/pages/1-introduction.

9   "Autonomic Nervous System" by CNX OpenStax is licensed under CC BY 4.0.

10   "The Synapse" by CNX OpenStax is licensed under CC BY 4.0 Access for free at https://openstax.org/books/anatomy-and-physiology/pages/12-5-communication-between-neurons.

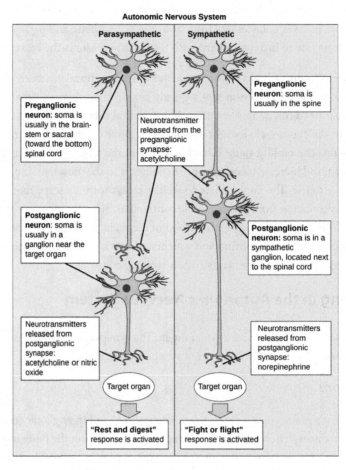

Figure 4.4 Autonomic System neurons conduct signals via the preganglionic neurons to postganglionic neurons to the target organs

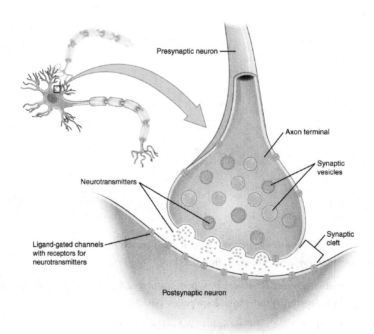

Figure 4.5 The synapse is the connection between a neuron and its target cell where neurotransmitters are released

Postganglionic Neurons

There are different types of postganglionic neurons in the SNS and PNS branches of the autonomic nervous system. Postganglionic neurons of the PNS branch are classified as **cholinergic**, meaning that acetylcholine (ACh) is released, whereas postganglionic neurons of the SNS are classifed as **adrenergic**, meaning that norepinephrine (NE) is released. The terms cholinergic and adrenergic refer not only to the signal that is released, but also to the class of neuroreceptors that each binds. (See Figure 4.6 for an image of the release of ACh and NE and their attachment to the corresponding adrenergic or nicotinic receptors.)

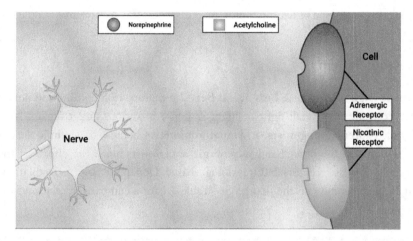

Figure 4.6 Sympathetic and Parasympathetic Pre-and Postganglionic Fibers and Neuroreceptors

The cholinergic system of the PNS includes two classes of postganglionic neuroreceptors: the nicotinic receptor and the muscarinic receptor. Both receptor types bind to ACh and cause changes in the target cell. The situation is similar to locks and keys. Imagine two locks—one for a classroom and the other for an office—opened by two separate keys. The classroom key will not open the office door, and the office key will not open the classroom door. This is similar to the specificity of nicotine and muscarine for their receptors. However, a master key can open multiple locks, such as a master key for the biology department that opens both the classroom and the office doors. This is similar to ACh that binds to both types of receptors.

The adrenergic system of the SNS has two major types of neuroreceptors: the alpha (α)-adrenergic receptor and beta (β)-adrenergic receptor. There are two types of α-adrenergic receptors, termed $\alpha1$ and $\alpha2$, and there are two types of β-adrenergic receptors, termed $\beta1$ and $\beta2$. An additional aspect of the adrenergic system is that there is a second neurotransmitter in addition to norepinephrine. The second neurotransmitter is called epinephrine. The chemical difference between norepinephrine and epinephrine is the addition of a methyl group (CH3) in epinephrine. The prefix "nor-" actually refers to this chemical difference in which a methyl group is missing.[11]

The term adrenergic should remind you of the word adrenaline, which is associated with the fight-or-flight response described earlier. Adrenaline and epinephrine are two names for the same molecule. The adrenal gland (in Latin, ad- = "on top of"; renal = "kidney") secretes adrenaline. The ending "-ine" refers to the chemical being derived, or extracted, from the adrenal gland.[12]

---

11   "Sympathetic and Parasympathetic Pre-and Postganglionic fibers and neuroreceptors" by Dominic Slausen at Chippewa Valley Technical College is licensed under CC BY 4.0.

12   This work is a derivative of *Anatomy and Physiology* by OpenStax licensed under CC BY 4.0. Access for free at Access for free at https://openstax.org/books/anatomy-and-physiology/pages/1-introduction.

My Notes

ANS Neuroreceptors and Effects

The effects of stimulating each type of neuroreceptor are outlined in this section and sample uses of medications are provided.

Sympathetic Nervous System

SNS receptors include Alpha-1, Alpha-2, Beta-1, and Beta-2 receptors. Epinephrine and norepinephrine stimulate these receptors, causing the overall fight-or-flight response in various target organs. Medications causing similar effects are called **adrenergic agonists**, or **sympathomimetics**, because they mimic the effects of the body's natural SNS stimulation. On the other hand, **adrenergic antagonists** block the effects of the SNS receptors. Dopamine also stimulates these receptors, but it is dosage-based. Dopamine causes vasodilation of arteries in the kidney, heart, and brain, depending on the dosage. See Table 4.1 for a comparison of stimulation and inhibition of these SNS receptors.

Table 4.1: Comparison of Medication Effects of Adrenergic Receptor Stimulation and Inhibition

Receptor	Effects of Stimulation	Effects of Inhibition
Alpha-1	Contract smooth muscle CNS stimulation Blood vessels: vasoconstriction to nonessential organs GI: relax smooth muscle and decrease motility Liver: glycogenolysis Bladder: contraction Uterus: contraction Pupils: dilation Medication example: Pseudoephedrine to treat nasal congestion by vasoconstriction	Relax smooth muscle Vasodilation Bladder: Increase urine flow Medication example: Tamsulosin to improve urine flow
Alpha-2	Vasodilation Medication Example: Clonidine to treat hypertension	Not used clinically
Beta-1	Primarily stimulates heart with increased heart rate and contractility Also causes kidneys to release renin Medication example: Dobutamine to treat acute heart failure to increase cardiac output	"Selective Beta blocker" used to decrease heart rate and blood pressure Medication example: Metoprolol to decrease heart rate and blood pressure

Beta-2	Primarily relax smooth muscle Blood vessels: vasodilation Lungs: bronchodilation GI: decreased motility Liver: glycogenolysis Uterus: relaxation Medication example: Albuterol for bronchodilation	"Nonselective Beta Blockers" block Beta-1 and Beta-2 receptors so also cause bronchoconstriction Medication example: Propranolol blocks Beta-1 and Beta-2 receptor so lowers blood pressure but inadvertently causes bronchoconstriction

Interactive Activity

 An interactive or media element has been excluded from this version of the text. You can view it online here: https://wtcs.pressbooks.pub/pharmacology/?p=822

Adrenergic Agonists

Adrenergic agonists stimulate Alpha-1, Alpha-2, Beta-1, or Beta-2 receptors. Stimulation of each type of receptor has different effects and are further explained below.

Alpha-1 receptor agonists: Stimulation of Alpha-1 receptors causes vasoconstriction in the periphery, which increases blood pressure. Vasoconstriction also occurs in mucus membranes, which decreases swelling and secretions for patients experiencing upper respiratory infections. Examples of Alpha-1 agonist medications are pseudoephedrine or phenylephrine, used to treat nasal congestion.

Alpha-2 receptor agonists: Stimulation of Alpha-2 receptors reduces CNS stimulation and is primarily used as an antihypertensive or a sedative. An example of an Alpha-2 agonist medication is clonidine, which is used to treat hypertension and is also used to treat attention deficit hyperactivity disorder.

Beta-1 receptor agonists: Stimulation of Beta-1 receptors primarily affects the heart by increasing heart rate and contractility. It also causes the kidneys to release renin. Effects on the heart are described as having a positive **chronotropic** (increases heart rate), positive **inotropic** (increases force of contraction), and positive **dromotropic** (increases speed of conduction between SA and AV node) properties. Medications that stimulate Beta-1 receptors are primarily used during cardiac arrest, acute heart failure, or shock. An example of a Beta-1 receptor agonist medication is dobutamine, which is used to increase cardiac output in someone experiencing acute heart failure or shock. See Figure 4.7[13] illustrating dromotropic properties of stimulating Beta-1 receptors.

---

13   "2018 Conduction System of Heart.jpg" by OpenStax College is licensed under CC BY 3.0.

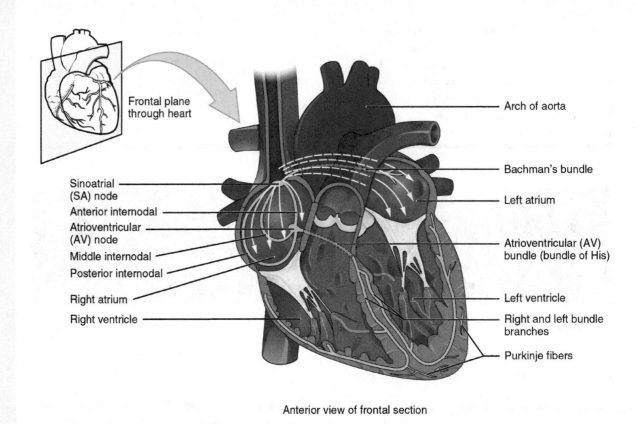

Anterior view of frontal section

Figure 4.7 Dromotropic Properties Affect the Speed of Conduction Between SA and AV Nodes

Beta-2 receptor agonists: Stimulation of Beta-2 receptors causes relaxation in smooth muscle in the lungs, GI, uterus, and liver. Medications that stimulate Beta-2 receptors are primarily used to promote bronchodilation, which opens the airway, and are often used to treat patients with asthma or chronic obstructive pulmonary disease (COPD). An example of a Beta-2 receptor agonist medication used in asthma is albuterol. See Figure 4.8[14] for an illustration of the effects of stimulating Beta-2 receptors in the lungs.

Side effects of Beta-2 receptor agonists are related to stimulation of Beta-2 receptors in other locations in the body. For example, albuterol can cause tachycardia by stimulating Beta-2 receptors in the heart. Stimulation of Beta-2 receptors can also inadvertently cause **hyperglycemia** in patients with diabetes because of activation of Beta-2 receptors in the liver, causing glycogenolysis.

---

14   "Bronchodilators" by BruceBlaus is licensed under CC BY 4.0.

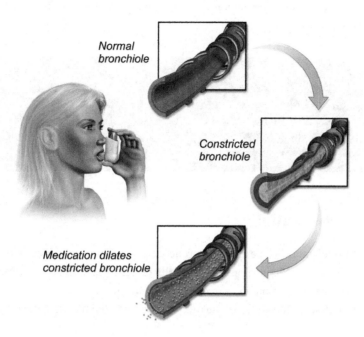

Figure 4.8 Effects of Medications Stimulating Beta-2 Receptors in the Lungs

Adrenergic Antagonists

Adrenergic antagonist medications inhibit the Alpha-1, Alpha-2, Beta-1, and Beta-2 receptors. The effects of inhibition of each receptor are explained further below.

Alpha-1 antagonists: Alpha-1 antagonists are primarily used to relax smooth muscle in the bladder and cause vasodilation.

Examples include:

- Tamsulosin is used to decrease resistance of an enlarged prostate gland and improve urine flow.
- Prazosin is used to cause vasodilation and decrease blood pressure in patients with hypertension.

Alpha-2 antagonists: This classification is used in research, but has limited clinical application.

Beta Antagonists: There are two types of beta antagonists: **selective beta blockers**, which inhibit Beta-1 receptors and affect the heart only, and **nonselective beta blockers,** that block both Beta-1 and Beta-2 receptors, thus affecting both the heart and lungs. Beta blockers are also referred to as having negative chronotropic (decreased heart rate), negative inotropic (decreased force of contraction), and negative dromotropic (decreased speed of conduction between SA and AV nodes) properties. It is also important for a nurse to remember that beta blockers can mask the usual hypoglycemic symptoms of tremor, tachycardia, and nervousness in patients with diabetes.

Beta-1 antagonists: Beta-1 antagonists primarily block receptors in the heart, causing decreased heart rate and decreased blood pressure. An example is metoprolol, a selective beta blocker used to treat high blood pressure, chest pain due to poor blood flow to the heart, and several conditions involving an abnormally fast heart rate.

Beta-2 antagonists: Nonselective beta blockers block Beta-1 receptors and Beta-2 receptors in the lungs. An example is propranolol, which is used to lower blood pressure by decreasing the heart rate and cardiac output.

However, it can also cause bronchoconstriction by inadvertently blocking Beta-2 receptors, so it must be used cautiously in patients with asthma or COPD.

> ## Interactive Activity
>
> An interactive or media element has been excluded from this version of the text. You can view it online here: https://wtcs.pressbooks.pub/pharmacology/?p=822

Parasympathetic Nervous System

Acetylcholine (ACh) stimulates nicotinic and muscarinic receptors. Drugs that stimulate nicotinic and muscarinic receptors are called cholinergics. Medications are primarily designed to stimulate muscarinic receptors. Nicotine stimulates pre- and post-ganglionic nicotinic receptors, causing muscle relaxation and other CNS effects. An example of a medication designed to stimulate nicotinic receptors is the nicotine patch, used to assist with smoking cessation.

Muscarinic agonists are also called **parasympathomimetics** and primarily cause smooth muscle contraction, resulting in decreased heart rate, bronchoconstriction, increased gastrointestinal/genitourinary tone, and pupillary constriction. There are two types of muscarinic agonists: direct-acting and indirect-acting. Direct-acting agonists bind to the muscarinic receptor. Indirect-acting muscarinic agonists work by preventing the breakdown of ACh, thus increasing the amount of acetylcholine available to bind receptors.

Examples of direct-acting muscarinic agonist medications include:

- Pilocarpine: Used to treat glaucoma by causing the ciliary muscle to contract and allow for the drainage of aqueous humor
- Bethanechol: Used for urinary retention by stimulating the bladder causing urine output

Examples of indirect-acting muscarinic agonist medications include:

- Pyridostigmine: Used to reverse muscle weakness in patients with myasthenia gravis
- Physostigmine: Used to treat organophosphate insecticide poisoning
- Donepezil: Enhances memory in some patients with early Alzheimer's disease

Muscarinic antagonists are referred to as **anticholinergics** or "parasympatholytics." Anticholinergics inhibit ACh and allow the SNS to dominate, creating similar effects as adrenergics. Their overall use is to relax smooth muscle. "SLUDGE" is a mnemonic commonly used to recall the effects of anticholinergics: **S**alivation decreased, **L**acrimation decreased, **U**rinary retention, **D**rowsiness/dizziness, **G**I upset, **E**yes (blurred vision/dry eyes). Anticholinergics may also cause confusion and constipation and must be used cautiously in the elderly. See Figure 4.9[15] for an illustration of the **"SLUDGE"** effects of anticholinergics.

---

15   ""SLUDGE" effects of Anticholinergics" by Dominic Slausen at Chippewa Valley Technical College is licensed under CC BY 4.0.

Examples of anticholinergic medications include:

- Atropine: Specific anticholinergic responses are dose-related. Small doses of atropine inhibit salivary and bronchial secretions and sweating; moderate doses dilate the pupil, inhibit accommodation, and increase the heart rate (vagolytic effect); larger doses will decrease motility of the gastrointestinal (GI) and urinary tracts; very large doses will inhibit gastric acid secretion

- Oxybutynin: Relaxes overactive bladder

- Benztropine: Reduces tremor and muscle rigidity in Parkinson's disease or in treatment of extrapyramidal reactions from antipsychotic medications

- Scopolamine: Decreases GI motility and GI secretions; used for motion sickness and postoperative nausea and vomiting[16, 17, 18, 19]

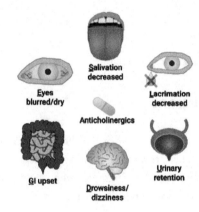

Figure 4.9 "SLUDGE" Effects of Anticholinergics: Salivation decreased, Lacrimation decreased, Urinary retention, Drowsiness/Dizziness, GI upset, Eyes (blurred vision/dry eyes). Also may cause confusion and constipation

16   McCuistion, L., Vuljoin-DiMaggio, K., Winton, M, and Yeager, J. (2018). *Pharmacology: A patient-centered nursing process approach*. Elsevier.

17   Gersch, C., Heimgartner, N., Rebar, C., and Willis, L. (Eds.). (2017). *Pharmacology made incredibly easy*. Wolters Kluwer.

18   Lilley, L., Collins, S., and Snyder, J. (2014). *Pharmacology and the Nursing Process*. Elsevier.

19   This work is a derivative of *Principles of Pharmacology* by LibreTexts licensed under CC BY-NC-SA 4.0.

My Notes

4.3   USING THE NURSING PROCESS WITH ANS MEDICATIONS

Assessment

Many types of medications stimulate or inhibit specific ANS receptors. By memorizing the effects, it becomes easy for the nurse to recognize side effects resulting from the stimulation or inhibition of ANS neuroreceptors. Medications that stimulate ANS receptors often impact the heart, lungs, and blood vessels, so the nurse must often monitor blood pressure, heart rate, and lung sounds carefully for expected therapeutic effects and side effects. Anticholinergics cause muscle relaxation and can cause urinary retention, constipation, and dry mouth. The nurse should anticipate and assess for these side effects, and manage them as needed for patient comfort.

Planning

Common goals include:

Patient will adhere to the drug regimen.

Patient's vital signs will be within the desired range.

Implementation of Interventions

A nurse should be aware of parameters to administer or withhold medications affecting the autonomic nervous system. If the order parameters are unclear, the nurse should withhold the medication following safe administration guidelines, and notify the prescriber. For example, when no parameters are provided, blood pressure medications should not be administered if the patient's apical heart rate is less than 60 beats per minute and/or the systolic blood pressure is less than 100 mmHg.

Report any marked vital signs changes or suspected adverse effects.

Implement fall precautions, when needed, based on anticipated side effects of ANS medications.

Evaluation

It is always important for nurses to know the reason why a medication is ordered for a specific patient, so evaluation of therapeutic effectiveness can be documented. For example, if the purpose of medication is to improve urine flow, then improvement should be seen and documented. Otherwise, the side effects may not warrant the use of the medication.

4.4 ANS MEDICATION CLASSES AND NURSING CONSIDERATIONS

Classes of medication, categorized according to neuroreceptor, are further discussed in more detail below. Table 4.2[20] contrasts agonist and antagonist medications for each ANS neuroreceptor.

Table 4.2: Comparison of Prototype Medications that Stimulate Versus Inhibit PNS and SNS Receptors

Receptor	Stimulation (Agonist)	Inhibition (Antagonist)
Nicotine	Nicotine is a muscle relaxant with CNS effects. **Nicotine patch** is used for nicotine addiction by slowly reducing dose and avoiding withdrawal effects	Not clinically applicable
Muscarinic	**Pilocarpine** causes muscle contraction; assists with glaucoma by contracting ciliary muscle and draining fluid	**Atropine** in small doses inhibits secretions; in moderate doses increases heart rate; in large doses decreases gastrointestinal motility
Alpha-1	**Pseudoephedrine** and **Phenylephrine** cause vasoconstriction, decreased swelling of mucus membranes, and decreased secretions	**Tamsulosin** relaxes smooth muscle in bladder/prostate to improve urine flow and also decreases blood pressure due to vasodilation
Alpha-2	**Clonidine** decreases CNS outflow to treat ADHD and also reduces blood pressure and heart rate	Limited clinical use
Beta-1	**Dobutamine** increases heart rate, force of heart contraction, and speed of conduction between SA to AV nodes	**Selective B blocker: Metoprolol** works on Beta-1 receptors to decrease blood pressure and heart rate
Beta-2	**Albuterol** used for bronchodilation	**Nonselective B blocker: Propranolol** works on Beta-2 and Beta-1 receptors; decreases blood pressure but can also cause bronchoconstriction
Catecholamines stimulate multiple adrenergic receptors	**Epinephrine** and **Norepinephrine**: stimulate alpha- and beta-receptors on target organs, causing increased heart rate and vasoconstriction for improved blood flow to essential organs **Dopamine** has dose-dependent effects that target arteries in the kidneys, heart, and brain	Not clinically applicable

Supplementary Videos: See the supplementary videos below related to sympathetic and parasympathetic nervous system medications.

---

20   This work is a derivative of *Daily Med* by U.S. National Library of Medicine in the public domain.

My Notes

Sympathetic Nervous System Drugs[21]

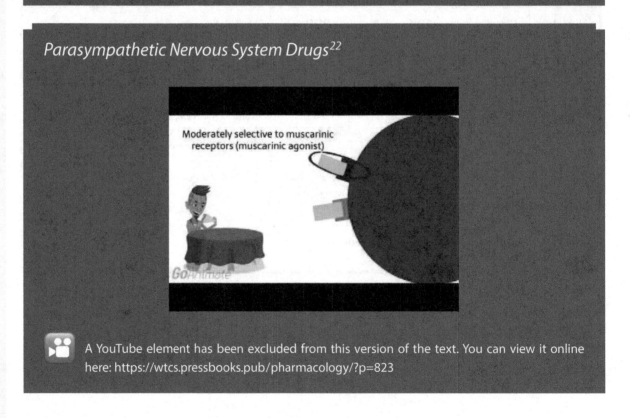

A YouTube element has been excluded from this version of the text. You can view it online here: https://wtcs.pressbooks.pub/pharmacology/?p=823

Parasympathetic Nervous System Drugs[22]

A YouTube element has been excluded from this version of the text. You can view it online here: https://wtcs.pressbooks.pub/pharmacology/?p=823

21 Forciea, B. (2018, January 12). *Sympathetic nervous system drugs.* [Video]. YouTube. All rights reserved. Video used with permission. https://youtu.be/-e_s-jTPtm4.

22 Forciea, B. (2018, February 2). *Parasympathetic nervous system drugs.* [Video]. YouTube. All rights reserved. Video used with permission. https://youtu.be/ZSRk_NkbBPg.

4.5   NICOTINE RECEPTOR AGONISTS

Nicotine binds to and activates nicotinic acetylcholine receptors, mimicking the effect of acetylcholine at these receptors.

Indications: Nicotine patches are used as an aid to smoking cessation and for the relief of nicotine withdrawal signs and symptoms as part of a comprehensive behavioral smoking cessation program.

Nursing Considerations: Nicotine is a hazardous drug; use safe handling and disposal precautions. Apply one new patch every 24 hours on skin that is dry, clean, and hairless. Remove backing from patch and immediately press onto skin. Hold for 10 seconds. Wash hands after applying or removing the patch. Save pouch to use for patch disposal. Dispose of the used patches by folding sticky ends together and putting in pouch. The used patch should be removed and a new one applied to a different skin site at the same time each day. Do not wear more than one patch at a time. Discontinue use and call provider if an allergic reaction occurs, such as difficulty breathing or rash, or symptoms of nicotine overdose occur, such as nausea, vomiting, dizziness, weakness, and rapid heartbeat. It may also cause vivid dreams or sleep disturbances. If these occurrences occur, patients should be counseled to remove the patch at bedtime and apply a new one in the morning.

Patient Teaching and Education: Emphasize that the patient should stop smoking completely while on nicotine replacement therapy to avoid additive nicotine levels higher than smoking alone. Advise patients that participating in a comprehensive smoking cessation program improves success. If using a nicotine patch, patients should be aware that skin sensitivity at the site of patch placement typically resolves within one hour.[23]

Alert: Advise patient to keep all nicotine products, including used inhaler cartridges, nasal spray bottles, and patches out of the reach of children and pets.

Now let's take a closer look at the medication grid on nicotine patch in Table 4.5.[24] Medication grids assist students to learn key points about each medication class. Basic information related to a common generic medication in this class is outlined, including administration considerations, therapeutic effects, and side effects/adverse effects. Prototype/generic medication listed in the medication grid is also hyperlinked directly to a free resource from the U.S. National Library of Medicine called *Daily Med*. Because information about medication is constantly changing, nurses should always consult evidence-based resources to review current recommendations before administering specific medication.

---

23   uCentral from Unbound Medicine. https://www.unboundmedicine.com/ucentral.

24   This work is a derivative of *Daily Med* by U.S. National Library of Medicine in the public domain.

Table 4.5: Nicotine Patch Medication Grid

Class/ Subclass	Prototype/ Generic	Administration Considerations	Therapeutic Effects	Side/Adverse Effects
Nicotinic Agonist	**nicotine patch**	Hazardous drug; use safe handling and disposal precautions Check for allergy to adhesives See administration guidelines in packaging Use cautiously in patients with recent myocardial infarction, serious arrhythmias, coronary artery disease, severe or worsening angina, hypertension, vasospastic diseases, or peripheral vascular disease Patients taking monoamine oxidase inhibitors (MAOIs) require lower dosage Can cause fetal harm	Used for nicotine addiction by slowly reducing dose and avoiding withdrawal effects	Discontinue use and call provider if: ■ Allergic reaction such as difficulty breathing or rash ■ Irregular heartbeat or palpitations ■ Symptoms of nicotine overdose such as nausea, vomiting, dizziness, weakness, and rapid heartbeat

4.6   MUSCARINIC RECEPTOR AGONISTS

Pilocarpine is a muscarinic receptor agonist.

Mechanism of Action: Pilocarpine causes the ciliary muscle to contract, allowing for the drainage of aqueous humor from the anterior chamber of the eye and reducing intraocular pressure related to glaucoma.

Indication: Pilocarpine is used to treat glaucoma.

Nursing Considerations: Remove contact lens before administration. Apply light finger pressure on lacrimal sac for 2 minutes after instilling to minimize systemic absorption.

Patient Teaching and Education: Advise the patient to use caution with night driving. Additionally, use of this medication can cause hypotension.[25]

Now let's take a closer look at the medication grid on pilocarpine in Table 4.6.[26]

Table 4.6: Pilocarpine Medication Grid				
Class/ Subclass	**Prototype/ Generic**	**Administration Considerations**	**Therapeutic Effects**	**Side/Adverse Effects**
Muscarinic Agonist	pilocarpine	Remove contact lens before administration Apply light finger pressure on lacrimal sac for 2 minutes after instilling to minimize systemic absorption	Controls intraocular pressure in glaucoma	Caution with night driving

---

25   uCentral from Unbound Medicine. https://www.unboundmedicine.com/ucentral.

26   This work is a derivative of *Daily Med* by U.S. National Library of Medicine in the public domain.

4.7 MUSCARINIC ANTAGONISTS

Atropine is a muscarinic antagonist.

Mechanism of Action: Specific anticholinergic responses are dose-related. Small doses of atropine inhibit salivary and bronchial secretions and sweating. Moderate doses dilate the pupil, inhibit accommodation, and increase the heart rate (vagolytic effect). Large doses decrease motility of the gastrointestinal and urinary tracts, and very large doses will inhibit gastric acid secretion.

Indications: Varying dosages are used preoperatively to diminish secretions, to stimulate the heart rate in conditions causing bradycardia, or to treat muscarinic symptoms of insecticide (organophosphorus or carbamate) poisoning or mushroom poisoning.

Nursing Considerations: As with all anticholinergics, use with caution with the elderly, because elderly patients may react with agitation or drowsiness. Heat stroke may occur in the presence of high temperatures. Immediately report symptoms of overdose: urine retention, abnormal heartbeat, dizziness, passing out, difficulty breathing, weakness, or tremors. Physostigmine has been used to reverse anticholinergic effects.

Patient Teaching and Education: Advise patients that use of these medications may cause dizziness and drowsiness, so patients should be aware of potential impact on their level of alertness. Additionally, use of medications may cause dry mouth, and frequent oral hygiene is encouraged. The use of atropine may cause urinary retention in males with benign prostatic hypertrophy (BPH).[27]

Now let's take a closer look at the medication grid on atropine in Table 4.7.[28]

Table 4.7: Atropine Medication Grid

Class/ Subclass	Prototype/ Generic	Administration Considerations	Therapeutic Effects	Side/Adverse Effects
Muscarinic Antagonist	atropine	Use with caution with elderly Contraindicated in high environmental temperatures	Dose dependent: small dose inhibits secretions; moderate dose increases heart rate; large dose decreases gastrointestinal motility	Immediately report symptoms of overdose: urine retention, abnormal heartbeat, dizziness, passing out, difficulty breathing, weakness, or tremors

---

27 uCentral from Unbound Medicine. https://www.unboundmedicine.com/ucentral.

28 This work is a derivative of *Daily Med* by U.S. National Library of Medicine in the public domain.

4.8   ALPHA-1 AGONISTS

Pseudoephedrine and phenylephrine are Alpha-1 agonists.

Mechanism of Action: Alpha-1 agonists stimulate alpha receptors in the respiratory tract, causing constriction of blood vessels and shrinkage of swollen nasal mucous membranes, thus increasing airway patency and reducing nasal congestion.

Indication: These drugs are commonly used for symptomatic relief in upper respiratory infections.

Nursing Considerations: Pseudoephedrine has had recent limitations placed on its use because it is a common ingredient in the illicit manufacturing of the drug methamphetamine. Pharmacies now require individuals to provide identification to purchase pseudoephedrine and must track the number of purchases. As a result, most over-the-counter decongestants now contain phenylephrine. Both should be used cautiously in patients with glaucoma, hypertension, or an enlarged prostate gland and are contraindicated in patients taking monoamine oxidase inhibitors (MAOIs), an older class of medication used to treat depression. Monitor for elevated blood pressure, urinary retention, nervousness, or difficulty sleeping. Do not administer within 2 hours of bedtime.

Patient Teaching and Education: Patients should be instructed to take medication as prescribed and be careful not to double doses. If they experience nervousness, breathing difficulties, or heart rate changes, they should notify their healthcare provider.[29]

Now let's take a closer look at the medication grid on phenylephrine and pseudoephedrine in Table 4.8.[30]

Table 4.8: Phenylephrine and Pseudoephedrine Medication Grid				
Class/ Subclass	Prototype/ Generic	Administration Considerations	Therapeutic Effects	Side/Adverse Effects
Alpha-1 agonist	phenylephrine pseudoephedrine	Contraindicated with MAOIs Use cautiously in patients with glaucoma, hypertension, or enlarged prostate Do not administer within 2 hours of bedtime	Decreased swelling of mucous membranes and decreased secretions	Increased blood pressure Urinary retention Nervousness Difficulty sleeping

---

29   uCentral from Unbound Medicine. https://www.unboundmedicine.com/ucentral.

30   This work is a derivative of *Daily Med* by U.S. National Library of Medicine in the public domain.

4.9 ALPHA-1 ANTAGONISTS

Tamsulosin is an Alpha-1 antagonist.

Mechanism of Action: Tamsulosin selectively blocks alpha receptors in the prostate, leading to the relaxation of smooth muscles in the bladder, neck, and prostate, thus improving urine flow and reducing symptoms of benign prostatic hypertrophy (BPH).

Indications: Tamsulosin is used to treat BPH.

Nursing Considerations: Avoid using with other alpha-blockers. Tamsulosin is contraindicated with strong CYP3A4 inhibitors such as ketoconazole. Assess and monitor blood pressure, especially after first dose because tamsulosin may cause orthostatic hypotension.

Patient Teaching and Education: Advise patients to change positions slowly because the drug may cause orthostatic blood pressure changes. Additionally, the patient should take the medication at the same time each day. The patient should follow up with their healthcare provider to assess the effectiveness of the medication.[31]

Now let's take a closer look at the medication grid on tamsulosin in Table 4.9.[32]

Table 4.9: Tamsulosin Medication Grid				
Class/ Subclass	**Prototype/ Generic**	**Administration Considerations**	**Therapeutic Effects**	**Side/Adverse Effects**
Alpha-1 antagonist	**tamsulosin**	Avoid using with other alpha-blockers Assess and monitor blood pressure, especially after first dose	Relaxes smooth muscle in bladder/ prostate to improve urine flow	Hypotension, especially after first dose. Advise patient to change positions slowly

---

31   uCentral from Unbound Medicine. https://www.unboundmedicine.com/ucentral.

32   This work is a derivative of *Daily Med* by U.S. National Library of Medicine in the public domain.

4.10 ALPHA-2 AGONISTS

Clonidine is an Alpha-2 Agonist.

Mechanism of Action: Clonidine reduces sympathetic outflow from the central nervous system and decreases peripheral resistance and renal vascular resistance.

Indications: Clonidine is used to treat hypertension (HTN) and attention deficit hyperactivity disorder (ADHD).

Nursing Considerations: Monitor blood pressure and pulse rate frequently. Dosage is usually adjusted to the patient's blood pressure and can cause hypotension, bradycardia, and sedation. Rebound hypertension may occur if stopped abruptly.

Patient Teaching and Education: Patients should be taught the importance of adhering to the same dosing schedule each day. Patients may experience orthostatic blood pressure changes and should be cautioned against the use of alcohol while taking this medication. Additionally, patients may experience increased susceptibility to blood pressure changes when exercising and exposed to hot environments. If the patient experiences mental depression as a side effect of the medication, a different medication therapy may be needed. [33]

Now let's take a closer look at the medication grid on clonidine in Table 4.10. [34]

Table 4.10: Cloinidine Medication Grid				
Class/ Subclass	**Prototype/ Generic**	**Administration Considerations**	**Therapeutic Effects**	**Side/Adverse Effects**
Alpha-2 agonist	clonidine	Monitor blood pressure and pulse rate frequently Dosage is usually adjusted to patient's BP and tolerance	Treat hypertension or ADHD	Hypotension Bradycardia Sedation Rebound hypertension if stopped abruptly

Alpha-2 Antagonists

A2 antagonists are used in research with limited clinical application. [35]

---

33 uCentral from Unbound Medicine. https://www.unboundmedicine.com/ucentral.

34 This work is a derivative of *Daily Med* by U.S. National Library of Medicine in the public domain.

35 This work is a derivative of *Daily Med* by U.S. National Library of Medicine in the public domain.

4.11 BETA-1 AGONISTS

Dobutamine is a Beta-1 agonist.

Mechanism of Action: Dobutamine stimulates Beta-1 receptors to increase heart rate, force of contraction, and conduction velocity.

Indications: Dobutamine is used to treat cardiogenic shock and severe heart failure to increase contractility and cardiac output.

Nursing Considerations: In IV administration, dilute concentration before administering. Continuously monitor electrocardiogram (ECG), blood pressure, cardiac output, and urine output during therapy. This drug can cause a marked increase in heart rate and blood pressure. Report all adverse reactions promptly, especially labored breathing, angina, palpitations, and dizziness.

Patient Teaching and Education: The patient should be instructed to inform the nurse immediately if they notice chest pain, shortness of breath, or numbness or tingling in the extremities.[36]

Now let's take a closer look at the dobutamine medication grid in Table 4.11.[37]

Table 4.11: Dobutamine Medication Grid

Class/ Subclass	Prototype/ Generic	Administration Considerations	Therapeutic Effects	Side/Adverse Effects
Beta-1 agonist	dobutamine	Continuously monitor ECG, blood pressure, cardiac output, and urine output during therapy	Increases heart rate, force of heart contraction, and speed of conduction between SA to AV nodes	Marked increase in heart rate and blood pressure Report all adverse reactions promptly, especially labored breathing, angina, palpitations, and dizziness

---

36   uCentral from Unbound Medicine. https://www.unboundmedicine.com/ucentral.

37   This work is a derivative of *Daily Med* by U.S. National Library of Medicine in the public domain.

4.12 BETA-1 ANTAGONISTS

Metoprolol is a selective Beta-1 antagonist.

Mechanism of Action: Metoprolol primarily blocks Beta-1 receptors in the heart, causing decreased heart rate and decreased blood pressure. However, higher doses can also block Beta-2 receptors in the lungs, causing bronchoconstriction.

Indications: Metoprolol is commonly used to treat high blood pressure, chest pain due to poor blood flow to the heart, as an early intervention during a myocardial infarction (MI), and in several heart conditions involving an abnormally fast heart rate.

Nursing Considerations: Don't crush extended-release (ER) formulations. Always check patient's apical pulse rate before giving drug. Withhold the drug and call the prescriber immediately if the heart rate is slower than 60 beats/minute, unless other parameters are provided. In diabetic patients, monitor glucose level closely because the drug masks common signs and symptoms of hypoglycemia. The most serious potential adverse effects are shortness of breath, bradycardia, and worsening heart failure. Other adverse effects include fatigue, dizziness, depression, insomnia, nightmares, gastrointestinal upset, erectile dysfunction, dyspnea, and wheezing.

Black Box Warning: When stopping therapy, the dosage should be tapered over 1 to 2 weeks because abrupt discontinuation may cause chest pain or myocardial infarction (MI).

Patient Teaching and Education: Patients should be instructed to take the medication as prescribed. They should be advised that abrupt cessation of medication therapy may result in life-threatening cardiac arrhythmias. Patients should also be taught how to self-check pulse and blood pressure to assess the effectiveness of medication therapy. Additionally, they should be cautioned against sudden changes in position due to orthostatic blood pressure changes. Patients may experience increase sensitivity to cold and should be cautioned to avoid caffeinated substances.[38]

---

38   uCentral from Unbound Medicine. https://www.unboundmedicine.com/ucentral.

Now let's take a closer look at the medication grid on metoprolol in Table 4.12.[39]

Table 4.12: Metoprolol Medication Grid

Class/ Subclass	Prototype/ Generic	Administration Considerations	Therapeutic Effects	Side/Adverse Effects
Beta-1 antagonist	Selective B blocker: **metoprolol**	Do not crush extended-release (ER) formulations Always assess apical HR and if less than 60, do not administer and call the prescriber unless other parameters are provided Monitor blood sugar in diabetic patients because drug can mask symptoms of hypoglycemia	Decreases blood pressure or controls rapid heart rate	Decreased blood pressure or heart rate Most serious: ■ Hypotension ■ Bradycardia ■ Worsening heart failure (HF) Other: ■ CNS: fatigue, dizziness, depression, insomnia, nightmares ■ GI upset ■ GU: erectile dysfunction ■ Respiratory: dyspnea and wheezing

---

39 This work is a derivative of *Daily Med* by U.S. National Library of Medicine in the public domain.

4.13 BETA-2 AGONISTS

Albuterol is a Beta-2 agonist.

Mechanism of Action: Albuterol is a selective Beta-2 agonist primarily used to cause bronchodilation in the lungs. However, Beta-2 receptors in the heart can also be stimulated, causing cardiovascular side effects.

Indications: Albuterol is commonly used to treat asthma and chronic obstructive pulmonary disease (COPD).

Nursing Considerations: Monitor respiratory rate, oxygen saturation, and lungs sounds before and after administration. If more than one inhalation is ordered, wait at least 2 minutes between inhalations. Use a spacer device to improve drug delivery, if appropriate.

Adverse Effects: Albuterol can cause hypersensitivity or paradoxical bronchospasm. It can also produce a clinically significant cardiovascular effect in some patients by causing increased heart rate and blood pressure, which may require the drug to be discontinued.

Patient Teaching and Education: Patients should remain compliant with the medication dosing regimen. Individuals should contact their healthcare provider if they experience ongoing shortness of breath unrelieved with medication therapy. If using an inhaler, the patient should be sure to prime the inhaler prior to administering the dose of medication. The medication can cause an unusual taste in the mouth, so patients should rinse their mouth with water after each use. [40]

Now let's take a closer look at the medication grid on albuterol in Table 4.13. [41]

Table 4.13: Albuterol Medication Grid

Class/ Subclass	Prototype/ Generic	Administration Considerations	Therapeutic Effects	Side/Adverse Effects
Beta-2 agonist	albuterol	If more than 1 inhalation is ordered, wait at least 2 minutes between inhalations Use spacer device to improve drug delivery, if appropriate	Bronchodilation in asthma or COPD	Hypersensitivity Can cause paradoxical bronchospasm Report significantly increased heart rate and blood pressure, which may require the drug to be discontinued

40   uCentral from Unbound Medicine. https://www.unboundmedicine.com/ucentral.

41   This work is a derivative of *Daily Med* by U.S. National Library of Medicine in the public domain.

4.14 BETA-2 ANTAGONISTS

Propranolol is a Beta-2 antagonist.

Mechanism of Action: Propranolol is a nonselective beta blocker because of its inhibition of both Beta-1 and Beta-2 receptors.

Indications: Propranolol is used to treat high blood pressure, angina, various heart dysrhythmias (to lower the heart rate), and essential tremors. It is also used after a myocardial infarction to reduce mortality by decreasing heart workload, and in migraine prevention.

Nursing Considerations: Nonselective beta blockers must be used cautiously with patients who have co-existing asthma or chronic obstructive pulmonary disease (COPD) because of the effects on Beta-2 receptors that could potentially cause bronchoconstriction. It can also mask symptoms of hypoglycemia in diabetics. Use with caution in patients with impaired hepatic or renal function. Give immediate-release (IR) formulations on an empty stomach. Do not crush extended-release (ER) formulations. Propranolol ER is not considered a simple milligram-for-milligram substitute for conventional propranolol. Check blood pressure and apical pulse before giving drug; withhold and notify prescriber if apical pulse is less than 60 beats per minute or systolic blood pressure is less than 100 mm Hg, unless other parameters are provided. During IV administration, monitor blood pressure, ECG, and heart rate frequently. The most serious adverse effects include bronchoconstriction, hypotension, bradycardia, and signs of worsening heart failure. Other adverse effects are similar to selective beta blockers like metoprolol. Black Box Warning: Abrupt withdrawal of this drug may cause exacerbation of angina or a myocardial infarction. To discontinue this drug, gradually reduce dosage over 1 to 2 weeks.

Patient Teaching and Education: Patients should be instructed to follow the medication dosing regimen. Stopping medication therapy abruptly may cause life-threatening arrhythmias. Patients should be instructed on how to self-assess pulse and blood pressure to evaluate medication effectiveness. The medication may cause increased susceptibility to orthostatic blood pressure changes and increased sensitivity to cold.[42]

Now let's take a closer look at the medication grid on propranolol in Table 4.14.[43]

---

42 uCentral from Unbound Medicine. https://www.unboundmedicine.com/ucentral.

43 This work is a derivative of *Daily Med* by U.S. National Library of Medicine in the public domain.

Table 4.14: Propranolol Medication Grid

Class/ Subclass	Prototype/ Generic	Administration Considerations	Therapeutic Effects	Side/Adverse Effects
Beta-2 Antagonist	Nonselective B-blocker: **propranolol**	Contraindicated in patients with asthma, COPD, or bradycardia Use cautiously in patients who have diabetes mellitus because drug masks some symptoms of hypoglycemia Use with caution in patients with impaired hepatic or renal function Give immediate release formulations on an empty stomach Do not crush ER formulations Check BP and apical pulse before giving drug; withhold and notify prescriber if apical pulse is less than 60 or systolic blood pressure is less than 100 unless other parameters are provided During IV administration, monitor blood pressure, ECG, and heart rate frequently	Decrease blood pressure and heart rate Prevent migraines Manage tremors	Most serious: ■ Bronchocon-striction ■ Hypotension ■ Bradycardia ■ Worsening heart failure Black Box Warning: Abrupt withdrawal of drug may cause exacerbation of angina or myocardial infarction. To discontinue drug, gradually reduce dosage over 1 to 2 weeks Other adverse effects similar to metoprolol

4.15   ALPHA AND BETA RECEPTOR AGONISTS (CATECHOLAMINES)

Catecholamines

Epinephrine and norepinephrine (NE) are adrenergics that stimulate the beta and alpha receptors on the target cell. Dopamine has dose-dependent effects on targeted arteries in the kidneys, heart, and brain.

Epinephrine (Alpha and Beta Receptor Agonist): Epinephrine acts on both alpha- and beta-adrenergic receptors and is used in several routes including intravenously (IV), subcutaneously, intramuscularly, and via inhalation. Epinephrine decreases vasodilation and increases vascular permeability through its alpha-adrenergic receptor action, which can lead to loss of intravascular fluid volume and hypotension. Through its action on beta-adrenergic receptors, epinephrine causes bronchial smooth muscle relaxation and helps alleviate bronchospasm, wheezing, and dyspnea that may occur during anaphylaxis.

Indications: Epinephrine is used for severe allergic reactions, acute bronchospasm during asthma attacks, cardiac resuscitation, hypotension in severe shock, or for local injection to control superficial bleeding.

Nursing Considerations: Epinephrine is contraindicated for use in fingers, toes, ears, nose, or genitalia when used with local anesthetic due to the vasoconstrictive action. Contraindicated in patients with narrow angle glaucoma. Administer with caution to the elderly and those with pre-existing cardiovascular disease. When administering IV, monitor vitals (blood pressure, heart rate, and respiratory rate) and cardiovascular and respiratory systems closely; if blood pressure increases sharply, give rapid-acting vasodilators. Monitor IV site for extravasation. Discard IV solution if discolored.

Patient Teaching and Education with EpiPen: Epinephrine formulated in a pen for injection is known as EpiPen. EpiPen is used for severe allergic reactions after exposure to an allergen like a bee sting. Check expiration date, store at room temperature, and protect from light. Effects fade after 15-20 minutes, so seek medical care immediately.[44]

Norepinephrine is another catecholamine and is used as a peripheral vasoconstrictor (due to alpha-adrenergic action) and as an inotropic stimulator of the heart and dilator of coronary arteries (due to beta-adrenergic action) in patients with critically low blood pressure.

Now let's take a closer look at the medication grid on epinephrine and norepinephrine in Table 4.15a.[45]

44   uCentral from Unbound Medicine. https://www.unboundmedicine.com/ucentral.

45   This work is a derivative of *Daily Med* by U.S. National Library of Medicine in the public domain.

Table 4.15a: Epinephrine and Norepinephrine Medication Grid

Class/ Subclass	Prototype/ Generic	Administration Considerations	Therapeutic Effects	Side/Adverse Effects
Catechol-amine	epinephrine norepinephrine	Contraindicated for use in fingers, toes, ears, nose, or genitalia when used with local anesthetic Monitor vitals (blood pressure, heart rate, respiratory rate), cardiovascular and respiratory systems closely when administering IV If administering IV, monitor IV site for extravasation Discard IV solution if discolored	Reversal of severe allergic reaction, bronchodilation, increased blood pressure, cardiac resuscitation, or control of superficial bleeding	Hypertension Tachycardia

Dopamine is another type of catecholamine specifically used to improve perfusion of organs, improve cardiac output, and increase blood pressure.

Mechanism of Action: In low doses, dopamine mainly stimulates dopamine receptors and dilates the renal vasculature. Moderate doses of dopamine stimulate beta receptors for a positive inotropic effect. Higher doses also stimulate alpha receptors, constricting blood vessels and increasing blood pressure.

Indications: Dopamine is used to treat shock, improve perfusion to vital organs, increase cardiac output, and correct hypotension.

Nursing Considerations: During infusion, frequently monitor blood pressure, cardiac output, urine output, and color and temperature of limbs. If urine flow decreases without hypotension, notify prescriber because dosage may need to be reduced. Concurrent alpha or beta blockers can antagonize dopamine. Adverse effects include hypotension, tachycardia, palpitations, and decreased blood flow to the extremities.

Patient Teaching and Education: Patients should contact their health care provider immediately if experiencing unusual sweating, dizziness, heart palpitations, or chest pain.

Now let's take a closer look at the medication grid on dopamine in Table 4.15b.[46]

---

46   This work is a derivative of *Daily Med* by U.S. National Library of Medicine in the public domain.

Table 4.15b: Dopamine Medication Grid

Class/ Subclass	Prototype/ Generic	Administration Considerations	Therapeutic Effects	Side/Adverse Effects
Catechol- amine	Dopamine	During infusion, frequently monitor ECG, blood pressure, cardiac output, pulse rate, urine output, and color and temperature of limbs Check urine output often	Increased blood flow to kidneys causing increased urine output Increased cardiac output and elevated blood pressure	Hypotension Tachycardia Palpitations Dyspnea Decreased blood flow to extremities If urine flow decreases without hypotension, notify prescriber because dosage may need to be reduced

4.16 MODULE LEARNING ACTIVITIES

Light Bulb Moment

Test your knowledge and application.

Practice applying your knowledge regarding ANS neuroreceptors to the following patient scenarios where a nurse must use clinical judgment for a solution:

1. A patient begins a nicotine patch in an attempt to stop smoking. The patient reports feelings of nausea, weakness, and a rapid heartbeat. What is the likely cause of these symptoms, and what is the nurse's best response?

2. A patient with benign prostatic hyperplasia (BPH) has a new order for tamsulosin. He asks, "How will tamsulosin help me? I already take so many pills."

    a) What is the nurse's best response?

    b) What does the nurse plan to monitor carefully, especially after administering the first dose of tamsulosin?

3. A patient with asthma is taking albuterol to help when she feels increased shortness of breath.

    a) How will albuterol assist in her breathing?

The patient states, "After I take albuterol, it feels like my heart is racing."

    b) What is the likely cause of this symptom?

    c) What is the nurse's best response to the patient's concern?

4. A patient with high blood pressure is prescribed propranolol.

    a) How will propranolol help to lower his blood pressure?

    b) What will the nurse assess before administering the propranolol?

The nurse listens to the patient's lungs a few hours after administering propranolol and notices new wheezing.

    c) What could be a potential cause of this new finding?

    d) What is the nurse's next best response?

5. A patient is prescribed metoprolol to help control his atrial fibrillation, an irregular heart rhythm.

    a) What will the nurse assess before administering the metoprolol?

    b) What findings would cause the nurse to call the provider before administering the metoprolol?

Upon reassessment the next day, the nurse notices a new finding of edema in the patient's feet and lower legs.

    c) What could be a potential cause of this new finding?

    d) What is the nurse's next best response?

6. A patient with an acute episode of heart failure is admitted and is prescribed dobutamine.

    a) How will dobutamine improve the patient's condition?

    b) What will the nurse monitor carefully during administration?

Note: Answers to the Light Bulb Moment can be found in the "Answer Key" sections at the end of the book.

GLOSSARY

Acetylcholine (ACh): Binds to both nicotinic receptors and muscarinic receptors in the PNS.

Adrenergic: Postganglionic neuron where neurotransmitters norepinephrine and epinephrine are released. Includes alpha (α) receptors and beta (β) receptors.

Adrenergic Agonist: Mimics the effects of the body's natural SNS stimulation on alpha (α) and beta (β) receptors. Also called sympathomimetics.

Adrenergic Antagonist: Blocks the effects of the SNS receptors.

Anticholinergics: Inhibit acetylcholine (ACh), which allows the SNS to dominate. Also called parasympatholytics or muscarinic antagonists. Overall use is to relax smooth muscle.

Autonomic Nervous System: Controls cardiac and smooth muscle, as well as glandular tissue; associated with involuntary responses.

Catecholamines: Include norepinephrine, epinephrine, and dopamine. Stimulate the adrenergic receptors.

Central Nervous System (CNS): Anatomical division of the nervous system located within the cranial and vertebral cavities, namely the brain and spinal cord.

Cholinergic: Postganglionic neuron where acetylcholine (ACh) is released that stimulates nicotinic receptors and muscarinic receptors. Also relating to drugs that inhibit, enhance, or mimic the action of ACh.

Chronotropic: Drugs may change the heart rate and rhythm by affecting the electrical conduction system of the heart and the nerves that influence it, such as by changing the rhythm (increasing) produced by the sinoatrial node. Positive chronotropes increase heart rate; negative chronotropes decrease heart rate.

Dromotropic: Stimulation causes increases speed of conduction between SA and AV node.

Fight-or-Flight Response: The response when the SNS is stimulated, causing the main effects of increased heart rate, increased blood pressure, and bronchodilation.

Glycogenolysis: The breakdown of glycogen into glucose, causing elevated blood glucose.

Homeostasis (in ANS): Balance between the SNS and PNS. At each target organ, dual innervation determines activity. For example, SNS stimulation causes the heart rate to increase, whereas PNS stimulation causes the heart rate to decrease.

Hyperglycemia: Elevated blood glucose.

Inotropic: Stimulation causes increased force of contraction.

Involuntary Responses: Responses that the brain controls without the need for conscious thought.

Motor Neurons: Consist of the somatic nervous system that stimulates voluntary movement of muscles and the autonomic nervous system that controls involuntary responses.

Muscarinic Agonists: Also called parasympathomimetics. Primarily cause smooth muscle contraction, resulting in decreased HR, bronchoconstriction, increased gastrointestinal/genitourinary tone, and pupil constriction.

Neurons: Cells that carry electrical impulses to the synapse of a target organ.

Nonselective Beta Blockers: Medications that block both Beta-1 and Beta-2 receptors, thus affecting both the heart and lungs.

Parasympathetic Division (PNS): Includes nerves outside the brain and spinal cord. Associated with the "rest and digest" response. Stimulation of PNS causes decreased heart rate, decreased blood pressure via vasodilation, bronchial constriction, and stimulates intestinal motility, salivation, and relaxation of the bladder.

Parasympatholytics: Inhibit acetylcholine (ACh), which allows the SNS to dominate. Also called anticholinergics or muscarinic antagonists.

Parasympathomimetics: Also called muscarinic agonists. Primarily cause smooth muscle contraction, resulting in decreased HR, bronchoconstriction, increased GI/GU tone, and pupil constriction.

Peripheral Nervous System (PNS): An anatomical division of the nervous system that is largely outside the cranial and vertebral cavities, namely all parts except the brain and spinal cord.

Postganglionic Neurons: Differ for the SNS and PNS branches. Postganglionic neurons of the autonomic system are classified as either cholinergic, meaning that acetylcholine (ACh) is released, or adrenergic, meaning that norepinephrine is released.

Preganglionic Neurons: All preganglionic neurons (in the SNS and PNS) release acetylcholine (ACh).

Selective Beta Blocker: Medications that mostly inhibit B1 receptors.

Sensory Neurons: Sense the environment and conduct signals to the brain that become a conscious perception of that stimulus.

"SLUDGE": Mnemonic for the effects of anticholinergics: **S**alivation decreased, **L**acrimation decreased, **U**rinary retention, **D**rowsiness/dizziness, **GI** upset, **E**yes (blurred vision/dry eyes).

Somatic Nervous System: Causes contraction of skeletal muscles; associated with voluntary responses.

Sympathetic Division (SNS): Associated with the "fight-or-flight response." Stimulation causes the main effects of increased heart rate, increased blood pressure via the constriction of blood vessels, and bronchodilation.

Sympathomimetics: Mimic the effects of the body's natural SNS stimulation of adrenergic receptors. Also called adrenergic agonists.

Synapse: The connection between the neuron and its target cell.

Chapter V

Respiratory

5.1   RESPIRATORY INTRODUCTION

Learning Objectives

- Identify the classifications and actions of respiratory system drugs
- Give examples of when, how, and to whom respiratory system drugs may be administered
- Identify the side effects and special considerations associated with respiratory system drugs
- Include considerations and implications of using respiratory system drugs across the life span
- Include evidence-based concepts when using the nursing process related to medications that affect the respiratory system
- Identify and interpret related laboratory tests

Every year millions of Americans visit their health care provider for respiratory diseases such as allergies, asthma, bronchitis, common cold, chronic obstructive pulmonary disease (COPD), and pneumonia. Currently more than 25 million people in the United States have asthma. Approximately 14.8 million adults have been diagnosed with COPD, and approximately 12 million people have not yet been diagnosed. The burden of respiratory diseases affects individuals and their families, schools, workplaces, neighborhoods, cities, and states. Because of the cost to the health care system, the burden of respiratory diseases also falls on society; it is paid for with tax dollars, higher health insurance rates, and lost productivity. Annual health care expenditures for asthma alone are estimated at $20.7 billion.[1]

Before we learn about medications that are used to treat respiratory conditions in our patients, let's review the respiratory system.

---

1   This work is a derivative of Respiratory Diseases by Office of Disease Prevention and Health Promotion in the public domain.

5.2 RESPIRATORY BASICS

Basic Concepts Related to Respiratory Medications

Overview of the Respiratory System

The purpose of the respiratory system is to perform gas exchange. Pulmonary ventilation provides air to the alveoli for this gas exchange process. At the respiratory membrane where the alveolar and capillary walls meet, gases move across the membranes, with oxygen entering the bloodstream and carbon dioxide exiting. It is through this mechanism that blood is oxygenated and carbon dioxide, the waste product of cellular respiration, is removed from the body.

The major organs of the respiratory system function primarily to provide oxygen to body tissues for cellular respiration, remove the waste product carbon dioxide, and help maintain acid-base balance. Portions of the respiratory system are also used for non-vital functions, such as sensing odors, speech production, and for straining, such as during childbirth or coughing.[2]

See Figure 5.1[3] illustrating major respiratory structures.

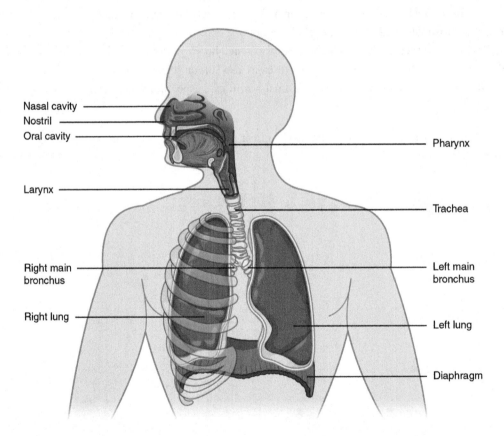

Figure 5.1 Major Respiratory Structures: The major respiratory structures span the nasal cavity to the diaphragm

---

2   This work is a derivative of *Anatomy and Physiology* by OpenStax licensed under CC BY 4.0. Access for free at https://openstax.org/books/anatomy-and-physiology/pages/1-introduction.

3   "2301 Major Respiratory Organs.jpg" by OpenStax College is licensed under CC BY 4.0 Access for free at https://openstax.org/books/anatomy-and-physiology/pages/22-1-organs-and-structures-of-the-respiratory- system.

Functionally, the respiratory system can be divided into a conducting zone and a respiratory zone. The conducting zone of the respiratory system includes the organs and structures not directly involved in gas exchange. The gas exchange occurs in the respiratory zone.

Conducting Zone

The major functions of the conducting zone are to provide a route for incoming and outgoing air, remove debris and pathogens from the incoming air, and warm and humidify the incoming air. Several structures within the conducting zone perform other functions as well. The epithelium of the nasal passages, for example, is essential to sensing odors, and the bronchial epithelium that lines the lungs can metabolize some airborne carcinogens.

The cilia of the respiratory epithelium help remove the mucus and debris from the nasal cavity with a constant beating motion, thus sweeping materials toward the throat to be swallowed. Interestingly, cold air slows the movement of the cilia, resulting in the accumulation of mucus that may, in turn, lead to a runny nose during cold weather. This moist epithelium functions to warm and humidify incoming air. Capillaries located just beneath the nasal epithelium warm the air by convection.

Bronchial Tree

The trachea branches into the right and left primary bronchi at the carina. A bronchial tree (or respiratory tree) is the collective term used for these multiple-branched bronchi. The main function of the bronchi, like other conducting zone structures, is to provide a passageway for air to move into and out of each lung. In addition, the mucous membrane traps debris and pathogens.

A bronchiole branches from the tertiary bronchi. Bronchioles, which are about 1 mm in diameter, further branch until they become the tiny terminal bronchioles, which lead to the structures of gas exchange. There are more than 1,000 terminal bronchioles in each lung. The muscular walls of the bronchioles do not contain cartilage like those of the bronchi. This muscular wall can change the size of the tubing to increase or decrease airflow through the tube.

Respiratory Zone

In contrast to the conducting zone, the respiratory zone includes structures that are directly involved in **gas exchange**. See Figure 5.2[4] for an illustration of the respiratory zone. The respiratory zone begins where the terminal bronchioles join a respiratory bronchiole, the smallest type of bronchiole, which then leads to an alveolar duct, opening into a cluster of alveoli.

---

4   "2309 The Respiratory Zone.jpg" by OpenStax College is licensed under CC BY 3.0 Access for free at https://openstax .org/books/anatomy-and-physiology/pages/22-1-organs-and-structures-of-the-respiratory- system.

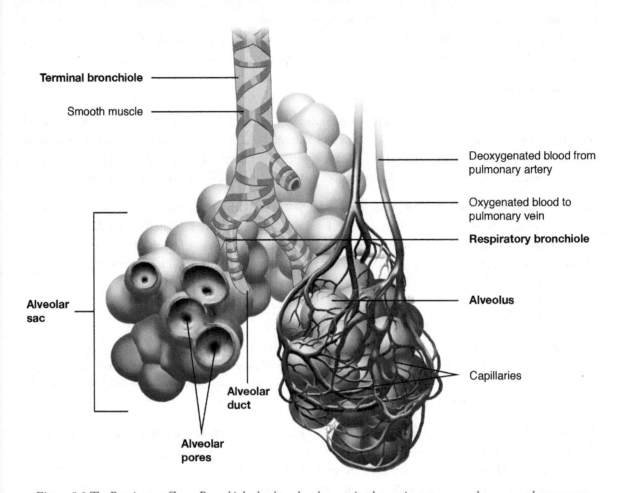

Figure 5.2 The Respiratory Zone. Bronchioles lead to alveolar sacs in the respiratory zone where gas exchange occurs

Alveoli

An alveolar duct is a tube composed of smooth muscle and connective tissue, which opens into a cluster of alveoli. An alveolus is one of the many small, grape-like sacs that are attached to the alveolar ducts.

An alveolar sac is a cluster of many individual alveoli that are responsible for gas exchange. See Figure 5.3[5] for an illustration of the structures of the respiratory zone.

5 "2310 Structures of the Respiratory Zone.jpg" by OpenStax College is licensed under CC BY 3.0 Access for free at https://openstax.org/books/anatomy-and-physiology/pages/22-1-organs-and-structures-of-the-respiratory- system.

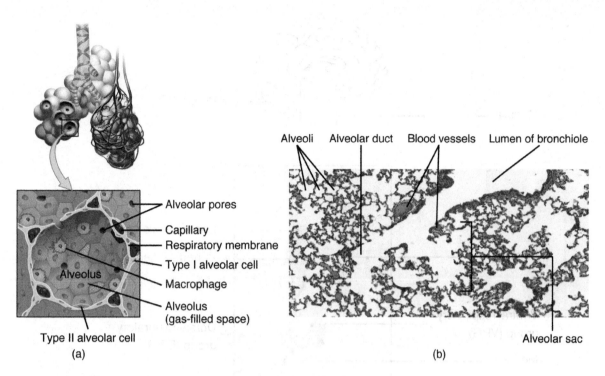

Figure 5.3 Structures of the Respiratory Zone. The alveolus is responsible for gas exchange

Respiratory Rate and Control of Ventilation

Breathing usually occurs without thought, although at times you can consciously control it, such as when you swim under water, sing a song, or blow bubbles. The **respiratory rate** is the total number of breaths, or respiratory cycles, that occur each minute. Respiratory rate can be an important indicator of disease, as the rate may increase or decrease during an illness. The respiratory rate is controlled by the respiratory center located within the medulla oblongata in the brain, which responds primarily to changes in carbon dioxide, oxygen, and pH levels in the blood.

The normal respiratory rate of a child decreases from birth to adolescence. A child under 1 year of age has a normal respiratory rate between 30 and 60 breaths per minute, but by the time a child is about 10 years old, the normal rate is closer to 18 to 30. By adolescence, the normal respiratory rate is similar to that of adults, 12 to 18 breaths per minute.

Neurons that stimulate the muscles of the respiratory system are responsible for controlling and regulating pulmonary ventilation. The major brain centers involved in pulmonary ventilation are the medulla oblongata and the pontine respiratory group. (See Figure 5.4[6] for an illustration of the respiratory centers of the brain.)

---

6   "2327 Respiratory Centers of the Brain.jpg" by OpenStax College is licensed under CC BY 3.0 .Access for free at https://openstax.org/books/anatomy-and-physiology/pages/22-3-the-process-of-breathing.

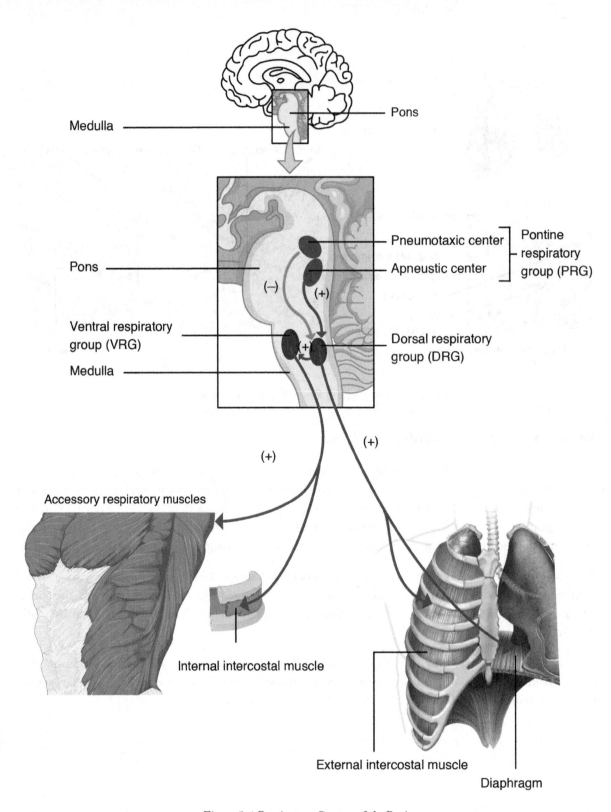

Figure 5.4 Respiratory Centers of the Brain

Supplementary Videos: See the supplementary videos below related to respiratory anatomy and physiology.

Anatomy of Respiratory System[7]

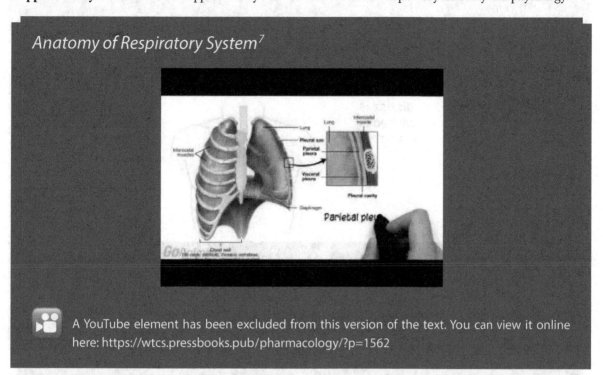

A YouTube element has been excluded from this version of the text. You can view it online here: https://wtcs.pressbooks.pub/pharmacology/?p=1562

Inhalation and Exhalation[8]

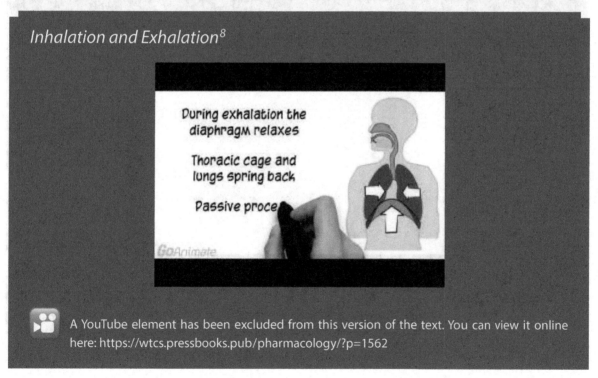

A YouTube element has been excluded from this version of the text. You can view it online here: https://wtcs.pressbooks.pub/pharmacology/?p=1562

---

7   Forciea, B. (2015, May 13). *Repiratory System Anatomy (v2.0).* [Video]. YouTube. All rights reserved. Video used with permission. https://youtu.be/aqTwrdMS6CE.

8   Forciea, B. (2015, May 12). *Anatomy and Physiology: Respriratory System: Breathing Mechanics* (v2.0). [Video]. YouTube. All rights reserved. Video used with permission. https://youtu.be/X-J5Xgg3l6s.

Carbon Dioxide Transport[9]

A YouTube element has been excluded from this version of the text. You can view it online here: https://wtcs.pressbooks.pub/pharmacology/?p=1562

Surface Tension[10]

A YouTube element has been excluded from this version of the text. You can view it online here: https://wtcs.pressbooks.pub/pharmacology/?p=1562

---

9   Forciea, B. (2015, May 12). *Repiratory System: C02 Transport (v2.0)*. [Video]. YouTube. All rights reserved. Video used with permission. https://youtu.be/BmrvqZoxHYI.

10   Forciea, B. (2015, May 13). *Anatomy and Physiology: Respiratory System: Surface Tension (v2.0)*. [Video]. YouTube. All rights reserved. Video used with permission. https://youtu.be/YHTAausYA94.

5.3   DISEASES OF THE RESPIRATORY SYSTEM

Allergies

Allergies occur when your immune system reacts to a foreign substance—such as pollen, bee venom, pet dander, or food—that doesn't cause a reaction in most people.

Your immune system produces substances known as antibodies. When you have allergies, your immune system makes antibodies that identify a particular allergen as harmful, even though it isn't. When you come into contact with the allergen, your immune system's reaction can inflame your skin, sinuses, airways, or digestive system.

The severity of allergies varies from person to person and can range from minor irritation to a potentially life-threatening emergency. While most allergies can't be cured, treatments can help relieve allergy symptoms.

Allergy symptoms, which depend on the substance involved, can affect airways, sinuses, and nasal passages, skin, and the digestive system.[11]

Hay fever, also called allergic rhinitis, can cause:

- Sneezing
- Itching of the nose, eyes, or roof of the mouth
- Runny, stuffy nose
- Watery, red or swollen eyes (conjunctivitis)

A food allergy can cause:

- Tingling in the mouth
- Swelling of the lips, tongue, face, or throat
- Hives
- Anaphylaxis

An insect sting allergy can cause:

- Large area of swelling (edema) at the sting site
- Itching or hives all over the body
- Cough, chest tightness, wheezing, or shortness of breath
- Anaphylaxis

A drug allergy can cause:

- Hives
- Itchy skin
- Rash

---

11   Mayo Clinic Staff. (2018, January 6). *Allergies*. https://www.mayoclinic.org/diseases-conditions/allergies/symptoms-causes/syc-20351497.

- Facial swelling
- Wheezing
- Anaphylaxis

Atopic dermatitis, an allergic skin condition also called eczema, can cause skin to:

- Itch
- Redden
- Flake or peel

Anaphylaxis

Some types of allergies, including allergies to foods and insect stings, can trigger a severe reaction known as **anaphylaxis.** As a life-threatening medical emergency, anaphylaxis can cause a patient to go into shock. Signs and symptoms of anaphylaxis include:

- Loss of consciousness
- Drop in blood pressure
- Severe shortness of breath
- Skin rash
- Lightheadedness
- Rapid, weak pulse
- Nausea and vomiting

Asthma

Asthma is a common condition that affects the lungs in both adults and children. Approximately 8.2 percent of adults (18.7 million) and 9.4 percent of children (7 million) in the United States suffer from asthma. In addition, asthma is the most frequent cause of hospitalization in children.

Asthma is a chronic disease characterized by inflammation, edema, and bronchospasm of the airways, which inhibits air from entering the lungs. In addition, excessive mucus secretion can occur, which further contributes to airway blockage. Cells of the immune system, such as eosinophils and mononuclear cells, may also be involved in infiltrating the walls of the bronchi and bronchioles.

Bronchospasms occur periodically and lead to an "asthma attack." An attack may be triggered by environmental factors such as dust, pollen, pet hair, or dander; changes in the weather; mold; tobacco smoke; respiratory infections; exercise; and stress.[12]

See Figure 5.5[13] for an illustration of how asthma affects the airways.

---

12 This work is a derivative of *Anatomy and Physiology* by OpenStax licensed under CC BY 4.0. Access for free at https://openstax.org/books/anatomy-and-physiology/pages/1-introduction.

13 "Asthma and Your Airways" by unknown, is licensed under CC BY-NC-SA 3.0 Access for free at https://humannhealth.com/what-you-need-to-know-about-asthma/341/.

Asthma and Your Airways

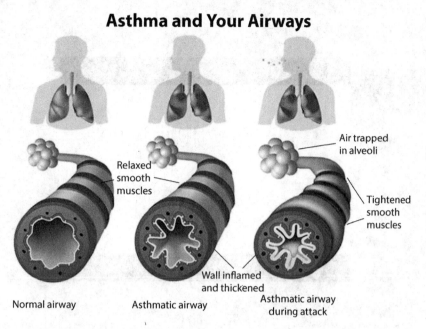

Figure 5.5 How Asthma Affects the Airways

Symptoms of an asthma attack involve coughing, shortness of breath, wheezing, and tightness of the chest. Symptoms of a severe asthma attack that requiring immediate medical attention include difficulty breathing that results in **cyanotic** lips or face, confusion, drowsiness, a rapid pulse, sweating, and severe anxiety.

The severity of the condition, frequency of attacks, and identified triggers influence the type of medication that an individual may require. Long-term treatments are used for patients with severe asthma. Short-term, fast-acting drugs are used to treat an asthma attack and are typically administered via an inhaler or nebulizer. View the following video for additional insight into how asthma works.[14]

---

14   This work is a derivative of *Anatomy and Physiology* by OpenStax licensed under CC BY 4.0. Access for free at https://openstax.org/books/anatomy-and-physiology/pages/1-introduction.

How Does Asthma Work?[15]

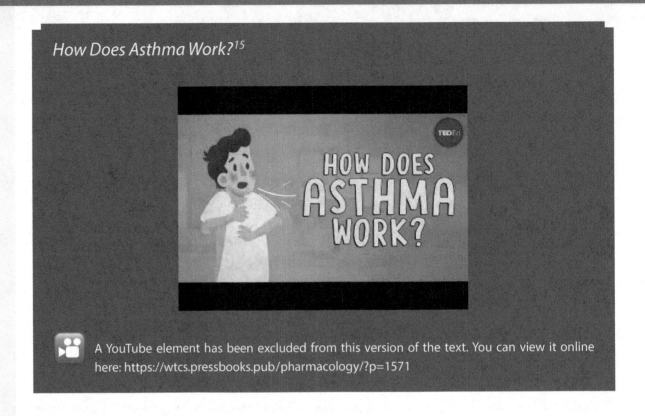

A YouTube element has been excluded from this version of the text. You can view it online here: https://wtcs.pressbooks.pub/pharmacology/?p=1571

Bronchitis

Bronchitis is an inflammation of the lining of the bronchial tubes, which carry air to and from the lungs. People who have bronchitis often cough up thickened mucus, which can be discolored. Bronchitis may be either acute or chronic.

Often developing from a cold or other respiratory infection, acute bronchitis is very common. Acute bronchitis, also called a chest cold, usually improves within a week to 10 days without lasting effects, although the cough may linger for weeks.

Chronic bronchitis, a more serious condition, is a constant irritation or inflammation of the lining of the bronchial tubes, often due to smoking. Chronic bronchitis is one of the conditions included in COPD.[16]

Symptoms for either acute bronchitis or chronic bronchitis may include:

- Cough
- Production of mucus (sputum), which can be clear, white, yellowish-gray, or green in color—rarely, it may be streaked with blood
- Fatigue
- Shortness of breath

---

15   TED-Ed. (2017, May 11). *How does asthma work? - Christopher E. Gaw*. [Video]. YouTube. https://youtu.be/PzfLDi-sL3w.

16   Mayo Clinic Staff. (2017, April 11). *Bronchitis*. https://www.mayoclinic.org/diseases-conditions/bronchitis/symptoms-causes/syc-20355566.

- Slight fever and chills
- Chest discomfort

Cold

The common cold is a viral infection of the upper respiratory tract. Many types of viruses can cause a common cold. Children younger than 6 are at greatest risk of colds, but healthy adults can also expect to have two or three colds annually. Most people recover from a common cold in a week or 10 days. Symptoms might last longer in people who smoke.

Symptoms of a common cold usually appear one to three days after exposure to a cold-causing virus. Signs and symptoms, which can vary from person to person, might include:

- Runny or stuffy nose
- Sore throat
- Cough
- Congestion
- Slight body aches or a mild headache
- Sneezing
- Low-grade fever
- Generally feeling unwell (malaise)[17]

Chronic Obstructive Pulmonary Disease

Chronic Obstructive Pulmonary Disease (COPD) is a chronic inflammatory lung disease that causes obstructed airflow out of the lungs. Symptoms include breathing difficulty, cough, mucus (sputum) production, and wheezing. It is often caused by long-term exposure to irritating gases or dust, and most often occurs due to smoking. People with COPD are at increased risk of developing heart disease, lung cancer, and a variety of other conditions.

Emphysema and chronic bronchitis are the two types of COPD. Emphysema is a condition in which the alveoli at the end of the smallest air passages (bronchioles) of the lungs are destroyed and hyperinflated. Chronic bronchitis is inflammation of the lining of the bronchial tubes, characterized by daily cough and mucus (sputum) production. See Figure 5.6 for an illustration of normal lungs compared to lungs with COPD.[18]

---

17   Mayo Clinic Staff. (2019, April 20). *Common cold*. https://www.mayoclinic.org/diseases-conditions
/common- cold/symptoms-causes/syc-20351605.

18   "Copd 2010Side.JPG" by National Heart Lung and Blood Institute is licensed under CC0.

My Notes

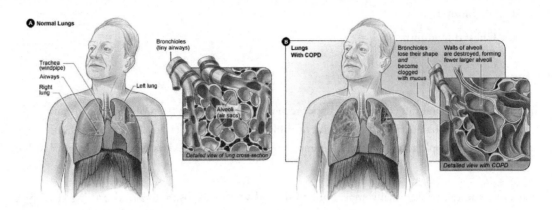

Figure 5.6 Normal lungs compared with lungs in a person with COPD

COPD is treatable but not curable. COPD symptoms often don't appear until significant lung damage has occurred, and they usually worsen over time, particularly if smoke exposure continues.

Other signs and symptoms of COPD may include:

- Shortness of breath, especially during physical activities
- Wheezing
- Chest tightness
- Chronic cough that may produce mucus (sputum) that may be clear, white, yellow, or greenish
- Cyanosis
- Frequent respiratory infections
- Lack of energy
- Unintended weight loss (in later stages)

Unlike some diseases, COPD has a clear cause and a clear path of prevention. The majority of cases are directly related to cigarette smoking, and the best way to prevent COPD is to never smoke—or to teach patients to stop smoking now.[19]

Interactive Activity

 An interactive or media element has been excluded from this version of the text. You can view it online here: https://wtcs.pressbooks.pub/pharmacology/?p=1571

---

19   Mayo Clinic Staff. (2017, August 11). *COPD*. https://www.mayoclinic.org/diseases-conditions/copd /symptoms- causes/syc-20353679.

Everyday Connection

The Effects of Second-Hand Tobacco Smoke

The burning of a tobacco cigarette creates multiple chemical compounds that are released through mainstream smoke, which is inhaled by the smoker, and through sidestream smoke, which is the smoke that is given off by the burning cigarette. Second-hand smoke, which is a combination of sidestream smoke and the mainstream smoke that is exhaled by the smoker, has been demonstrated by numerous scientific studies to cause disease. At least 40 chemicals in sidestream smoke have been identified that negatively impact human health, leading to the development of cancer or other conditions, such as immune system dysfunction, liver toxicity, cardiac arrhythmias, pulmonary edema, and neurological dysfunction. Furthermore, second- hand smoke has been found to harbor at least 250 compounds that are known to be toxic, carcinogenic, or both. Some major classes of carcinogens in second-hand smoke are polyaromatic hydrocarbons (PAHs), N-nitrosamines, aromatic amines, formaldehyde, and acetaldehyde.

Tobacco and second-hand smoke are considered to be carcinogenic. Exposure to second-hand smoke can cause lung cancer in individuals who are not tobacco users themselves. It is estimated that the risk of developing lung cancer is increased by up to 30 percent in nonsmokers who live with an individual who smokes in the house, as compared to nonsmokers who are not regularly exposed to second-hand smoke. Children are especially affected by second-hand smoke. Children who live with an individual who smokes inside the home have a larger number of lower respiratory infections, which are associated with hospitalizations, and higher risk of sudden infant death syndrome (SIDS). Second-hand smoke in the home has also been linked to a greater number of ear infections in children, as well as worsening symptoms of asthma.[20]

---

20   This work is a derivative of *Anatomy and Physiology* by OpenStax licensed under CC BY 4.0. Access for free at https://openstax.org/books/anatomy-and-physiology/pages/1-introduction.

5.4   NURSING PROCESS CONSIDERATIONS

Nursing Process Related to Respiratory Medications

Now that we have reviewed the respiratory system and common respiratory disorders, let's apply the nursing process to the administration of respiratory medications.

Nursing Process: Assessment

Although there are numerous details to consider when administering medications, it is always important to first think about what you are giving and why?

First, let's think of why?

Respiratory medications are often given to alleviate allergies, cold symptoms, or to decrease/eliminate shortness of breath (SOB). An important piece of your nursing assessment should be to assess the patient's respiratory status. The respiratory assessment includes observing the respiratory rate and quality of respirations (shallow, deep), obtaining a pulse oximetry reading, and auscultating lung sounds. Other pieces of the assessment include inspecting skin color, such as observing for **pallor**, or cyanosis, and determining if there is a cough or **sputum** present. If sputum is present, it should be assessed for color, odor, consistency, and amount (COCA).

Additional baseline information to collect prior to the administration of any respiratory medication includes any history of allergy or previous adverse drug response.

Nursing Process: Implementation of Interventions

Respiratory medications are available in many different formulations, such as nasal spray, inhalations, oral tablets or liquids, injections, or intravenous route, so it is always important to verify the correct route and anticipate the associated side effects. For example, inhalations deliver the required medicine or medicines directly to the lungs, which means the medicine(s) can act directly on the lung tissues, minimizing systemic side effects. On the other hand, intravenous medications are administered to act quickly, but can cause systemic side effects. Additionally, some products contain more than one medicine with different dosages (for example, inhalers that combine a long-acting bronchodilator with a glucocorticoid).

During the administration of respiratory medications, it is important to anticipate the expected outcome of the medication and any common side effects. For example, albuterol is a short acting Beta-2 agonist that is given for bronchodilation. The nurse should plan to perform a respiratory assessment before and after administration of albuterol to document the effectiveness of the medication, as well as monitor for tachycardia, a common side effect.

Additionally, the nurse should also ensure the proper use of the inhalers by the patient. Observe the patient self-administering the medication, and further instruct the patient in proper use.[21]

Nursing Process: Evaluation

Finally, it is important to always evaluate the patient's response to a medication. With respiratory medications, the nurse should assess decrease in allergy symptoms (cough, runny nose, tearing eyes) and any decrease in shortness of breath. The nurse should complete a respiratory assessment (respirations, pulse oximetry, and lung auscultation) before and after the medications have been administered and compare the results. If the symptoms are not improving or the clinical assessment is worsening, prompt intervention is required (such as notification of the health care provider for further orders) to prevent further clinical deterioration.

---

21   Drugs.com. (n.d.). *Respiratory agents.* https://www.drugs.com/drug-class/respiratory-agents.html.

5.5   RESPIRATORY MEDICATION CLASSES

Now that we have reviewed basic concepts, we will take a closer look at specific respiratory classes and specific administration considerations, therapeutic effects, adverse/side effects, and teaching needed for each class of medications.

5.6 ANTIHISTAMINES

Diphenhydramine is an example of a first-generation antihistamine. (See Figures 5.7[22] and 5.8.[23]) Second-generation antihistamines were developed to have fewer side effects. An example of a second-generation antihistamine is cetirizine.

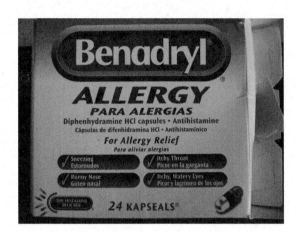

Figure 5.7 Diphenhydramine is a first-generation antihistamine that is available orally or as an IV medication

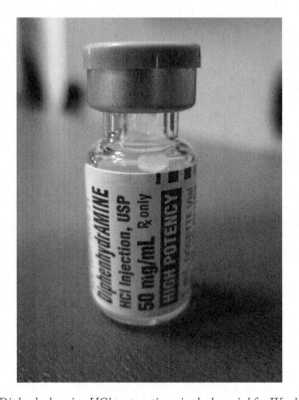

Figure 5.8 Diphenhydramine HCl preparation, single dose vial for IV administration

---

22 "Benadryl Allergy USA" by ZenBenjamin is licensed under CC BY-NC-SA 2.0.

23 "diphenhydramine (1)" by Intropin is licensed under CC BY-NC 2.0.

Mechanism of Action

Antihistamines have the following mechanisms of action: blocks histamine at H1 receptors; inhibits smooth muscle constriction in blood vessels and the respiratory and GI tracts; and decreases capillary permeability, salivation, and tear formation.

Indications for Use

Antihistamines are used for relief of allergy or cold symptoms.

Nursing Considerations Across the Life Span

This medication is not safe for children under the age of 2 years without a healthcare provider's order.

Adverse/Side Effects

First-generation medications can cause anticholinergic effects (such as dry mouth, urinary retention, constipation and blurred vision). CNS depression or CNS stimulation with excessive doses can occur, especially in children. Therefore, first-generation antihistamines should be used with caution in the elderly.

Second-generation medications may cause headache, nausea, vomiting, dysmenorrhea, and fatigue.

Patient Teaching and Education

Patients should be advised that antihistamines may cause drowsiness, and concurrent use of alcohol or other CNS depressants should be avoided. Patients should take only the recommended amount of medication and not to exceed dosing recommendations. Some patients may experience side effects such as dry mouth, and frequent oral hygiene may assist in alleviating discomfort.[24]

Now let's take a closer look at the medication grid for diphenhydramine and cetirizine in Table 5.6.[25, 26, 27, 28] Medication grids are intended to assist students to learn key points about each medication class. Basic information related to a common generic medication in this class is outlined, including administration considerations, therapeutic effects, and side effects/adverse effects. Prototype/generic medication listed in the medication grid is also hyperlinked to a free resource from the U.S. National Library of Medicine called *Daily Med*. Because information about medication is constantly changing, nurses should always consult evidence-based resources to review current recommendations before administering specific medication.

24   Frandsen, G. and Pennington, S. (2018). *Abrams' clinical drug: Rationales for nursing practice* (11th ed.). Wolters Kluwer.

25   uCentral from Unbound Medicine. https://www.unboundmedicine.com/ucentral.

26   This work is a derivative of *Pharmacology Notes: Nursing Implications for Clinical Practice* by Gloria Velarde licensed under CC BY-NC-SA 4.0.

27   Frandsen, G. and Pennington, S. (2018). *Abrams' clinical drug: Rationales for nursing practice* (11th ed.). Wolters Kluwer.

28   This work is a derivative of *Daily Med* by U.S. National Library of Medicine in the public domain.

Table 5.6: Diphenhydramine and Cetirizine Medication Grid

Class/ Subclass	Prototype/ Generic	Administration Considerations	Therapeutic Effects	Adverse/Side Effects
First-generation antihistamine	diphenhydramine	Take as directed Avoid allergens Avoid alcohol or CNS depressants due to sedation	Temporarily relieves symptoms due to hay fever or other upper respiratory allergies: runny nose; sneezing; itchy, watery eyes; itching of the nose or throat Temporarily relieves symptoms due to the common cold such as runny nose and sneezing	Sedation Anticholinergic effects Gastrointestinal: Nausea/ Vomiting Paradoxical effect: excitation in children
Second-generation antihistamine	cetirizine	Take as directed Avoid allergens Avoid alcohol or CNS depressants due to sedation	Temporarily relieves symptoms due to hay fever or other upper respiratory allergies: runny nose; sneezing; itchy, watery eyes; itching of the nose or throat	Non-sedating Anticholinergic effects Gastrointestinal: Nausea/ vomitting Paradoxical effect: excitation in children

5.7   DECONGESTANTS

Pseudoephedrine is an over-the-counter (OTC) decongestant (see Figure 5.9[29]). More details regarding pseudoephedrine are described in the "Autonomic Nervous System" chapter.

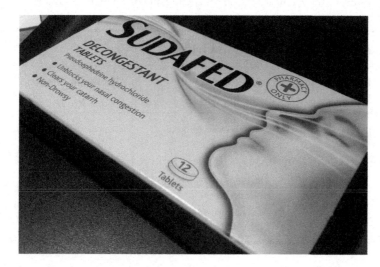

Figure 5.9 Pseudoephedrine (Sudafed) is a decongestant that is available OTC

Mechanism of Action

Pseudoephedrine acts directly on the adrenergic receptors and acts indirectly by releasing norepinephrine from its storage sites. The drug produces vasoconstriction, which shrinks nasal mucosa membranes.

Indications for Use

Decongestants relieve nasal obstruction due to inflammation.

Nursing Considerations Across the Life Span

This medication is not safe for children under the age of 4 years.

Adverse/Side Effects

Common adverse/side effects include hypertension, dysrhythmia, dizziness, headache, insomnia, and restlessness. Some patients may experience blurred vision, tinnitus, chest tightness, dry nose, and nasal congestion.

Decongestants are contraindicated in patients with severe hypertension, coronary artery disease (CAD), narrow-angle glaucoma, and some antidepressant use. Also, use with caution in patients who have cardiac dysrhythmias, hyperthyroidism, DM (diabetes mellitus), prostatic hypertrophy, and glaucoma.[30]

---

29   "Project 366 #165: 130612 Helping Hand?" by Pete is licensed under public domain.

30   Frandsen, G. and Pennington, S. (2018). *Abrams' clinical drug: Rationales for nursing practice* (11th ed.). Wolters Kluwer.

Patient Teaching and Education

Patients must take care to follow dosing recommendations. If dosing standards are surpassed, some patients may experience side effects such as increased nervousness, breathing difficulties, heart rate changes, and hallucinations.[31]

Now let's take a closer look at the medication grid on Pseudoephedrine in Table 5.7.[32, 33, 34]

Table 5.7: Pseudoephedrine Medication Grid				
Class/ Subclass	**Prototype/ Generic**	**Administration Considerations**	**Therapeutic Effects**	**Adverse/ Side Effects**
Decongestant	pseudoephedrine	Administration (drops, sprays) Avoid prolonged use > 7 days Use cautiously with cardiovascular disease Maintain hydration (2-3 liters/day)	Temporarily relieves nasal congestion due to the common cold, hay fever, or other upper respiratory allergies Temporarily relieves sinus congestion and pressure	Cardiovascular stimulation Rebound congestion with nasal route

31   uCentral from Unbound Medicine. https://www.unboundmedicine.com/ucentral.

32   This work is a derivative of *Pharmacology Notes: Nursing Implications for Clinical Practice* by Gloria Velarde is licensed under CC BY-NC-SA 4.0.

33   Frandsen, G. and Pennington, S. (2018). Abrams' clinical drug: Rationales for nursing practice (11th ed.). Wolters Kluwer.

34   This work is a derivative of *Daily Med* by U.S. National Library of Medicine in the public domain.

5.8   ANTITUSSIVES

Dextromethorphan is an example of an antitussive (see Figure 5.10[35]).

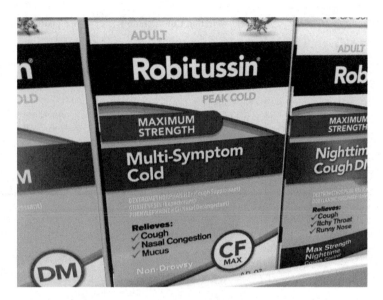

Figure 5.10 Robitussin DM is an OTC medication that contains dextromethorphan and guaifenesin

Mechanism of Action

Dextromethorphan suppresses a cough by depressing the cough center in the medulla oblongata or the cough receptors in the throat, trachea, or lungs, effectively elevating the threshold for coughing.

Indication for Use

Antitussives are used for a dry, hacking, nonproductive cough that interferes with rest and sleep.

Nursing Considerations Across the Life Span

This medication is not safe for children under the age of 4 years.

Adverse/Side Effects

The most common side effects include nausea and drowsiness. Some patients may experience a rash or difficulty breathing. High doses may cause hallucinations and disassociation, and the drug has been reported to be used as a recreational drug.[36]

Patient Teaching and Education: Patients should take care to avoid irritants that stimulate their cough. Additionally, antitussive medications can cause drowsiness, and patients should avoid taking them with other CNS depressants or alcohol.[37]

---

35   "Robitussin Cough Cold Flu Congestion decongestant Relief Medicine" by Mike Mozart is licensed under CC BY 2.0.

36   Frandsen, G. and Pennington, S. (2018). *Abrams' clinical drug: Rationales for nursing practice* (11th ed.). Wolters Kluwer.

37   uCentral from Unbound Medicine. https://www.unboundmedicine.com/ucentral.

Now let's take a closer look at the medication grid on dextromethorphan in Table 5.8.[38, 39, 40]

Table 5.8: Dextromethorphan Medication Grid

Class/ Subclass	Prototype/ Generic	Administration Considerations	Therapeutic Effects	Adverse/ Side Effects
Antitussive	dextromethorphan	Take as directed Administer undiluted No alcohol due to CNS depression Use with caution in patients with respiratory disease and with those taking monoamine oxidase inhibitors (MAOIs)	Temporarily relieves coughing due to minor throat and bronchial irritation as may occur with the common cold	CNS: sedation and dizziness Mild gastrointestinal effects

38   This work is a derivative of *Pharmacology Notes: Nursing Implications for Clinical Practice* by Gloria Velarde licensed under CC BY-NC-SA 4.0.

39   Frandsen, G. and Pennington, S. (2018). *Abrams' clinical drug: Rationales for nursing practice* (11th ed.). Wolters Kluwer.

40   This work is a derivative of *Daily Med* by U.S. National Library of Medicine in the public domain.

5.9   EXPECTORANTS

Guaifenesin is an example of an expectorant.

Mechanism of Action

Expectorants reduce the viscosity of tenacious secretions by irritating the gastric vagal receptors that stimulate respiratory tract fluid, thus increasing the volume but decreasing the viscosity of respiratory tract secretions.

Indication for Use

Expectorants are used for a productive cough and for loosening mucus from the respiratory tract.

Nursing Considerations Across the Life Span

The medication is safe for all ages. Guaifenesin is only recommended for use during pregnancy and breastfeeding when benefit outweighs the risk.

Adverse/Side Effects

Guaifenesin may cause a skin rash, headache, nausea, and vomiting.[41]

Patient Teaching and Education

Patients should take care to avoid irritants that stimulate their cough.

Additionally, the medication can cause drowsiness. Patients should avoid taking them with other CNS depressants or alcohol.[42]

---

41   Frandsen, G. and Pennington, S. (2018). *Abrams' clinical drug: Rationales for nursing practice* (11th ed.). Wolters Kluwer.

42   uCentral from Unbound Medicine. https://www.unboundmedicine.com/ucentral.

Now let's take a closer look at the medication grid for guaifenesin in Table 5.9.[43, 44, 45]

Table 5.9: Guaifenesin Medication Grid				
Class/ Subclass	**Prototype/ Generic**	**Administration Considerations**	**Therapeutic Effects**	**Adverse/ Side Effects**
Expectorant	guaifenesin	No eating or drinking for 30 minutes after syrup Encourage patient to cough and deep breath Stay hydrated (2-3 liters/day)	Helps loosen sputum (mucus) and thin bronchial secretions to make coughs more productive	Increased drowsiness in large doses Gastrointestinal: Nausea, vomiting, diarrhea

43   This work is a derivative of *Pharmacology Notes: Nursing Implications for Clinical Practice* by Gloria Velarde licensed under CC BY-NC-SA 4.0.

44   Frandsen, G. and Pennington, S. (2018). *Abrams' clinical drug: Rationales for nursing practice* (11th ed.). Wolters Kluwer.

45   This work is a derivative of *Daily Med* by U.S. National Library of Medicine in the public domain.

5.10 BETA-2 AGONIST

Albuterol is an example of a short-acting Beta-2 agonist. See Figures 5.11[46] and 5.12[47] for images of an albuterol inhaler and nebulizer.

Salmeterol is an example of a long-acting Beta-2 agonist.

See the "Autonomic Nervous System" chapter for more information regarding Beta-2 agonists.

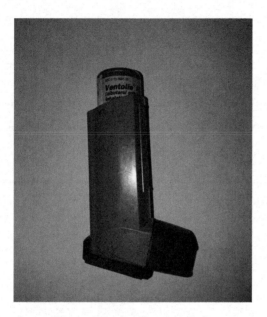

Figure 5.11 An albuterol inhaler

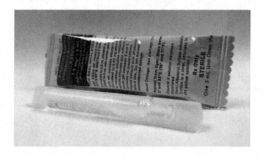

Figure 5.12 A vial of albuterol sulfate for inhalation

Mechanism of Action

Albuterol and salmeterol stimulate Beta 2-adrenergic receptors in the smooth muscle of bronchi and bronchioles producing bronchodilation. Beta-1 receptors can also be inadvertently stimulated, causing tachycardia.

---

46   "Ventolin® HFA (Albuterol Sulfate) Inhaler.jpg" by MisterNarwhal is licensed under CC BY SA 4.0.

47   "Albuterol 2.jpg" by Mark Oniffrey is licensed under CC BY SA 4.0.

Indications for Use

Short-acting albuterol is used to prevent or treat bronchospasms in people with asthma, reversible obstructive airway disease, or exercise-induced bronchospasm. Long-acting salmeterol is used to prevent bronchospasm.

Adverse/Side Effects

Beta-2 agonists can cause muscle tremor, excessive cardiac stimulation, and CNS stimulation.[48]

Patient Teaching and Education

Patients should be instructed to take medication as directed and report any sustained or worsening symptoms to their healthcare provider. When first using an inhaler, patients should be instructed to prime the inhaler unit prior to administering their medication. Use of medications like albuterol can cause an unusual taste in the mouth and rinsing the mouth with water after use is permitted. Patients should have an understanding of medication onset and use short-acting and long-acting inhalers appropriately.[49]

Now let's take a closer look at the medication grid for albuterol and salmeterol in Table 5.10.[50, 51, 52, 53, 54]

Table 5.10: Albuterol and Salmeterol Medication Grid

Class/ Subclass	Prototype/ Generic	Administration Consideration	Therapeutic Effects	Adverse/Side Effects
Short-acting Beta-2 agonist (SABA)	albuterol	Fast onset of action	Rapid bronchodilation	CNS stimulation (excitability) Cardiovascular stimulation (tachycardia)
Long-acting Beta-2 agonist (LABA)	salmeterol	Has a slow onset of action and will not abort an acute bronchospasm Increased risk of death with use during an "asthma attack" due to slow onset of action	Prevention of bronchospasm	Tachycardia, dysrhythmias, hypokalemia, hyperglycemia, paradoxical bronchoconstriction, and increased risk for asthma- related death

48   Frandsen, G. and Pennington, S. (2018). *Abrams' clinical drug: Rationales for nursing practice* (11th ed.). Wolters Kluwer.

49   uCentral from Unbound Medicine. https://www.unboundmedicine.com/ucentral.

50   This work is a derivative of *Pharmacology Notes: Nursing Implications for Clinical Practice* by Gloria Velarde licensed under CC BY-NC-SA 4.0.

51   This work is a derivative of *Daily Med* by U.S. National Library of Medicine in the public domain.

52   Frandsen, G. and Pennington, S. (2018). *Abrams' clinical drug: Rationales for nursing practice* (11th ed.). Wolters Kluwer.

53   This work is a derivative of *Daily Med* by U.S. National Library of Medicine in the public domain.

54   Adams, M., Holland, N., and Urban, C. (2020). *Pharmacology for nurses: A pathophysiologic approach* (6th ed.). pp. 622–63 and 626. Pearson.

5.11   ANTICHOLINERGICS

Ipratropium is an example of a short-acting anticholinergic. Tiotropium is an example of a long-acting anticholinergic. Additional information regarding anticholinergics can be found in the "Autonomic Nervous System" chapter. (See Figure 5.13[55] for an image of tiotropium.)

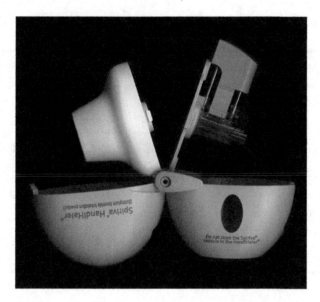

Figure 5.13 Tiotropium, a long-acting anticholinergic

Mechanism of Action

Anticholinergics block the action of acetylcholine in bronchial smooth muscle, which reduces bronchoconstrictive substance release.

Indications for Use

Anticholinergics are used for maintenance therapy of bronchoconstriction associated with asthma, chronic bronchitis, and emphysema.

Adverse/Side Effects

Anticholinergics should be used with caution with the elderly and can cause cough, drying of the nasal mucosa, nervousness, nausea, GI upset, headaches, and dizziness.[56]

---

55   "Spiriva HandiHaler"-brand dry powder inhaler (open).png" by RonEJ at English Wikipedia is licensed under CC0 1.0.

56   Frandsen, G. and Pennington, S. (2018). Abrams' clinical drug: Rationales for nursing practice (11th ed.). Wolters Kluwer.

Patient Teaching and Education

Patients should be instructed to use the inhaler as directed and be careful not to exceed dosage recommendations. They should receive education regarding the onset of medication and differences in usage for short- and long-acting anticholinergics. Some long-acting anticholinergics may cause signs of angioedema and the healthcare provider should be notified if this occurs.[57]

Now let's take a closer look at the medication grid for ipratropium and tiotropium in Table 5.11.[58, 59, 60, 61]

Table 5.11: Ipratropium and Tiotropium Medication Grid

Class/ Subclass	Prototype/ Generic	Administration Considerations	Therapeutic Effects	Adverse/ Side Effects
Anticholinergics (short acting)	ipratropium	Long-term management of pulmonary disease Slower onset of action	Rapid bronchodilation	Cough and drying of the nasal mucosa
Anticholinergics (long acting)	tiotropium	Long-term management of pulmonary disease Slower onset of action	Prevention of bronchospasm and reduces exacerbations in COPD patients	Cough and drying of the nasal mucosa

57   uCentral from Unbound Medicine. https://www.unboundmedicine.com/ucentral.

58   This work is a derivative of *Pharmacology Notes: Nursing Implications for Clinical Practice* by Gloria Velarde licensed under CC BY-NC-SA 4.0.

59   Frandsen, G. and Pennington, S. (2018). Abrams' clinical drug: Rationales for nursing practice (11th ed.). Wolters Kluwer.

60   This work is a derivative of *Daily Med* by U.S. National Library of Medicine in the public domain.

61   Adams, M., Holland, N., and Urban, C. (2020). *Pharmacology for nurses: A pathophysiologic approach* (6th ed.). pp. 622–63 and 626. Pearson.

5.12 CORTICOSTERIODS

Corticosteroids can be prescribed in a variety of routes. Fluticasone is an example of a commonly used inhaled corticosteroid; prednisone is an example of a commonly used oral corticosteroid; and methylprednisolone is a commonly used IV corticosteroid. Additional information about corticosteroids and potential adrenal effects is located in the "Endocrine" chapter.

Mechanism of Action

Fluticasone is a locally acting anti-inflammatory and immune modifier. The nasal spray is used for allergies, and the oral inhaler is used for long-term control of asthma. Fluticasone is also used in a combination product with salmeterol. It decreases the frequency and severity of asthma attacks and improves overall asthma symptoms. See Figures 5.14-16[62, 63, 64] for images of different formulations of fluticasone.

Oral prednisone prevents the release of substances in the body that cause inflammation. It also suppresses the immune system.

Methylprednisolone IV prevents the release of substances in the body that cause inflammation. It also suppresses the immune system. Methylprednisolone requires reconstitution before administration. See Figure 5.17[65] for an image of methylprednisolone.

Indications for Use

Fluticasone inhalers are used to prevent asthma attacks. In respiratory conditions, oral prednisone is used to control severe or incapacitating allergic conditions that are unresponsive to adequate trials of conventional treatment for seasonal or perennial allergic rhinitis, bronchial asthma, contact dermatitis, atopic dermatitis, serum sickness, and drug hypersensitivity reactions. Methylprednisolone IV is used to rapidly control these same conditions.

Nursing Considerations Across the Life Span

Fluticasone is safe for 4 years and older. Prednisone and methylprednisolone are safe for all ages.

Adverse/Side Effects

Fluticasone can cause hoarseness, dry mouth, cough, sore throat, and oropharyngeal candidiasis. Patients should rinse their mouths after use to prevent candidiasis (thrush).

Prednisone and methylprednisolone: See more information about adverse effects of corticosteroids in the "Endocrine" chapter. Cardiovascular symptoms can include fluid retention, edema, and hypertension. Imbalances such as hypernatremia ($\uparrow$Na), hypokalemia ($\downarrow$K+), and increased blood glucose with associated weight gain can occur. CNS symptoms include mood swings and euphoria. GI symptoms can include nausea, vomiting, and GI bleed. In long- term therapy, bone resorption occurs, which increases the risk for fractures; the skin may bruise

---

62   "Fluticasone Propionate Nasal Spray" by _BuBBy_ is licensed under CC BY 2.0.

63   "Fluticasone.JPG" by James Heilman, MD is licensed under CC BY-SA 4.0.

64   "Asthmatic Control" by David Camerer is licensed under CC BY-NC-ND 2.0.

65   "Methylprednisolone vial.jpg" by Intropin is licenced under CC BY 3.0.

easily and become paper thin; wound healing is delayed; infections can be masked; and the risk for infection increases. Long-term corticosteroid therapy should never be stopped abruptly because adrenal insufficiency may occur.[66]

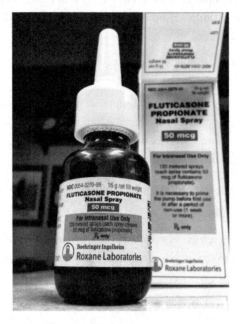

Figure 5.14 Fluticasone nasal spray formulation

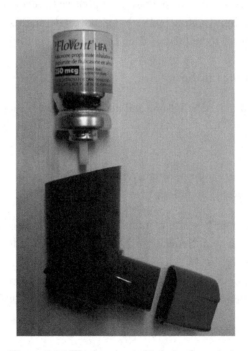

Figure 5.15 Fluticasone oral inhaler formulation

66   Frandsen, G. and Pennington, S. (2018). *Abrams' clinical drug: Rationales for nursing practice* (11th ed.). Wolters Kluwer.

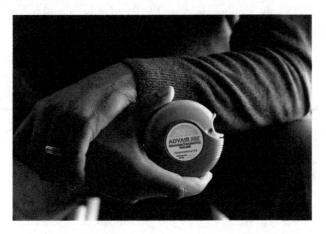

Figure 5.16 Fluticasone combination formulation

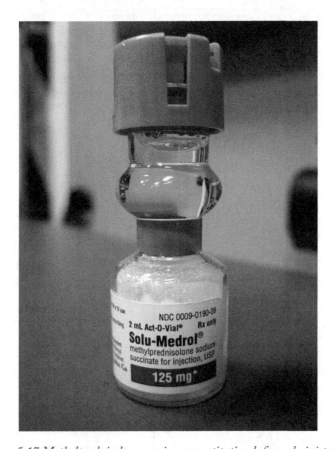

Figure 5.17 Methylprednisolone requires reconstitution before administration

Patient Teaching and Education

Patients should be advised that corticosteroids are not used to treat an acute asthma attack. They can cause immunosuppression and suppress signs of infection. Corticosteroids can also cause an increase in blood glucose levels.

Patients may experience weight gain, swelling, increased fatigue, bruising, and behavioral changes. These occurrences should be reported to one's healthcare provider.[67]

Now let's take a closer look at the medication grid for fluticasone, prednisone, and methylprednisolone in Table 5.12.[68, 69, 70]

Table 5.12: Fluticasone, Prednisone, and Methylprednisolone Medication Grid

Class/ Subclass	Prototype/ Generic	Administration Considerations	Therapeutic Effects	Adverse/Side Effects
Corticosteroids	fluticasone	Rinse mouth after use Do not use as a "rescue" medication	Nasal spray: Used for management of the nasal symptoms of perennial nonallergic rhinitis Inhaler: Used to improve the control of asthma by reducing inflammation in the airways	Hoarseness, dry mouth, cough, sore throat, and oropharyngeal candidiasis
Corticosteroids	prednisone	Do not use if signs of a systemic infection When using more than 10 days, the dose must be slowly tapered May increase blood glucose levels	Used to control severe or incapacitating allergic or respiratory conditions	CV: fluid retention, edema, and hypertension Electrolytes: ↑Na, ↓K+, ↑Ca, ↑BG CNS: mood swings and euphoria in high doses GI: Nausea/Vomiting, GI bleed MS: bone resorption Skin: acne, paper thin, bruises, infections, and delayed healing Weight gain Adrenal suppression Increased risk for infection and infections can be masked Long-term use may result in Cushing's syndrome
Corticosteroids	methylpred-nisolone	May increase blood glucose levels	Used to rapidly control severe or incapacitating allergic or respiratory conditions, in sepsis to reduce systemic inflammation, and to treat adrenal insufficiency	Same as prednisone

67   uCentral from Unbound Medicine. https://www.unboundmedicine.com/ucentral.

68   This work is a derivative of *Pharmacology Notes: Nursing Implications for Clinical Practice* by Gloria Velarde licensed under CC BY-NC-SA 4.0.

69   Frandsen, G. and Pennington, S. (2018). *Abrams' clinical drug: Rationales for nursing practice* (11th ed.). Wolters Kluwer.

70   This work is a derivative of *Daily Med* by U.S. National Library of Medicine in the public domain.

5.13 LEUKOTRIENE RECEPTOR ANTAGONISTS

Montelukast is a leukotriene antagonist medication with a distinctly shaped tablet. See Figure 5.18.[71]

Mechanism of Action

Montelukast blocks leukotriene receptors and decreases inflammation.

Indications for Use

Montelukast is used for the long-term control of asthma and for decreasing the frequency of asthma attacks. It is also indicated for exercise-induced bronchospasm and allergic rhinitis.

Nursing Considerations Across the Life Span

The medication is safe for children 12 months and older. It is available in granule packets and chewable tablets, as well as regular tablets.

Adverse/Side Effects

Montelukast can cause headache, cough, nasal congestion, nausea, and hepatotoxicity.[72]

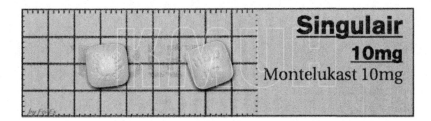

Figure 5.18 Montelukast Tablets

Patient Teaching and Education

Patients should be instructed to take medications at the same time each day and at least two hours prior to exercise. They should not discontinue medications without notifying the healthcare provider.[73]

Now let's take a closer look at the medication grid on montelukast in Table 5.13.[74, 75, 76, 77]

---

71   "Singulair 10mg" by FedEx is licenced under CC BY-NC-ND 2.0.

72   Frandsen, G. and Pennington, S. (2018). *Abrams' clinical drug: Rationales for nursing practice* (11th ed.). Wolters Kluwer.

73   uCentral from Unbound Medicine. https://www.unboundmedicine.com/ucentral.

74   This work is a derivative of *Pharmacology Notes: Nursing Implications for Clinical Practice* by Gloria Velarde licensed under CC BY-NC-SA 4.0.

75   Frandsen, G. and Pennington, S. (2018). *Abrams' clinical drug: Rationales for nursing practice* (11th ed.). Wolters Kluwer.

76   This work is a derivative of *Daily Med* by U.S. National Library of Medicine in the public domain.

77   Adams, M., Holland, N., and Urban, C. (2020). *Pharmacology for nurses: A pathophysiologic* approach (6th ed.). pp. 622–63 and 626. Pearson.

Table 5.13: Montelukast Medication Grid

Class/ Subclass	Prototype/ Generic	Administration Considerations	Therapeutic Effects	Adverse/ Side Effects
Leukotriene inhibitor	montelukast	Use as directed; not to be used as "rescue" medication Typically 3-7 days to reach effectiveness	Prevention and treatment of asthma and exercise-induced bronchoconstriction	Headache Cough Nasal congestion Nausea Hepatotoxicity

5.14 XANTHINE DERIVATIVES

Theophylline is a xanthine derivative.

Mechanism of Action

Theophylline relaxes bronchial smooth muscle by inhibition of the enzyme phosphodiesterase and suppresses airway responsiveness to stimuli that cause bronchoconstriction.

Indications for Use

Theophylline is used for the long-term management of persistent asthma that is unresponsive to beta agonists or inhaled corticosteroids.

Adverse/Side Effects

Theophylline can cause nausea, vomiting, CNS stimulation, nervousness, and insomnia.[78]

Patient Teaching and Education

Patients should be sure to take medications as prescribed at appropriate intervals. They should avoid irritants and drink fluids to help thin secretions. Patients will need serum blood levels tested every six to twelve months.[79]

Now let's take a closer look at the medication grid on theophylline in Table 5.14.[80, 81, 82]

Table 5.14: Theophylline Medication Grid				
Class/ Subclass	Prototype/ Generic	Administration Considerations	Therapeutic Effects	Adverse/ Side Effects
Xanthine	theophylline	Avoid caffeine Requires evaluation of therapeutic blood level to prevent toxicity	Long-term treatment of chronic asthma and COPD unresponsive to other treatment	GI: Nausea, vomiting CNS stimulation Nervousness and insomnia

78   Frandsen, G. and Pennington, S. (2018). *Abrams' clinical drug: Rationales for nursing practice* (11th ed.). Wolters Kluwer.

79   uCentral from Unbound Medicine. https://www.unboundmedicine.com/ucentral.

80   This work is a derivative of *Pharmacology Notes: Nursing Implications for Clinical Practice* by Gloria Velarde licensed under CC BY-NC-SA 4.0.

81   Frandsen, G. and Pennington, S. (2018). *Abrams' clinical drug: Rationales for nursing practice* (11th ed.). Wolters Kluwer.

82   This work is a derivative of *Daily Med* by U.S. National Library of Medicine in the public domain.

5.15 MODULE LEARNING ACTIVITIES

Light Bulb Moment

Let's apply what you have learned in the respiratory unit.

Asthma Scenario

An adult patient presents to the emergency department with complaints of shortness of breath and increased work of breathing. The patient is alert and oriented times 3, skin is pink, warm and dry, BP 148/88, T 98, P92, R 24, pulse oximetry 91% on room air.

Assessment of the lung reveals expiratory wheezing throughout the lung fields. The patient has a past medical history of asthma, hypertension, and diabetes.

1. The nurse anticipates which of the following medications will be initially administered to the patient?

   a. Theophylline

   b. Montelukast

   c. Albuterol

   d. Salmeterol

2. List the steps the nurse should take to safely administer the medication.

3. What assessments should the nurse plan to complete after administering the medication?

4. The nurse plans on teaching the patient about using the albuterol inhaler at home. What information should be included?

5. What is the best method for the nurse to use to ensure that the patient is correctly using an inhaler?

Allergy Scenario

A pediatric patient presents to the emergency department with complaints of shortness of breath, increased work of breathing, and a cough. The patient is alert and oriented times 3, skin is pink, warm and dry, BP 112/68, T 99, P106, R 32, pulse oximetry 90% on room air. Assessment of the lung sounds reveals diminished lung sounds throughout all lung fields. The patient has a past medical history of peanut allergy. The mother tells you that they were at a birthday party and after consumption of a cupcake, the symptoms started.

1. The nurse anticipates that which of the following medications will be likely ordered for this patient?

   a. Diphenhydramine

   b. Epinephrine

   c. Cetirizine

   d. Guaifenesin

Note: Answers to the Light Bulb Moment can be found in the "Answer Key" sections at the end of the book.

Interactive Activities

 An interactive or media element has been excluded from this version of the text. You can view it online here: https://wtcs.pressbooks.pub/pharmacology/?p=1551

GLOSSARY

Allergies: Allergies occur when the immune system reacts to a foreign substance and makes antibodies that identify a particular allergen as harmful, even though it isn't.

Anaphylaxis: A severe, potentially life-threatening allergic reaction. It can occur within seconds or minutes of exposure to something you're allergic to, such as peanuts or bee stings.

Cyanotic: A bluish or purplish discoloration (as of skin) due to deficient oxygenation of the blood.

Gas Exchange: The process at the alveoli level where blood is oxygenated and carbon dioxide, the waste product of cellular respiration, is removed from the body.

Pallor: A deficiency of color especially of the face; paleness.

Paradoxical Effect: An effect that is opposite to what is expected.

Respiratory Rate: The total number of breaths, or respiratory cycles, that occur each minute. A child under 1 year of age has a normal respiratory rate between 30 and 60 breaths per minute, but by the time a child is about 10 years old, the normal rate is closer to 18 to 30. By adolescence, the normal respiratory rate is similar to that of adults, 12 to 18 breaths per minute.

Sputum: Matter expectorated from the respiratory system and especially the lungs that is composed of mucus but may contain pus, blood, fibrin, or microorganisms (such as bacteria) in diseased states.

Chapter VI

Cardiovascular & Renal System

6.1   CARDIOVASCULAR AND RENAL SYSTEM INTRODUCTION

Learning Objectives

- Cite the classifications and actions of cardiovascular drugs
- Cite the classifications and actions of renal system drugs
- Give examples of when, how, and to whom cardiovascular system drugs may be administered
- Give examples of when, how, and to whom renal system drugs may be administered
- Identify the side effects and special considerations associated with cardiovascular and renal system drug therapy
- Identify considerations and implications of using cardiovascular system medications across the life span
- Identify considerations and implications of using renal system medications across the life span
- Apply evidence-based concepts when using the nursing process
- Identify and interpret related laboratory tests

The heart is the powerhouse of the body, providing oxygenated blood to organs so that they can conduct the vital processes needed to keep the body functioning. Without a properly functioning heart to ensure blood flow, cells are in jeopardy of oxygenation starvation, impairment, and subsequent death.

Did you know that the average adult human heart contracts approximately 108,000 times in one day, more than 39 million times in one year, and nearly 3 billion times during a 75-year life span? Each heartbeat ejects approximately 70 mL blood, resulting in 5.25 liters of fluid per minute and approximately 14,000 liters per day. Over one year, that means over 2.6 million gallons of blood are sent through roughly 60,000 miles of vessels in the adult body[1]. It is no wonder that the heart is the most important muscle of the body! This chapter will review important concepts and disorders related to the heart and cardiovascular system before discussing common medication classes. It is vital for nurses to understand how these cardiovascular medications work to provide safe, effective care to the patients who take them.

---

1   This work is a derivative of *Anatomy and Physiology* by OpenStax licensed under CC BY 4.0. Access for free at https://openstax.org/books/anatomy-and-physiology/pages/1-introduction.

OPEN RN
OPEN RESOURCES FOR NURSING

My Notes

6.2   REVIEW OF BASIC CONCEPTS

To understand the effects of various cardiovascular medications, it is important to first understand the basic anatomy and physiology of the cardiovascular and renal system.

Location of the Heart

The human heart is located within the thoracic cavity, medially between the lungs in the space known as the mediastinum. The great veins, the superior and inferior venae cavae, and the great arteries, the aorta and pulmonary trunk, are attached to the superior surface of the heart, called the base. The base of the heart is located at the level of the third costal cartilage, as seen in Figure 6.1.[2] The inferior tip of the heart, the apex, lies just to the left of the sternum between the junction of the fourth and fifth ribs. It is important to remember the position of the heart when placing a stethoscope on the chest of a patient and listening for heart sounds.[3]

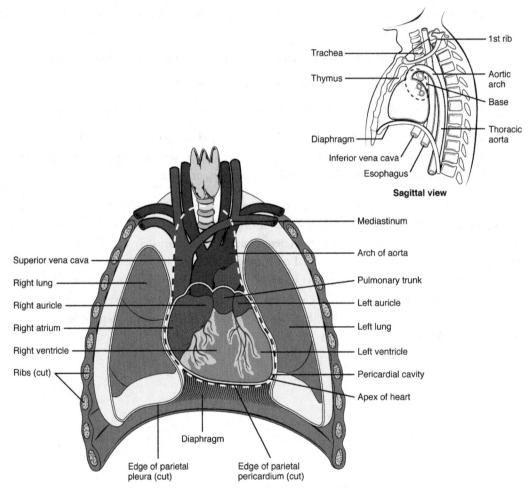

Figure 6.1 Position of the heart in the thoracic cavity

---

2   "Position of the Heart in the Thorax" by OpenStax College is licensed under CC BY 4.0. Access for free at https://openstax.org/books/anatomy-and-physiology/pages/19-1-heart-anatomy.

3   This work is a derivative of *Anatomy and Physiology* by OpenStax licensed under CC BY 4.0. Access for free at https://openstax.org/books/anatomy-and-physiology/pages/1-introduction.

Chambers and Circulation Through the Heart

The heart consists of four chambers: two atria and two ventricles. The right atrium receives deoxygenated blood from the systemic circulation, and the left atrium receives oxygenated blood from the lungs. The atria contract to push blood into the lower chambers, the right ventricle and the left ventricle. The right ventricle contracts to push blood into the lungs, and the left ventricle is the primary pump that propels blood to the rest of the body.

There are two distinct but linked circuits in the human circulation called the pulmonary and systemic circuits. The pulmonary circuit transports blood to and from the lungs, where it picks up oxygen and delivers carbon dioxide for exhalation. The systemic circuit transports oxygenated blood to virtually all of the tissues of the body and returns deoxygenated blood and carbon dioxide to the heart to be sent back to the pulmonary circulation. See Figure 6.2[4] for an illustration of blood flow through the heart and blood circulation throughout the body.[5]

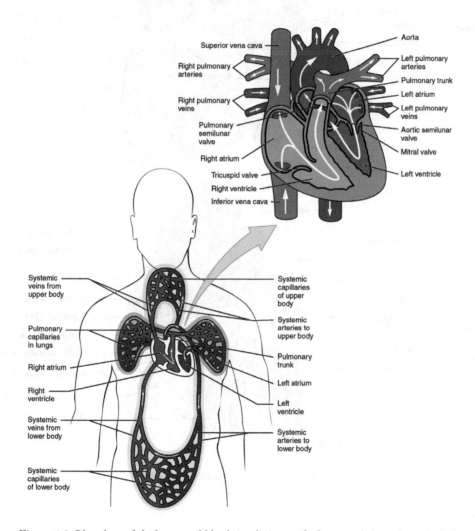

Figure 6.2 Chambers of the heart and blood circulation to the lungs and throughout the body

---

4   "Dual System of the Human Blood Circulation" by OpenStax College is licensed under CC By 4.0. Access for free at https://openstax.org/books/anatomy-and-physiology/pages/19-1-heart-anatomy.

5   This work is a derivative of *Anatomy and Physiology* by OpenStax licensed under CC BY 4.0. Access for free at https://openstax.org/books/anatomy-and-physiology/pages/1-introduction.

My Notes

Blood also circulates through the coronary arteries with each beat of the heart. The left coronary artery distributes blood to the left side of the heart, and the right coronary distributes blood to the right atrium, portions of both ventricles, and the heart conduction system. See Figure 6.3[6] for an illustration of the coronary arteries. When a patient has a myocardial infarction, a blood clot lodges in one of these coronary arteries that perfuse the heart tissue. If a significant area of muscle tissue dies from lack of perfusion, the heart is no longer able to pump.

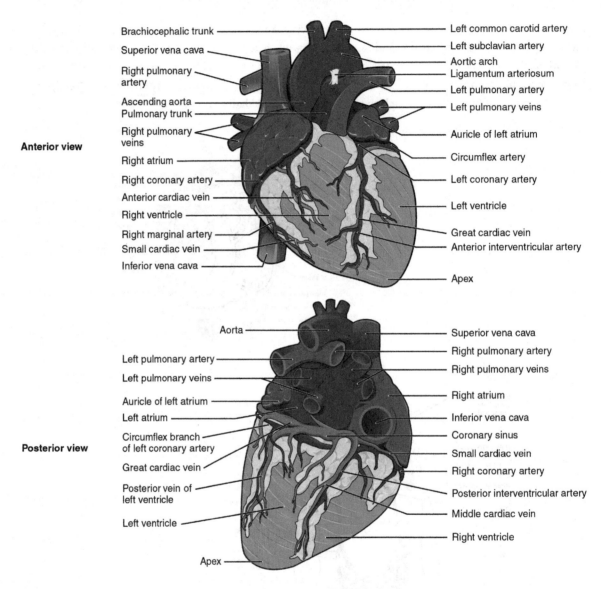

Figure 6.3 Coronary arteries of the heart

Conduction System of the Heart

Contractions of the heart are stimulated by the electrical conduction system. The components of the cardiac conduction system include the sinoatrial (SA) node, the atrioventricular (AV) node, the left and right bundle branches, and the Purkinje fibers. (See Figure 6.4 for an image of the conduction system of the heart.[7])

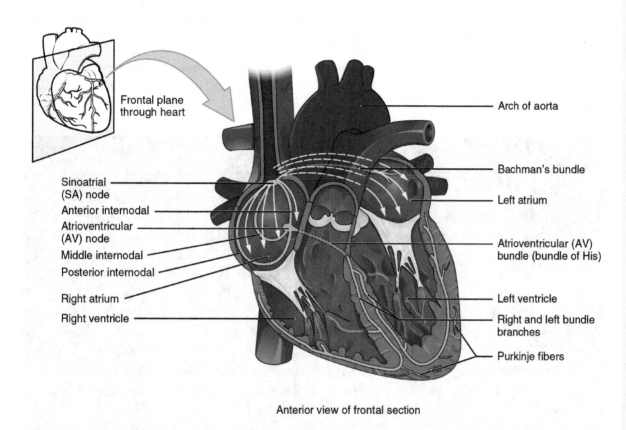

Figure 6.4 Components of the cardiac conduction system

Normal cardiac rhythm is established by the **sinoatrial (SA) node**. The SA node has the highest rate of depolarization and is known as the pacemaker of the heart. It initiates the **sinus rhythm** or normal electrical pattern followed by contraction of the heart. The SA node initiates the action potential, which sweeps across the atria through the AV node to the bundle branches and Purkinje fibers, and then spreads to the contractile fibers of the ventricle to stimulate the contraction of the ventricle.[8]

Cardiac Conductive Cells

Sodium (Na), potassium (K) and calcium (Ca2) ions play critical roles in cardiac conducting cells in the conduction system of the heart. Unlike skeletal muscles and neurons, cardiac conductive cells do not have a stable resting potential. Conductive cells contain a series of sodium ion channels that allow influx of sodium ions that cause

---

7 "2018 Conduction System of the Heart" by OpenStax College is licensed under CC BY 4.0 Access it for free at https://openstax.org/books/anatomy-and-physiology/pages/19-2-cardiac-muscle-and-electrical-activity.

8 This work is a derivative of *Anatomy and Physiology* by OpenStax licensed under CC BY 4.0. Access for free at https://openstax.org/books/anatomy-and-physiology/pages/1-introduction.

the membrane potential to rise slowly and eventually cause spontaneous depolarization. At this point, calcium ion channels open and Ca2 enters the cell, further depolarizing it. As the calcium ion channels then close, the K channels open, resulting in repolarization. When the membrane potential reaches approximately –60 mV, the K channels close and Na channels open, and the prepotential phase begins again. This phenomenon explains the autorhythmicity properties of cardiac muscle. Calcium ions play two critical roles in the physiology of cardiac muscle. In addition to depolarization, calcium ions also cause myosin to form cross bridges with the muscle cells that then provide the power stroke of contraction. Medications called calcium channel blockers thus affect both the conduction and contraction roles of calcium in the heart.

The autorhythmicity inherent in cardiac cells keeps the heart beating at a regular pace. However, the heart is regulated by other neural and endocrine controls, and it is sensitive to other factors, including electrolytes. These factors are further discussed in the homeostatic section below.[9]

Focus on Clinical Practice: The ECG

Surface electrodes placed on specific anatomical sites on the body can record the heart's electrical signals. This tracing of the electrical signal is called an electrocardiogram (ECG), also historically abbreviated EKG. Careful analysis of the ECG reveals a detailed picture of both normal and abnormal heart function and is an indispensable clinical diagnostic tool. A normal ECG tracing is presented in Figure 6.5.[10] Each component, segment, and the interval is labeled and corresponds to important electrical events.

There are five prominent components of the ECG: the P wave, the Q, R, and S components, and the T wave. The small P wave represents the depolarization of the atria. The large QRS complex represents the depolarization of the ventricles, which requires a much stronger impulse because of the larger size of the ventricular cardiac muscle. The ventricles begin to contract as the QRS reaches the peak of the R wave. Lastly, the T wave represents the repolarization of the ventricle. Several cardiac disorders can cause abnormal ECG readings called "dysrhythmias," also called "arrhythmias," and there are several types of antidysrhythmic medications used to treat these disorders that will be discussed later in this chapter.[11]

9   This work is a derivative of *Anatomy and Physiology* by OpenStax licensed under CC BY 4.0. Access for free at https://openstax.org/books/anatomy-and-physiology/pages/1-introduction.

10   "Electrocardiogram Depolarization.jpg" by OpenStax College is licensed under CC BY 4.0 Access for free at https://openstax.org/books/anatomy-and-physiology/pages/19-2-cardiac-muscle-and-electrical-activity.

11   This work is a derivative of *Anatomy and Physiology* by OpenStax licensed under CC BY 4.0. Access for free at https://openstax.org/books/anatomy-and-physiology/pages/1-introduction.

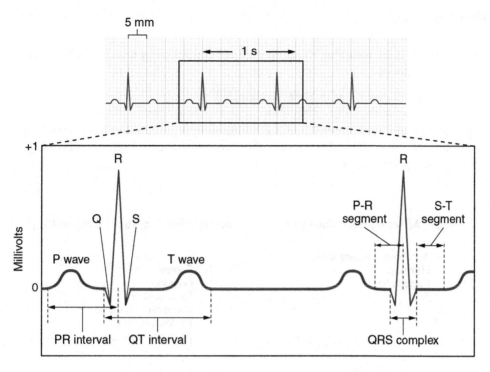

Figure 6.5 Components of an ECG reading

Cardiac Cycle

The period of time that begins with contraction of the atria and ends with ventricular relaxation is known as the cardiac cycle. The period of contraction that the heart undergoes while it pumps blood into circulation is called **systole**. The period of relaxation that occurs as the chambers fill with blood is called **diastole**.

Phases of the Cardiac Cycle

At the beginning of the cardiac cycle, both the atria and ventricles are relaxed (diastole). Blood is flowing into the right atrium from the superior and inferior venae cavae and into the left atrium from the four pulmonary veins. Contraction of the atria follows depolarization, which is represented by the P wave of the ECG. Just prior to atrial contraction, the ventricles contain approximately 130 mL blood in a resting adult. This volume is known as the end diastolic volume or **preload**. As the atrial muscles contract, pressure rises within the atria and blood is pumped into the ventricles.

Ventricular systole follows the depolarization of the ventricles and is represented by the QRS complex in the ECG. During the ventricular ejection phase, the contraction of the ventricular muscle causes blood to be pumped out of the heart. This quantity of blood is referred to as **stroke volume (SV)**. Ventricular relaxation, or diastole, follows repolarization of the ventricles and is represented by the T wave of the ECG.[12]

---

12   This work is a derivative of *Anatomy and Physiology* by OpenStax licensed under CC BY 4.0. Access for free at https:// openstax.org/books/anatomy-and-physiology/pages/1-introduction.

My Notes

Cardiac Output

Cardiac output (CO) is a measurement of the amount of blood pumped by each ventricle in one minute. To calculate this value, multiply stroke volume (SV), the amount of blood pumped by each ventricle, by the heart rate (HR) in beats per minute. It can be represented mathematically by the following equation: CO = HR × SV. Factors influencing CO are summarized in Figure 6.6[13] and include autonomic innervation by the sympathetic and parasympathetic nervous system, hormones such as epinephrine, preload, contractility, and afterload. Each of these factors is further discussed below.[14] SV is also used to calculate ejection fraction, which is the portion of the blood that is pumped or ejected from the heart with each contraction.

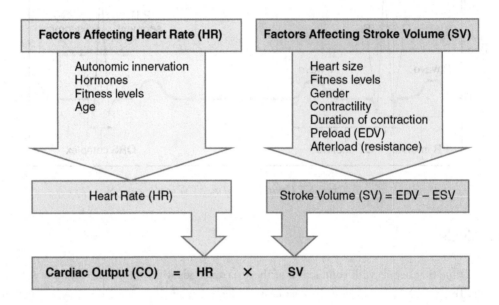

Figure 6.6 Factors affecting cardiac output

Heart Rate

Heart rate (HR) can vary considerably, not only with exercise and fitness levels, but also with age. Newborn resting HRs may be 120 -160 bpm. HR gradually decreases until young adulthood and then gradually increases again with age. For an adult, normal resting HR will be in the range of 60–100 bpm. Bradycardia is the condition in which resting rate drops below 60 bpm, and tachycardia is the condition in which the resting rate is above 100 bpm.

Correlation Between Heart Rates and Cardiac Output

Conditions that cause increased HR also trigger an initial increase in SV. However, as the HR rises, there is less time spent in diastole and, consequently, less time for the ventricles to fill with blood. As HR continues to increase,

---

13 "2031 Factors in Cardiac Output.jpg" by OpenStax College is licensed under CC BY 4.0 Access for free at https://openstax.org/books/anatomy-and-physiology/pages/19-4-cardiac-physiology.

14 This work is a derivative of *Anatomy and Physiology* by OpenStax licensed under CC BY 4.0. Access for free at https://openstax.org/books/anatomy-and-physiology/pages/1-introduction.

SV gradually decreases due to less filling time. In this manner, tachycardia will eventually cause decreased cardiac output.

Cardiovascular Centers

Sympathetic stimulation increases the heart rate and contractility, whereas parasympathetic stimulation decreases the heart rate. (See Figure 6.7 for an illustration of the ANS stimulation of the heart.[15]) Sympathetic stimulation causes the release of the neurotransmitter norepinephrine (NE), which shortens the repolarization period, thus speeding the rate of depolarization and contraction and increasing the HR. It also opens sodium and calcium ion channels, allowing an influx of positively charged ions.

NE binds to the Beta-1 receptor. Some cardiac medications (for example, beta blockers) work by blocking these receptors, thereby slowing HR and lowering blood pressure. However, an overdose of beta blockers can lead to bradycardia and even stop the heart.[16]

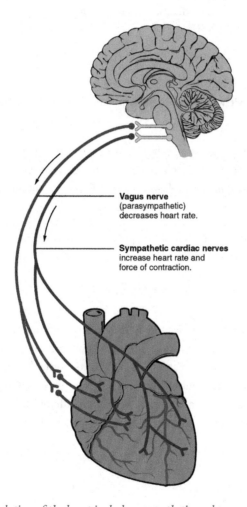

Vagus nerve
(parasympathetic)
decreases heart rate.

Sympathetic cardiac nerves
increase heart rate and
force of contraction.

Figure 6.7 ANS stimulation of the heart includes sympathetic and parasympathetic stimulation

---

15   "2032 Automatic Innervation.jpg" by OpenStax College is licensed under CC BY 4.0 Access for free at https://openstax.org/books/anatomy-and-physiology/pages/19-4-cardiac-physiology.

16   This work is a derivative of *Anatomy and Physiology* by OpenStax licensed under CC BY 4.0. Access for free at https://openstax.org/books/anatomy-and-physiology/pages/1-introduction.

Stroke Volume

Many of the same factors that regulate HR also impact cardiac function by altering SV. Three primary factors that affect stroke volume are preload, or the stretch on the ventricles prior to contraction; **contractility**, or the force or strength of the contraction itself; and **afterload**, the force the ventricles must generate to pump blood against the resistance in the vessels. Many cardiovascular medications affect cardiac output by affecting preload, contractility, or afterload.[17]

Preload

Preload is another way of expressing end diastolic volume (EDV). Therefore, the greater the EDV is, the greater the preload is. One of the primary factors to consider is filling time, the duration of ventricular diastole during which filling occurs. Any sympathetic stimulation to the venous system will also increase venous return to the heart, which contributes to ventricular filling and preload. Medications such as diuretics decrease preload by causing the kidneys to excrete more water, thus decreasing blood volume.

Contractility

Contractility refers to the force of the contraction of the heart muscle, which controls SV. Factors that increase contractility are described as **positive inotropic factors,** and those that decrease contractility are described as **negative inotropic factors**.

Not surprisingly, sympathetic stimulation is a positive inotrope, whereas parasympathetic stimulation is a negative inotrope. The drug digoxin is used to lower HR and increase the strength of the contraction. It works by inhibiting the activity of an enzyme (ATPase) that controls movement of calcium, sodium, and potassium into heart muscle. Inhibiting ATPase increases calcium in heart muscle and, therefore, increases the force of heart contractions.

Negative inotropic agents include hypoxia, acidosis, hyperkalemia, and a variety of medications such as beta blockers and calcium channel blockers.

Afterload

Afterload refers to the force that the ventricles must develop to pump blood effectively against the resistance in the vascular system. Any condition that increases resistance requires a greater afterload to force open the semilunar valves and pump the blood, which decreases cardiac output. On the other hand, any decrease in resistance reduces the afterload and thus increases cardiac output. Figure 6.8[18] summarizes the major factors influencing cardiac output. Calcium channel blockers such as amlodipine, verapamil, nifedipine, and diltiazem can be used to reduce afterload and thus increase cardiac output.[19]

---

17 This work is a derivative of *Anatomy and Physiology* by OpenStax licensed under CC BY 4.0. Access for free at https://openstax.org/books/anatomy-and-physiology/pages/1-introduction.

18 "2036 Summary of Factors in Cardiac Output.jpg" by OpenStax College is licensed under CC BY 4.0 Access for free at https://openstax.org/books/anatomy-and-physiology/pages/19-4-cardiac-physiology.

19 This work is a derivative of *Anatomy and Physiology* by OpenStax licensed under CC BY 4.0. Access for free at https://openstax.org/books/anatomy-and-physiology/pages/1-introduction.

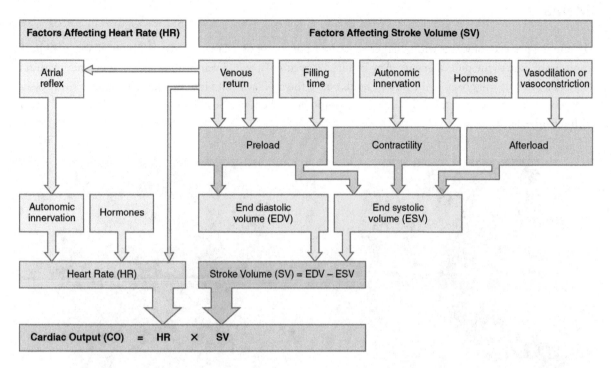

Figure 6.8 Factors affecting cardiac output

Systemic Circulation: Blood Vessels

After blood is pumped out of the ventricles, it is carried through the body via blood vessels. An **artery** is a blood vessel that carries blood away from the heart, where it branches into ever-smaller vessels and eventually into tiny **capillaries** where nutrients and wastes are exchanged at the cellular level. Capillaries then combine with other small blood vessels that carry blood to a **vein**, a larger blood vessel that returns blood to the heart. Compared to arteries, veins are thin-walled, low-pressure vessels. Larger veins are also equipped with valves that promote the unidirectional flow of blood toward the heart and prevent backflow caused by the inherent low blood pressure in veins as well as the pull of gravity.

In addition to their primary function of returning blood to the heart, veins may be considered blood reservoirs because systemic veins contain approximately 64 percent of the blood volume at any given time. Approximately 21 percent of the venous blood is located in venous networks within the liver, bone marrow, and integument. This volume of blood is referred to as **venous reserve**. Through venoconstriction, this reserve volume of blood can get back to the heart more quickly for redistribution to other parts of the circulation.

Nitroglycerin is an example of a medication that causes arterial and venous vasodilation. It is used for patients with angina to decrease cardiac workload and increase the amount of oxygen available to the heart. By causing vasodilation of the veins, nitroglycerin decreases the amount of blood returned to the heart, and thus decreases preload. It also reduces afterload by causing vasodilation of the arteries and reducing peripheral vascular resistance.[20]

---

20   This work is a derivative of *Anatomy and Physiology* by OpenStax licensed under CC BY 4.0. Access for free at https://openstax.org/books/anatomy-and-physiology/pages/1-introduction.

Edema

Despite the presence of valves within larger veins, over the course of a day, some blood will inevitably pool in the lower limbs, due to the pull of gravity. Any blood that accumulates in a vein will increase the pressure within it. Increased pressure will promote the flow of fluids out of the capillaries and into the interstitial fluid. The presence of excess tissue fluid around the cells leads to a condition called **edema**. See Figure 6.9[21] for an image of a patient with pitting edema.

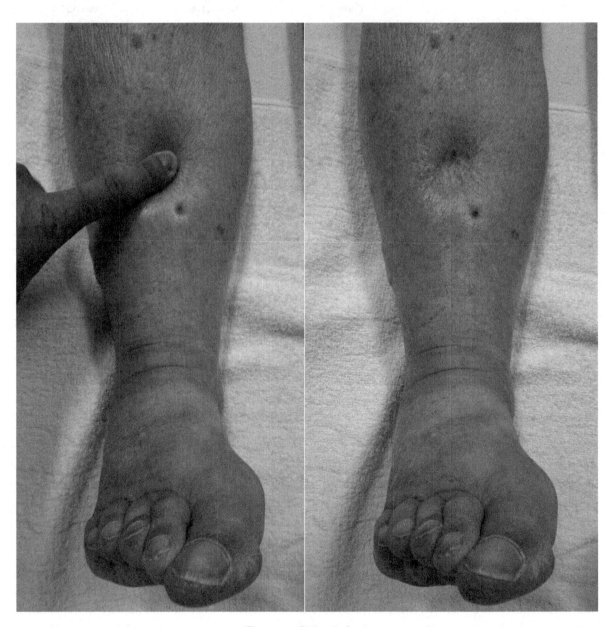

Figure 6.9 Pitting edema

Most people experience a daily accumulation of fluid in their tissues, especially if they spend much of their time on their feet (like most health professionals). However, clinical edema goes beyond normal swelling and requires

---

21 "Combinpedal.jpg" by James Heilman, MD is licensed under CC BY-SA 3.0.

medical treatment. Edema has many potential causes, including hypertension and heart failure, severe protein deficiency, and renal failure. Diuretics such as furosemide are used to treat edema by causing the kidneys to eliminate sodium and water.[22]

Blood Flow and Blood Pressure

Blood flow refers to the movement of blood through a vessel, tissue, or organ. **Blood pressure** is the force exerted by blood on the walls of the blood vessels. In clinical practice, this pressure is measured in mm Hg and is typically obtained using a sphygmomanometer (a blood pressure cuff) on the brachial artery of the arm. When systemic arterial blood pressure is measured, it is recorded as a ratio of two numbers expressed as systolic pressure over diastolic pressure (e.g., 120/80 is a normal adult blood pressure). The systolic pressure is the higher value (typically around 120 mm Hg) and reflects the arterial pressure resulting from the ejection of blood during ventricular contraction or systole. The diastolic pressure is the lower value (usually about 80 mm Hg) and represents the arterial pressure of blood during ventricular relaxation or diastole.

Three primary variables influence blood flow and blood pressure:

- Cardiac output
- Compliance
- Volume of the blood

Any factor that causes cardiac output to increase will elevate blood pressure and promote blood flow. Conversely, any factor that decreases cardiac output will decrease blood flow and blood pressure. See the previous section on cardiac output for more information about factors that affect cardiac output.

Compliance is the ability of any compartment to expand to accommodate increased content. A metal pipe, for example, is not compliant, whereas a balloon is. The greater the compliance of an artery, the more effectively it is able to expand to accommodate surges in blood flow without increased resistance or blood pressure. When vascular disease causes stiffening of arteries, called arteriosclerosis, compliance is reduced and resistance to blood flow is increased. The result is higher blood pressure within the vessel and reduced blood flow. Arteriosclerosis is a common cardiovascular disorder that is a leading cause of hypertension and coronary heart disease because it causes the heart to work harder to generate a pressure great enough to overcome the resistance.

There is a relationship between blood volume, blood pressure, and blood flow. As an example, water may merely trickle along a creek bed in a dry season, but rush quickly and under great pressure after a heavy rain. Similarly, as blood volume decreases, blood pressure and flow decrease, but when blood volume increases, blood pressure and flow increase.

Low blood volume, called **hypovolemia**, may be caused by bleeding, dehydration, vomiting, severe burns, or by diuretics used to treat hypertension. Treatment typically includes intravenous fluid replacement. Excessive fluid volume, called **hypervolemia**, is caused by retention of water and sodium, as seen in patients with heart failure, liver cirrhosis, and some forms of kidney disease. Treatment may include the use of diuretics that cause the kidneys to eliminate sodium and water.[23]

---

22 This work is a derivative of *Anatomy and Physiology* by OpenStax licensed under CC BY 4.0. Access for free at https://openstax.org/books/anatomy-and-physiology/pages/1-introduction.

23 This work is a derivative of *Anatomy and Physiology* by OpenStax licensed under CC BY 4.0. Access for free at https://openstax.org/books/anatomy-and-physiology/pages/1-introduction.

Homeostatic Regulation of the Cardiovascular System

To maintain homeostasis in the cardiovascular system and provide adequate blood to the tissues, blood flow must be redirected continually to the tissues as they become more active. For example, when an individual is exercising, more blood will be directed to skeletal muscles, the heart, and the lungs. On the other hand, following a meal, more blood is directed to the digestive system. Only the brain receives a constant supply of blood regardless of rest or activity. Three homeostatic mechanisms ensure adequate blood flow and ultimately perfusion of tissues: neural, endocrine, and autoregulatory mechanisms.

Neural Regulation

The nervous system plays a critical role in the regulation of vascular homeostasis based on baroreceptors and chemoreceptors. Baroreceptors are specialized stretch receptors located within the aorta and carotid arteries that respond to the degree of stretch caused by the presence of blood and then send impulses to the cardiovascular center to regulate blood pressure. In addition to the baroreceptors, chemoreceptors monitor levels of oxygen, carbon dioxide, and hydrogen ions (pH). When the cardiovascular center in the brain receives this input, it triggers a reflex that maintains homeostasis.

Endocrine Regulation

Endocrine control over the cardiovascular system involves catecholamines, epinephrine, and norepinephrine, as well as several hormones that interact with the kidneys in the regulation of blood volume.

Epinephrine and Norepinephrine

The catecholamines epinephrine and norepinephrine are released by the adrenal medulla and are a part of the body's sympathetic or fight-or-flight response. They increase heart rate and force of contraction, while temporarily constricting blood vessels to organs not essential for flight-or-fight responses and redirecting blood flow to the liver, muscles, and heart.

Antidiuretic Hormone

Antidiuretic hormone (ADH), also known as vasopressin, is secreted by the hypothalamus. The primary trigger prompting the hypothalamus to release ADH is increasing osmolarity of tissue fluid, usually in response to significant loss of blood volume. ADH signals its target cells in the kidneys to reabsorb more water, thus preventing the loss of additional fluid in the urine. This will increase overall fluid levels and help restore blood volume and pressure.

Renin-Angiotensin-Aldosterone System

The **renin-angiotensin-aldosterone system** (RAAS) has a major effect on the cardiovascular system. Specialized cells in the kidneys respond to decreased blood flow by secreting renin into the blood. Renin converts the plasma protein angiotensinogen into its active form—Angiotensin I. Angiotensin I circulates in the blood and is then converted into Angiotensin II in the lungs. This reaction is catalyzed by the enzyme called angiotensin-converting enzyme (ACE). Medications called ACE inhibitors such as lisinopril target this step in the RAAS in an effort to decrease blood pressure.

Angiotensin II is a powerful vasoconstrictor that greatly increases blood pressure. It also stimulates the release of ADH and aldosterone, a hormone produced by the adrenal cortex. Aldosterone then increases the reabsorption of sodium into the blood by the kidneys. Because water follows sodium, there is an increase in the reabsorption of water, which increases blood volume and blood pressure. See Figure 6.10 for an illustration of the renin-angiotensin-aldosterone system and Figure 6.11[24] for a summary of the effect of hormones involved in renal control of blood pressure.[25]

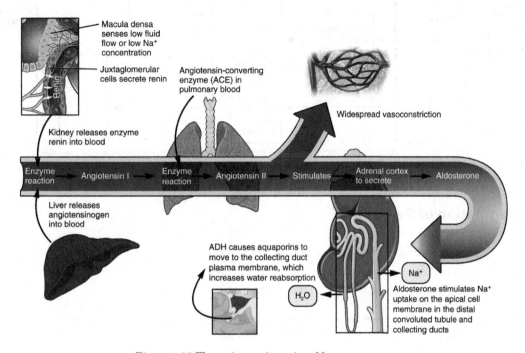

Figure 6.10 The renin-angiotensin-aldosterone system

---

24   "2626 Renin Aldosterone Angiotensin.jpg" by OpenStax College is licensed under CC BY 4.0 Access for free at https://openstax.org/books/anatomy-and-physiology/pages/25-4-microscopic-anatomy-of-the-kidney.

25   This work is a derivative of *Anatomy and Physiology* by OpenStax licensed under CC BY 4.0. Access for free at https://openstax.org/books/anatomy-and-physiology/pages/1-introduction.

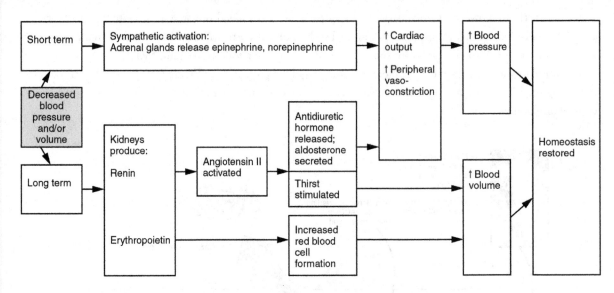

Figure 6.11 Hormones involved in renal control of blood pressure

Autoregulation of Perfusion

Local, self-regulatory mechanisms allow each region of tissue to adjust its blood flow—and thus its perfusion. These mechanisms are affected by sympathetic and parasympathetic stimulation, as well as endocrine factors. See Figure 6.12 for a summary of these factors and their effects.[26]

Control	Factor	Vasoconstriction	Vasodilation
Neural	Sympathetic stimulation	Arterioles within integument abdominal viscera and mucosa membrane; skeletal muscles (at high levels); varied in veins and venules	Arterioles within heart; skeletal muscles at low to moderate levels
	Parasympathetic	No known innervation for most	Arterioles in external genitalia; no known innervation for most other arterioles or veins
Endocrine	Epinephrine	Similar to sympathetic stimulation for extended flight-or-fight responses; at high levels, binds to specialized alpha (α) receptors	Similar to sympathetic stimulation for extended fight-or-flight responses; at low to moderate levels, binds to specialized beta (β) receptors
	Norepinephrine	Similar to epinephrine	Similar to epinephrine

---

26   This work is a derivative of *Anatomy and Physiology* by OpenStax licensed under CC BY 4.0. Access for free at https://openstax.org/books/anatomy-and-physiology/pages/1-introduction.

	Angiotensin II	Powerful generalized vaso-constrictor; also stimulates release of aldosterone and ADH	n/a
	ANH (peptide)	n/a	Powerful generalized vasodilator; also promotes loss of fluid volume from kidneys, hence reducing blood volume, pressure, and flow
	ADH	Moderately strong general-ized vasoconstrictor; also causes body to retain more fluid via kidneys, increasing blood volume and pressure	n/a
Other factors	Decreasing levels of oxygen	n/a	Vasodilation, also opens precapillary sphincters
	Decreasing pH	n/a	Vasodilation, also opens precapillary sphincters
	Increasing levels of carbon dioxide	n/a	Vasodilation, also opens precapillary sphincters
	Increasing levels of potassium ion	n/a	Vasodilation, also opens precapillary sphincters
	Increasing levels of prostaglandins	Vasoconstriction, closes precapillary sphincters	Vasodilation, opens precapillary sphincters
	Increasing levels of adenosine	n/a	Vasodilation
	Increasing levels of lactic acid and other metabolites	n/a	Vasodilation, also opens precapillary sphincters
	Increasing levels of endothelins	Vasoconstriction	n/a
	Increasing levels of platelet secretions	Vasoconstriction	n/a
	Increasing hypothermia	n/a	Vasodilation
	Stretching of vascular wall (myogenic)	Vasoconstriction	n/a
	Increasing levels of histamines from basophils and mast cells	n/a	Vasodilation

Figure 6.12 The effects of nervous, endocrine, and local controls on the vasoconstriction and vasodilation of arterioles

Kidney Function Review

As discussed earlier, the kidney helps to regulate blood pressure, along with the heart and blood vessels, primarily through the Renin-Angiotensin-Aldosterone System (RAAS). In addition to cardiovascular medications affecting the RAAS system, there are also medications called diuretics that reduce blood volume by working at the nephron level. This section will review the basic concepts of kidney function at the nephron level to promote understanding of the mechanism of action of various cardiovascular medications.

The kidney receives blood from the circulatory system via the renal artery. The renal artery branches into smaller and smaller arterioles until the smallest arteriole, the afferent arteriole, services the nephrons. There are about 1.3 million nephrons in each kidney. Nephrons filter the blood and modify it into urine by accomplishing three principal functions—filtration, reabsorption, and secretion. They also have additional secondary functions in regulating blood pressure (via the production of renin) and producing red blood cells (via the hormone erythropoietin).[27]

The initial filtering of the blood takes place in the glomerulus, a cluster of capillaries surrounded by the glomerular capsule. The rate at which this filtering occurs is called the glomerular filtration rate (GFR) and is used to gauge how well the kidneys are functioning. The rate at which blood flows into the glomerulus is controlled by afferent arterioles and the blood vessels flowing out of the glomerulus. These blood vessels are also called efferent arterioles.[28] See Figure 6.13[29] for an illustration of blood flow through the kidney and nephrons.

27 This work is a derivative of *Anatomy and Physiology* by OpenStax licensed under CC BY 4.0. Access for free at https://openstax.org/books/anatomy-and-physiology/pages/1-introduction.

28 McCuistion, L., Vuljoin-DiMaggio, K., Winton, M, and Yeager, J. (2018). *Pharmacology: A patient-centered nursing process approach*. pp. 443–454. Elsevier.

29 "2612 Blood Flow in the Kidneys.jpg" by OpenStax College is licensed under CC BY 4.0 Access for free at https://openstax.org/books/anatomy-and-physiology/pages/25-3-gross-anatomy-of-the-kidney.

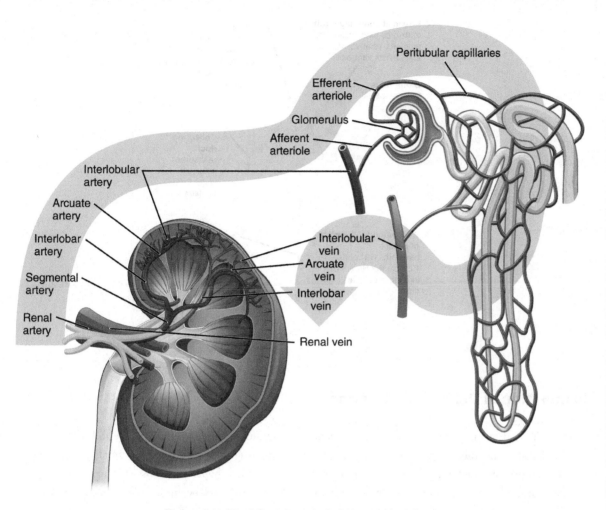

Figure 6.13 Blood flow through the kidney and nephrons

Lying just outside the glomerulus is the juxtaglomerular apparatus (JGA). One function of the JGA is to regulate renin release as part of the RAAS system discussed earlier in this chapter.

See Figure 6.14[30] for an illustration of nephron structure. From the glomerulus (1), the proximal tubule (2) returns 60-70% of the sodium and water back into the bloodstream. From the proximal tubule, the filtrate flows into the descending loop of Henle (3) and then the ascending loop of Henle (4). Another 20-25% of sodium is reabsorbed in the ascending loop of Henle, and this is the site of action of loop diuretics. Filtrate then enters the distal tubule (5), where sodium is actively filtered in exchange for potassium or hydrogen ions, a process regulated by the hormone aldosterone. This is the site of action for thiazide diuretics. The collecting duct (6) is the final pathway; this is where antidiuretic hormone (ADH) acts to increase the absorption of water back into the bloodstream, thereby preventing it from being lost in the urine.[31]

---

30   "Figure 41 03 04.jpg" by CNX OpenStax is licensed under CC BY 4.0.

31   McCuistion, L., Vuljoin-DiMaggio, K., Winton, M, and Yeager, J. (2018). *Pharmacology: A patient-centered nursing process approach*. pp. 443–454. Elsevier.

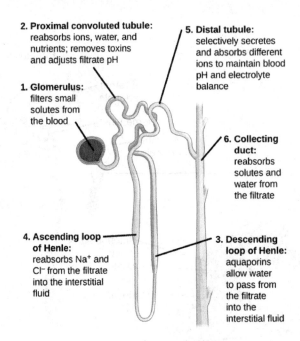

Figure 6.14 Nephron structure

Elimination of Drugs and Hormones

Water-soluble drugs may be excreted in the urine and are influenced by one or all of the following processes: glomerular filtration, tubular secretion, or tubular reabsorption. Drugs that are structurally small can be filtered by the glomerulus with the filtrate. However, large drug molecules such as heparin or those that are bound to plasma proteins cannot be filtered and are not readily eliminated. Some drugs can be eliminated by carrier proteins that enable secretion of the drug into the tubule (such as dopamine or histamine).[32]

Blood and Coagulation

Now that we have reviewed the functions of the heart, blood vessels, and kidneys, we will review coagulation. As we discussed, the primary function of blood as it moves through the blood vessels in the body is to deliver oxygen and nutrients and remove wastes as it is filtered by the kidney, but that is only the beginning of the story. Cellular elements of blood include red blood cells (RBCs), white blood cells (WBCs), and platelets, and each element has its own function. Red blood cells carry oxygen; white blood cells assist with the immune response; and platelets are key players in **hemostasis**, the process by which the body seals a small ruptured blood vessel and prevents further loss of blood. There are three steps to the hemostasis process: vascular spasm, the formation of a platelet plug, and coagulation (blood clotting). Failure of any of these steps will result in hemorrhage (excessive bleeding). Each of these steps will be further discussed below.[33]

---

32   This work is a derivative of *Anatomy and Physiology* by OpenStax licensed under CC BY 4.0. Access for free at https://openstax.org/books/anatomy-and-physiology/pages/1-introduction.

33   This work is a derivative of *Anatomy and Physiology* by OpenStax licensed under CC BY 4.0. Access for free at https://openstax.org/books/anatomy-and-physiology/pages/1-introduction.

Vascular Spasm

When a vessel is severed or punctured or when the wall of a vessel is damaged, vascular spasm occurs. In vascular spasm, the smooth muscle in the walls of the vessel contracts dramatically. The vascular spasm response is believed to be triggered by several chemicals called endothelins that are released by vessel-lining cells and by pain receptors in response to vessel injury. This phenomenon typically lasts for up to 30 minutes, although it can last for hours.

Formation of the Platelet Plug

In the second step, platelets, which normally float free in the plasma, encounter the area of vessel rupture with the exposed underlying connective tissue and collagenous fibers. The platelets begin to clump together, become spiked and sticky, and bind to the exposed collagen and endothelial lining. This process is assisted by a glycoprotein in the blood plasma called von Willebrand factor, which helps stabilize the growing platelet plug. As platelets collect, they simultaneously release chemicals from their granules into the plasma that further contribute to hemostasis. Among the substances released by the platelets are:

- adenosine diphosphate (ADP), which helps additional platelets to adhere to the injury site, reinforcing and expanding the platelet plug

- serotonin, which maintains vasoconstriction

- prostaglandins and phospholipids, which also maintain vasoconstriction and help to activate further clotting chemicals

A platelet plug can temporarily seal a small opening in a blood vessel, thus buying the body more time while more sophisticated and durable repairs are being made.[34]

Coagulation

The more sophisticated and more durable repairs are called **coagulation**, or the formation of a blood clot. The process is sometimes characterized as a cascade because one event prompts the next as in a multi-level waterfall. The result is the production of a gelatinous but robust clot made up of a mesh of fibrin in which platelets and blood cells are trapped. Figure 6.15[35] summarizes the three steps of hemostasis when an injury to a blood vessel occurs. First, vascular spasm constricts the flow of blood. Next, a platelet plug forms to temporarily seal small openings in the vessel. Coagulation then enables the repair of the vessel wall once the leakage of blood has stopped. The synthesis of fibrin in blood clots involves either an intrinsic pathway or an extrinsic pathway, both of which lead to a common pathway creating a clot.[36]

---

34   This work is a derivative of *Anatomy and Physiology* by OpenStax licensed under CC BY 4.0. Access for free at https://openstax.org/books/anatomy-and-physiology/pages/1-introduction.

35   "1909 Blood Clotting.jpg" by OpenStax College is licensed under CC BY 4.0 Access for free at https://openstax.org/books/anatomy-and-physiology/pages/18-5-hemostasis.

36   This work is a derivative of *Anatomy and Physiology* by OpenStax licensed under CC BY 4.0. Access for free at https://openstax.org/books/anatomy-and-physiology/pages/1-introduction.

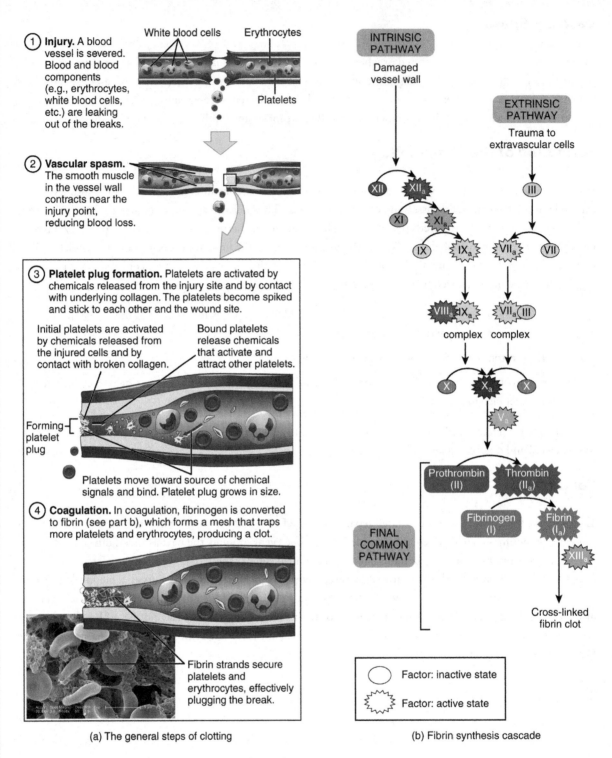

(a) The general steps of clotting

(b) Fibrin synthesis cascade

Figure 6.15 The steps of hemostasis

Extrinsic Pathway

The quicker responding and more direct extrinsic pathway (also known as the tissue factor pathway) begins when damage occurs to the surrounding tissues, such as in a traumatic injury. The events in the extrinsic pathway are completed in a matter of seconds.

Intrinsic Pathway

The intrinsic pathway is longer and more complex. In this case, the factors involved are intrinsic to (present within) the bloodstream. The pathway can be prompted by damage to the tissues or resulting from internal factors such as arterial disease. The events in the intrinsic pathway are completed in a few minutes.

Common Pathway

Both the intrinsic and extrinsic pathways lead to the common pathway, where fibrin is produced to seal off the vessel. Once Factor X has been activated by either the intrinsic or extrinsic pathway, Factor II, the inactive enzyme prothrombin, is converted into the active enzyme thrombin. Then thrombin converts Factor I, the soluble fibrinogen, into the insoluble fibrin protein strands. Factor XIII then stabilizes the fibrin clot.

Fibrinolysis

The stabilized clot is acted on by contractile proteins within the platelets. As these proteins contract, they pull on the fibrin threads, bringing the edges of the clot more tightly together, somewhat as we do when tightening loose shoelaces. This process also wrings out of the clot a small amount of fluid called serum, which is blood plasma without its clotting factors.

To restore normal blood flow as the vessel heals, the clot must eventually be removed. **Fibrinolysis** is the gradual degradation of the clot. Again, there is a fairly complicated series of reactions that involves Factor XII and protein-catabolizing enzymes. During this process, the inactive protein plasminogen is converted into the active plasmin, which gradually breaks down the fibrin of the clot. Additionally, bradykinin, a vasodilator, is released, reversing the effects of the serotonin and prostaglandins from the platelets. This allows the smooth muscle in the walls of the vessels to relax and helps to restore the circulation.

Plasma Anticoagulants

An anticoagulant is any substance that opposes coagulation. Several circulating plasma anticoagulants play a role in limiting the coagulation process to the region of injury and restoring a normal, clot-free condition of blood. For instance, antithrombin inactivates Factor X and opposes the conversion of prothrombin (Factor II) to thrombin in the common pathway. Basophils release heparin, a short-acting anticoagulant that also opposes prothrombin. A pharmaceutical form of heparin is often administered therapeutically to prevent or treat blood clots.

A **thrombus** is an aggregation of platelets, erythrocytes, and even WBCs typically trapped within a mass of fibrin strands. While the formation of a clot is normal following the hemostatic mechanism just described, thrombi can form within an intact or only slightly damaged blood vessel. In a large vessel, a thrombus will adhere to the vessel wall and decrease the flow of blood. In a small vessel, it may actually totally block the flow of blood and is termed an occlusive thrombus.

There are several medications that impact the coagulation cascade. For example, aspirin (acetylsalicylic acid) is very effective at inhibiting the aggregation of platelets. Patients at risk for cardiovascular disease often take a low dose of aspirin on a daily basis as a preventive measure. It is also routinely administered during a heart attack or stroke to reduce the formation of the platelet plug. Anticoagulant medications such as warfarin and heparin prevent the formation of clots by affecting the intrinsic or extrinsic pathways. Another class of drugs known as thrombolytic agents are used to dissolve an abnormal clot. If a thrombolytic agent is administered to a patient within a few hours following a thrombotic stroke or myocardial infarction, the patient's prognosis improves significantly. Tissue plasminogen activator (TPA) is an example of a medication that is released naturally by endothelial cells but is also used in clinical medicine to break down a clot.[37]

Video Review of Basic Concepts

For additional video review of the basic anatomy and physiology concepts of the cardiovascular and renal system, see the supplementary videos below.

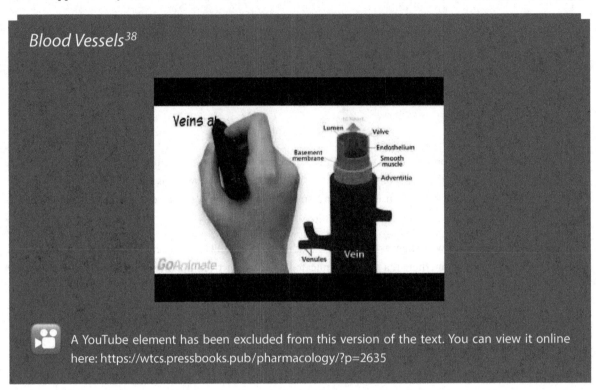

Blood Vessels[38]

A YouTube element has been excluded from this version of the text. You can view it online here: https://wtcs.pressbooks.pub/pharmacology/?p=2635

---

37   This work is a derivative of *Anatomy and Physiology* by OpenStax licensed under CC BY 4.0. Access for free at https://openstax.org/books/anatomy-and-physiology/pages/1-introduction.

38   Forciea, B. (2018, April 26). *Structure of Arteries and Veins V2.* [Video]. YouTube. All rights reserved. Video used with permission. https://youtu.be/HZAeua5JbrU.

Muscle Contraction[39]

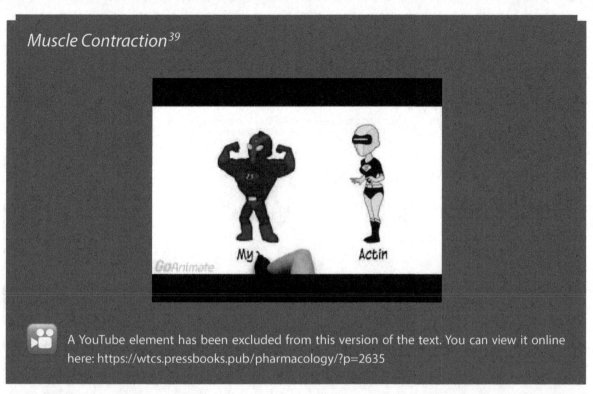

A YouTube element has been excluded from this version of the text. You can view it online here: https://wtcs.pressbooks.pub/pharmacology/?p=2635

Fluids and Electrolytes: Potassium and Aldosterone[40]

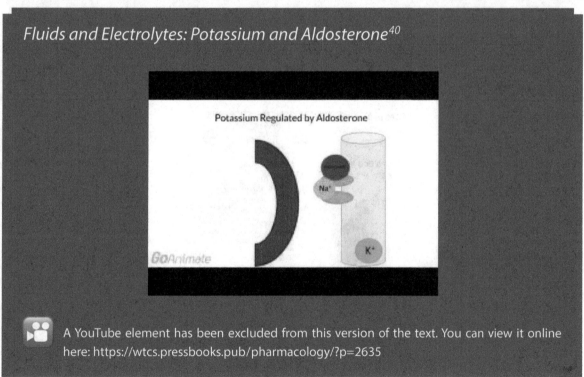

A YouTube element has been excluded from this version of the text. You can view it online here: https://wtcs.pressbooks.pub/pharmacology/?p=2635

---

39   Forciea, B. (2016, September 14). *Muscle Contraction Physiology.* [Video]. YouTube. All rights reserved. Video used with permission. https://youtu.be/TB7TypeksGk.

40   Forciea, B. (2017, April 26). *Fluids and Electrolytes Potassium.* [Video]. YouTube. All rights reserved. Video used with permission. https://youtu.be/SNAiGaaYkvs.

My Notes

Fluid and Electrolytes: Sodium[41]

A YouTube element has been excluded from this version of the text. You can view it online here: https://wtcs.pressbooks.pub/pharmacology/?p=2635

Anatomy of the Heart[42]

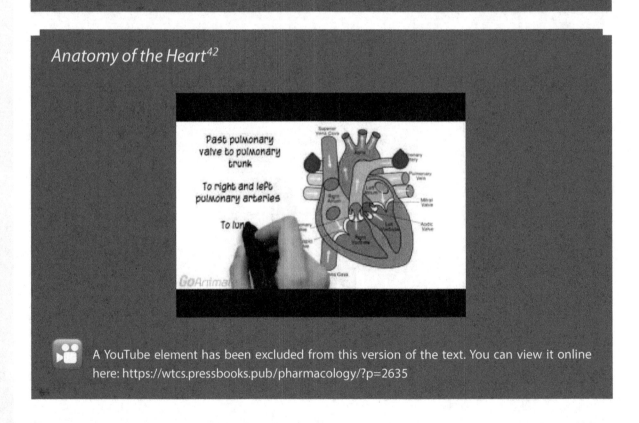

A YouTube element has been excluded from this version of the text. You can view it online here: https://wtcs.pressbooks.pub/pharmacology/?p=2635

41 Forciea, B. (2017, April 24). *Fluids and Electrolytes Sodium.* [Video]. YouTube. All rights reserved. Video used with permission. https://youtu.be/ar-WrfC7SJs.

42 Forciea, B. (2015, May 20). *Anatomy of the Heart* (v2.0). [Video]. YouTube. All rights reserved. Video used with permission. https://youtu.be/d8RSvcc8koo.

The Blood[43]

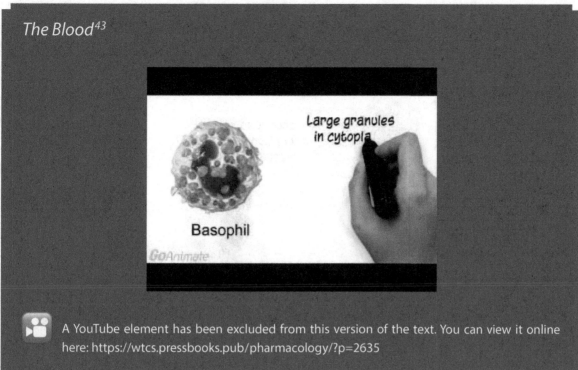

A YouTube element has been excluded from this version of the text. You can view it online here: https://wtcs.pressbooks.pub/pharmacology/?p=2635

Anatomy of Urinary System[44]

A YouTube element has been excluded from this version of the text. You can view it online here: https://wtcs.pressbooks.pub/pharmacology/?p=2635

---

43 Forciea, B. (2015, May 19). *Anatomy and Physiology: The Blood*. [Video]. YouTube. All rights reserved. Video used with permission. https://youtu.be/bjfcOSoDSzg.

44 Forciea, B. (2015, May 13). *Urinary System Anatomy (v2.0)* [Video]. YouTube. All rights reserved. Video used with permission. https://youtu.be/2Wd45Zmq_Ck.

Renin-Angiotensin System[45]

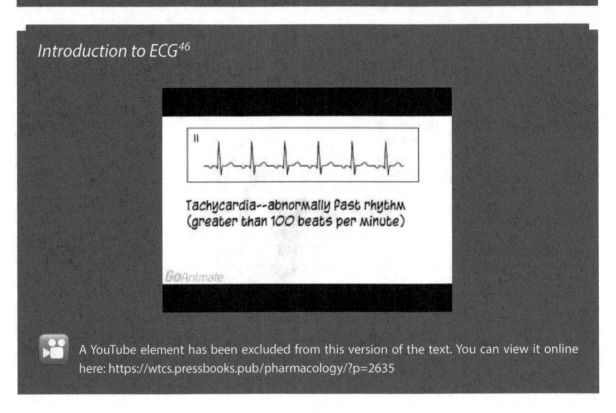

A YouTube element has been excluded from this version of the text. You can view it online here: https://wtcs.pressbooks.pub/pharmacology/?p=2635

Introduction to ECG[46]

A YouTube element has been excluded from this version of the text. You can view it online here: https://wtcs.pressbooks.pub/pharmacology/?p=2635

45 Forciea, B. (2015, May 13). *Renin-Angiotensin System for Anatomy and Physiology (v2.0)* [Video]. YouTube. All rights reserved. Video used with permission. https://youtu.be/iin4lbAKv7Q.

46 Forciea, B. (2015, May 12). *Introduction to the Electrocardiogram (ECG) V2.0.* [Video]. YouTube. All rights reserved. Video used with permission. https://youtu.be/mAN0GK7O9yU.

Circulatory System Anatomy[47]

A YouTube element has been excluded from this version of the text. You can view it online here: https://wtcs.pressbooks.pub/pharmacology/?p=2635

---

47   Forciea, B. (2015, May 12). *Circulatory System Anatomy (v2.0)*. [Video]. YouTube. All rights reserved. Video used with permission. https://youtu.be/nBSHhkOEKHA.

6.3   COMMON CARDIAC DISORDERS

Now that we have reviewed the basic anatomy and physiology concepts of the cardiovascular and renal system, let's discuss some common cardiac disorders.

Hyperlipidemia

Cholesterol is a fat (also called a lipid) that your body needs to work properly. However, too much bad cholesterol can increase the risk for heart disease, stroke, and peripheral vascular disease. The medical term for high blood cholesterol is **hyperlipidemia**. There are many types of cholesterol (see Figure 6.16 for basic types of cholesterol.[48])

- **Total cholesterol**: All the cholesterols combined

- **High density lipoprotein (HDL) cholesterol:** Often called "good" cholesterol because it promotes the excretion of cholesterol. Exercise helps to increase HDL and remove cholesterol from the bloodstream

- **Low density lipoprotein (LDL) cholesterol:** Often called "bad" cholesterol because it stores cholesterol in the bloodstream, which contributes to atherosclerosis

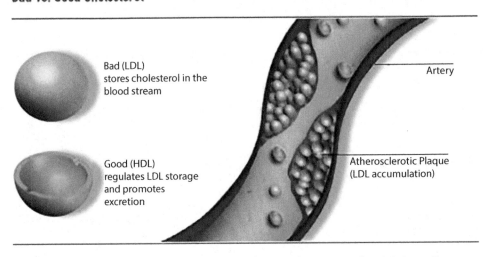

Figure 6.16 A comparison of LDL (bad cholesterol) and HDL (good cholesterol)

For many people, abnormal cholesterol levels are partly due to lifestyle choices, including a diet that is high in fat, being overweight, or lack of exercise. However, disorders can also be passed down through families that lead to abnormal cholesterol and triglyceride levels.[49] In addition to lifestyle modifications such as a low-fat diet and exercise, hyperlipidemia is treated with antilipidemic medication such as atorvastatin (Lipitor) to help prevent long-term complications.

---

48   "máu nhiễm mỡ - cholesterol" by LÊ VĂN THẢO is licensed under CC BY-SA 2.0.

49   A.D.A.M. Medical Encyclopedia [Internet]. Atlanta (GA): A.D.A.M., Inc.; c2019. High blood cholesterol levels; [reviewed 2018 February 22; updated 2018 March 28; cited 2019 November 29]. https://medlineplus.gov/ency/ article/000403. htm.

Hypertension

Chronically elevated blood pressure is known clinically as hypertension. High blood pressure is treated with lifestyle changes and medication. New American Heart Association guidelines state that hypertension should be treated at 130/80 mm Hg rather than the previous standard of 140/90.[50] See Figure 6.17[51] for an image of a health care professional obtaining an accurate blood pressure reading that will be used to determine a treatment plan for the patient.

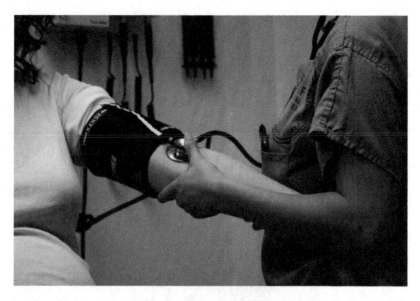

Figure 6.17 It is critical to obtain an accurate blood pressure that will be used for the development of a treatment plan for hypertension

About 68 million Americans currently suffer from hypertension. Unfortunately, hypertension is often a silent disorder, meaning no symptoms occur until complications happen, so patients may fail to recognize the seriousness of their condition and fail to follow their treatment plan. The result is often a heart attack or stroke. Hypertension may also lead to an aneurysm (ballooning of a blood vessel caused by a weakening of the wall), peripheral arterial disease (obstruction of vessels in peripheral regions of the body), myocardial infarction, chronic kidney disease, or heart failure.[52]

Many cardiovascular medications are commonly used to treat hypertension such as diuretics, ACE inhibitors, beta blockers, and calcium channel blockers.

50   Whelton, P.K., Carey R.M., Aronow W.S., et. al. (2018). 2017 Guideline for high blood pressure in adults. *Journal of the American College of Cardiology*, 71. https://www.acc.org/latest-in-cardiology/ten-points-to-remember/ 2017/11/09/11/41 /2017-guideline-for-high-blood-pressure-in-adults.

51   "Monthly check up." by Bryan Mason is licensed under CC BY 2.0.

52   This work is a derivative of *Anatomy and Physiology* by OpenStax licensed under CC BY 4.0. Access for free at https:// openstax.org/books/anatomy-and-physiology/pages/1-introduction.

My Notes

Thrombi and Emboli

Thrombi are most commonly caused by vessel damage to the endothelial lining, which activates the clotting mechanism. A thrombus can seriously impede blood flow to tissue or organs. Deep vein thrombosis (DVT) can occur when blood in the veins, particularly in the legs, remains stationary for long periods, such as during and after surgery. See Figure 6.18[53] for an image of a patient experiencing typical symptoms of a DVT, including unilateral edema and redness.[54]

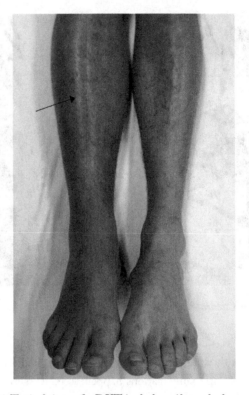

Figure 6.18 Typical signs of a DVT include unilateral edema and redness

When a portion of a thrombus breaks free from the vessel wall and enters the circulation, it is referred to as an embolus. An **embolus** that is carried through the bloodstream can be large enough to block a vessel critical to a major organ. When it becomes trapped, an embolus is called an embolism. In the heart, brain, or lungs, an embolism may cause a heart attack, a cerebrovascular accident (CVA) or otherwise known as a stroke, or a pulmonary embolism. These are medical emergencies.

Medications such as aspirin and warfarin are used to prevent the formation of clots in people who are at risk. Heparin is a medication that can be used to prevent or treat clots, and tPA is used to dissolve severe clots causing ischemia in the brain, heart, or lungs.[55]

---

53   This work is a derivative of "Deep vein thrombosis of the right leg.jpg" by James Heilman, MD is licensed under CC BY-SA 3.0.

54   This work is a derivative of *Anatomy and Physiology* by OpenStax licensed under CC BY 4.0. Access for free at https://openstax.org/books/anatomy-and-physiology/pages/1-introduction.

55   This pwork is a derivative of *Anatomy and Physiology* by OpenStax licensed under CC BY 4.0. Access for free at https://openstax.org/books/anatomy-and-physiology/pages/1-introduction.

Atherosclerosis

Arteriosclerosis begins with injury to the endothelium of an artery, which may be caused by irritation from high blood glucose, infection, tobacco use, excessive blood lipids, and other factors. Injured artery walls causes inflammation. As inflammation spreads into the artery wall, it weakens and scars it, leaving it stiff. Circulating triglycerides and cholesterol can seep between the damaged lining cells and become trapped within the artery wall, where they are joined by leukocytes, calcium, and cellular debris. Eventually, this buildup, called plaque, can narrow arteries enough to impair blood flow. The term for this condition, atherosclerosis, describes the plaque deposits. See Figure 6.19[56] for an illustration of atherosclerosis.[57]

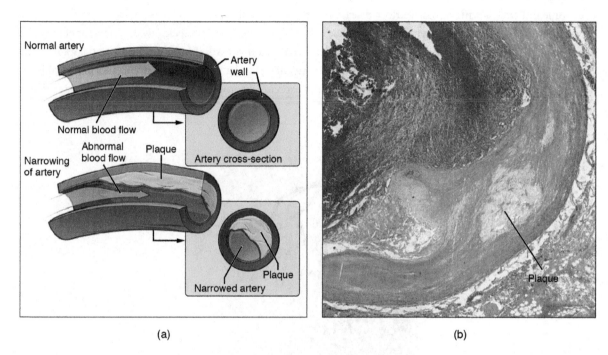

(a)   (b)

Figure 6.19 Atherosclerosis

Sometimes a plaque can rupture, causing microscopic tears in the artery wall that allow blood to leak into the tissue on the other side. When this happens, platelets rush to the site to clot the blood. This clot can further obstruct the artery and—if it occurs in a coronary or cerebral artery—cause a sudden heart attack or stroke. Alternatively, plaque can also break off and travel through the bloodstream as an **embolus** until it blocks a more distant, smaller artery.

Even without total blockage, narrowed vessels lead to **ischemia** (reduced blood flow to the tissue region "downstream" of the narrowed vessel).

Ischemia can lead to hypoxia (decreased supply of oxygen to the tissues), causing a myocardial infarction or cerebrovascular accident.

---

56   "2113ab Atherosclerosis.jpg" by OpenStax College is licensed under CC BY 4.0. Access for free at https://openstax.org /books/anatomy-and-physiology/pages/20-2-blood-flow-blood-pressure-and-resistance.

57   This work is a derivative of *Anatomy and Physiology* by OpenStax licensed under CC BY 4.0. Access for free at https:// openstax.org/books/anatomy-and-physiology/pages/1-introduction.

Treatment of atherosclerosis includes lifestyle changes, such as weight loss, smoking cessation, regular exercise, and adoption of a diet low in sodium and saturated fats. Antilipemic medications such as atorvastatin are prescribed to reduce cholesterol and help prevent atherosclerosis.

Coronary Artery Disease

Coronary artery disease is the leading cause of death worldwide. It occurs when atherosclerosis within the walls of the coronary arteries obstructs blood flow. As the coronary blood vessels become blocked with plaque, the flow of blood to the tissues is restricted, causing the cardiac cells to receive insufficient amounts of oxygen, which can cause pain called angina. Figure 6.20[58] shows the blockage of coronary arteries highlighted by the injection of dye. Some individuals with coronary artery disease report pain radiating from the chest called angina, but others, especially women, may remain asymptomatic or have alternative symptoms of neck, jaw, shoulder, upper back, or abdominal pain. If untreated, coronary artery disease can lead to a **myocardial infarction** (heart attack). Risk factors include smoking, family history, hypertension, obesity, diabetes, lack of exercise, stress, and hyperlipidemia. Treatments may include medication, changes to diet and exercise, a coronary angioplasty with a balloon catheter, insertion of a stent, or coronary bypass procedure.[59]

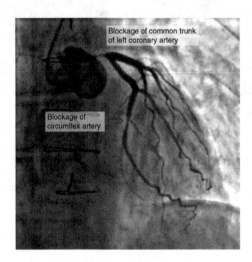

Figure 6.20 Image of blocked coronary arteries highlighted by the injection of dye during a coronary angiogram

Myocardial Infarction

Myocardial infarction (MI) is the medical term for what is commonly referred to as a "heart attack." It results from a lack of blood flow and oxygen to a region of the heart, resulting in death of the cardiac muscle cells. An MI often occurs when a coronary artery is blocked by the buildup of atherosclerotic plaque and becomes a thrombus or when a portion of an unstable atherosclerotic plaque travels through the coronary arterial system and lodges in one of the smaller vessels.

---

58 "2016 Occluded Coronay Arteries.jpg" by OpenStax College is licensed under CC BY 3.0.

59 This work is a derivative of *Anatomy and Physiology* by OpenStax licensed under CC BY 4.0. Access for free at https://openstax.org/books/anatomy-and-physiology/pages/1-introduction.

In the case of acute MI, there is often sudden pain beneath the sternum (retrosternal pain) called angina, often radiating down the left arm in male patients, but not as commonly in female patients (see Figure 6.21).[60] In addition, patients typically present with difficulty breathing and shortness of breath (dyspnea), irregular heartbeat (palpitations), nausea and vomiting, sweating (diaphoresis), anxiety, and fainting (syncope), although not all of these symptoms may be present. Many of the symptoms are shared with other medical conditions, including anxiety attacks and simple indigestion, so accurate diagnosis is critical for survival.

An MI can be confirmed by examining the patient's ECG, which frequently reveals alterations in the ST and Q components. Immediate treatments for MI are required and include administering supplemental oxygen, aspirin, and nitroglycerin. Longer-term treatments may include injections of thrombolytic agents such as tPA that dissolve the clot, along with the anticoagulant heparin, a balloon angioplasty with stents to open blocked vessels, or bypass surgery to allow blood to pass around the site of blockage.[61]

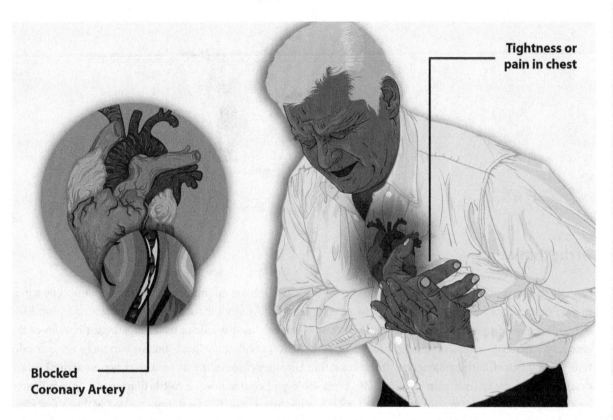

Tightness or pain in chest

Blocked Coronary Artery

Figure 6.21 Male patients often describe chest pain associated with MI "like something is sitting on my chest," but female patients may simply have feelings of GI upset

Cerebrovascular Accident (CVA)

The internal carotid arteries, along with the vertebral arteries, are the two primary suppliers of blood to the human brain. Given the central role and vital importance of the brain to life, it is critical that blood supply to this organ remains uninterrupted. However, blood flow may become obstructed due to atherosclerosis or an emboli that has

---

60   "A man having a Heart Attack.png" by https://www.myupchar.com/en is licensed under CC BY-SA 4.0.

61   This work is a derivative of *Anatomy and Physiology* by OpenStax licensed under CC BY 4.0. Access for free at https://openstax.org/books/anatomy-and-physiology/pages/1-introduction.

My Notes

traveled from elsewhere in the blood. For example, an arrhythmia called atrial fibrillation can cause clots to form in the heart that then move to the brain. When blood flow is interrupted, even for just a few seconds, a **transient ischemic attack (TIA)**, or mini-stroke, may occur, resulting in loss of consciousness or temporary loss of neurological function. Loss of blood flow for longer periods produces irreversible brain damage or a stroke, also called a **cerebrovascular accident (CVA)**.[62] There are two types of cerebrovascular accidents: ischemia and hemorrhagic. Ischemic strokes are caused by atherosclerosis or a blood clot that blocks the flow of blood to the brain (see Figure 6.22).[63] Eighty percent of strokes are ischemic. Hemorrhagic strokes are caused by a blood vessel that ruptures and bleeds into the brain. Risk factors for a stroke include smoking, high blood pressure, and cardiac arrhythmias. Treatment of a stroke depends on the cause.[64] Ischemic strokes are treated with thrombolytic medication such as tPA to dissolve the clot, whereas hemorrhagic strokes often require surgery to stop the bleeding.

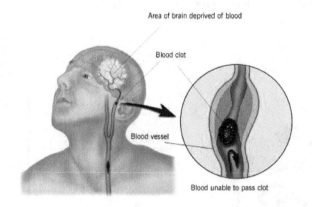

Figure 6.22 Ischemic Stroke

Arrhythmias

Occasionally, an area of the heart other than the SA node will initiate an impulse that will be followed by a premature contraction. Such an area is known as an ectopic focus. An ectopic focus may be stimulated by localized ischemia, exposure to certain drugs, elevated stimulation by both sympathetic or parasympathetic divisions of the autonomic nervous system, or several diseases or pathological conditions. Occasional occurrences are generally transitory and nonlife threatening, but if the condition becomes chronic, it may lead to either an **arrhythmia,** a deviation from the normal pattern of impulse conduction and contraction, or to **fibrillation,** an uncoordinated beating of the heart. Severe arrhythmias can lead to cardiac arrest, which is fatal if not treated within a few minutes. Abnormalities that may be detected by the ECGs are shown in Figure 6.23.[65] Antiarrhythmic medications such as sotalol, diltiazem, and amiodarone are used to treat arrhythmias.

62 This work is a derivative of *Anatomy and Physiology* by OpenStax licensed under CC BY 4.0. Access for free at https://openstax.org/books/anatomy-and-physiology/pages/1-introduction.

63 "Stroke Diagram" by ConstructionDealMkting is licensed under CC BY 2.0.

64 Anderson, P. and Townsend, T. (2015) Preventing high-alert medication errors in hospital patients. *Nurse Today, 10*(5). https://www.americannursetoday.com/wp-content/uploads/2015/05/ant5-CE-421.pdf.

65 "Common ECG Abnormalities" by CNX OpenStax is licensed under CC BY 4.0. Access for free at https://openstax.org/books/anatomy-and-physiology/pages/19-2-cardiac-muscle-and-electrical-activity.

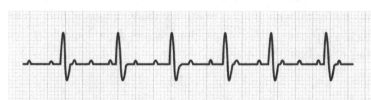

Note how half of the P waves are not followed by the QRS complex and T waves while the other half are.
Question: What would you expect to happen to heart rate (pulse)?

(a)   Second-degree (partial) block

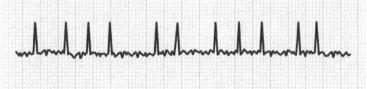

Note the abnormal electrical pattern prior to the QRS complexes. Also note how the frequency between the QRS complexes has increased.
Question: What would you expect to happen to heart rate (pulse)?

(b)   Atrial fibrillation

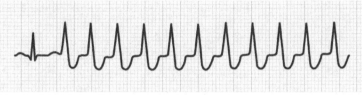

Note the unusual shape of the QRS complex, focusing on the "S" component.
Question: What would you expect to happen to heart rate (pulse)?

(c)   Ventricular tachycardia

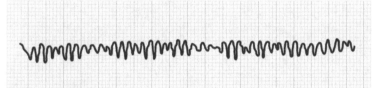

Note the total lack of normal electrical activity.
Question: What would you expect to happen to heart rate (pulse)?

(d)   Ventricular fibrillation

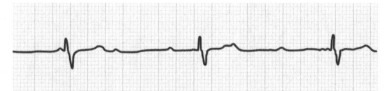

Note that in a third-degree block some of the impulses initiated by the SA node do not reach the AV node while others do. Also note that the P waves are not followed by the QRS complex.
Question: What would you expect to happen to heart rate (pulse)?

(e)   Third-degree block

Figure 6.23 Sample arrhythmias: a) In a second-degree or partial block, one-half of the P waves are pnot followed by the QRS complex and T waves while the other half are. (b) In atrial fibrillation, the electrical pattern is abnormal prior to the QRS complex, and the frequency between the QRS complexes has increased. (c) In ventricular tachycardia, the shape of the QRS complex is abnormal. (d) In ventricular fibrillation, there is no normal electrical activity. (e) In a third-degree block, there is no correlation between atrial activity (the P wave) and ventricular activity (the QRS complex)

Heart Failure

Heart failure is a condition in which the heart can't pump enough blood to meet the body's needs. Right-side heart failure occurs if the heart can't pump enough blood to the lungs to pick up oxygen, whereas left-side heart failure occurs if the heart can't pump enough oxygen-rich blood to the rest of the body. Heart failure is a very common condition with over 5.7 million people in the United States having this chronic condition. There is no cure, but the symptoms can be managed for several years with lifestyle modifications and several different types of medications. Causes of heart failure include hypertension, myocardial infarction, and other cardiac and respiratory

My Notes

diseases. Common symptoms of heart failure include peripheral edema and shortness of breath that occur as a result of fluid overload. Many patients are treated with diuretics to manage the symptoms of fluid overload and with antihypertensives to manage the blood pressure. Other medications such as digoxin and dobutamine may also be used to increase the contractility of the heart.[66]

66   National Heart, Lung, and Blood, National Institute of Health (2019). Heart failure. https://www.nhlbi.nih.gov/health-topics/heart-failure.

6.4   NURSING PROCESS RELATED TO CARDIOVASCULAR AND RENAL MEDICATIONS

Assessment

Understanding the mechanism of action of a cardiac medication will help a nurse choose the proper assessments to perform on a patient. It is important for a nurse to complete a full cardiac assessment to fully understand the health status of the patient, the safe implementation of the medication, and the expected effectiveness of the medication.

Many cardiovascular medications alter a patient's blood pressure or heart rate, such as antiarrhythmics, cardiac glycosides, antihypertensives, or diuretics. Therefore, it is important for a nurse to assess a patient's blood pressure and heart rate prior to administration. Medication parameters are often included in the order by a healthcare provider. For example, a common medication parameter is to hold a beta blocker if a patient's heart rate is less than 60 beats per minute. Additionally, antiarrhythmic medication will alter the electrical conduction of the heart, so intermittent or continuous ECG monitoring may be required during initial therapy or dose changes.

Electrolytes can play a large role in cardiac conduction and muscle function. Medications that alter electrolytes, such as loop diuretics, require a review of laboratory values before administration. Loop diuretics such as furosemide (Lasix) often cause a depletion of potassium. If a nurse administers a loop diuretic to a patient who already has low serum potassium levels (called hypokalemia), worsening symptoms of hypokalemia will occur, which can cause a life-threatening arrhythmia.

Monitoring kidney function is also important when administering many cardiovascular medications. For example, diuretics can cause renal injury. A nurse should be aware of cardiovascular medications that are affected by impaired renal function or cause renal injury. In addition, a nurse must appropriately assess and report abnormal laboratory values such as worsening serum creatinine and glomerular filtration rates (GFR). It is also important to assess for signs of dehydration, as well as intake and output in patients taking diuretics.

Anticoagulant medications cause serious risk for bleeding that can be life threatening. Prior to administering medication that alters a patient's coagulation, it is important to assess for signs and symptoms of unusual bleeding or bruising. Laboratory values, such as INR, PTT, or platelets, may also require review prior to administering an anticoagulant medication. Any new abnormal lab values or signs of increased bleeding and internal bleeding should be immediately reported.

Implementation

Before administration of any cardiovascular medication, it is vital for the nurse to determine if this particular cardiac medication is safe for this patient at this time. For example, if the patient's heart rate or blood pressure is below the anticipated parameters, the medication should be withheld and the prescribing provider notified.

It is also important to consider the effect of the medication before administering it at the ordered time. For example, if a diuretic is prescribed before a patient is sent to a diagnostic test, the test may be disrupted by the need for the patient to urinate, and the dosage should be rescheduled for a later time. A more significant safety concern arises when a patient who is scheduled for surgery is prescribed aspirin or an anticoagulant. The nurse should consider these types of upcoming events before administering medications as they are ordered.

Evaluation

It is always important to evaluate the patient's response to a medication compared to what is expected. Many medications require dose adjustments to produce desired effect. For example, IV heparin is administered based on a protocol that requires dose adjustment based on PTT or aPTT lab results to achieve therapeutic range (and avoid overdosage that can cause life-threatening bleeding).

It is also important to evaluate the patient's understanding of the purpose and proper use of their cardiac medications, as well as when they should notify their provider of changing symptoms. Additional patient education before discharge home is often required, especially if new medications are prescribed.

Nurses should continue to monitor a patient's blood pressure, heart rate, intake and output, edema, or other cardiac assessments to evaluate if ordered cardiac agents are effective or if further treatment or dosage adjustment is required. The patient should be continually monitored for potential adverse effects of medication, some of which can be life threatening and require prompt notification to the prescribing provider.

6.5   CARDIOVASCULAR AND RENAL SYSTEM MEDICATIONS

If you have not done so already, be sure to read the "Review of Basic Concepts" section earlier in this chapter. To truly understand the mechanism of actions of various cardiovascular and renal system medications and their potential adverse effects, it is vital to have a solid understanding of the anatomy and physiology underlying the cardiovascular system.

The remaining sections of this chapter will review classes of medications related to the cardiovascular and renal systems, including administration considerations, therapeutic effects, adverse/side effects, and patient education.

6.6 ANTIARRHYTHMICS

Antiarrhythmics

An arrhythmia is any deviation from the normal rate or pattern of a heartbeat. This includes heart rates that are too slow (bradycardia), too fast (tachycardia), or are irregular. The terms dysrhythmia (disturbed heart rhythm) and arrhythmia (absence of heart rhythm) are traditionally used interchangeably in clinical practice despite their difference in meaning.

The ECG is used to identify and monitor an arrhythmia. See more information about ECGs in the "Review of Basic Concepts" section and an overview of arrhythmias in the "Common Cardiac Disorders" section.

Antiarrhythmic medications regulate heart rate and rhythm by manipulating the conduction of electrical signals to change the heart rate or to attempt to revert an arrhythmia to a normal sinus rhythm. All antiarrhythmic medications have a risk of producing an arrhythmia. Some antiarrhythmic medications are used during emergency situations such as cardiac arrest, whereas others are used long-term, such as those used to control atrial fibrillation. Monitoring electrolytes and the ECG patterns are very important assessments for the nurse administering these types of medications.

Class I – Sodium Channel Blockers

Class I antidysrhythmic medications slow conduction and prolong depolarization by decreasing sodium influx into cardiac cells. There are three subgroups of sodium channel blockers: Class IA, IB, and IC. Quinidine is an example of a Class IA antidysrhythmic. Lidocaine is an example of a Class IB medication that is also used as a local anesthetic. Flecainide is an example of a class IC antidysrhythmic.

Mechanism of Action

Quinidine slows conduction and prolongs depolarization by decreasing sodium influx into cardiac cells. The conduction rate and automaticity are decreased. This medication also has alpha-antagonistic properties that cause peripheral vasodilation.

Indications for Use

This medication is typically used for life-threatening ventricular dysrhythmias such as ventricular tachycardia or for conversion of atrial fibrillation that has not responded to other therapy.

Nursing Considerations Across the Life Span

Sodium channel blockers are contraindicated in patients who have a history of thrombocytopenia or myasthenia gravis. Use cautiously with patients who have a serious heart block rhythm and do not have an artificial pacemaker, such as a 2nd degree heart block.

There is an increased risk for toxicity with patients who have heart failure and renal or hepatic dysfunction due to drug accumulation. This medication's safety has not been thoroughly evaluated in children and geriatric patients.

Grapefruit juice should be avoided by patients taking this medication.

Adverse/Side Effects

Quinidine may prolong QT interval leading to ventricular arrhythmias, such as ventricular tachycardia or torsades de pointes.

Quinidine may induce thrombocytopenia. Routine lab work may be evaluated by a patient's health care provider. Common side effects of this medication are nausea, vomiting, diarrhea, fever, chills, abnormal ECG/ arrhythmias, and headache.

In many research trials, use of antiarrhythmic therapy for non-life-threatening arrhythmias actually resulted in increased risk of death compared to placebo.[67]

Patient Teaching and Education

Patients should be instructed regarding the significance of compliance with therapeutic drug regimen and take medications as prescribed, even if not symptomatic. Patients or family members may need instruction on how to take pulse rate and parameters regarding reporting to their healthcare provider.

Some antiarrhythmic medications may cause dizziness and may increase sensitivity to light.[68]

Now let's take a closer look at the medication grid for quinidine in Table 6.6a.[69] Medication grids are intended to assist students to learn key points about each medication class. Basic information related to a common generic medication in this class is outlined, including administration considerations, therapeutic effects, and side effects/adverse effects. Prototype/generic medication listed in the medication grid is also hyperlinked directly to a free resource from the U.S. National Library of Medicine called *Daily Med*. Because information about medication is constantly changing, nurses should always consult evidence-based resources to review current recommendations before administering specific medication.

Table 6.6a: Quinidine Medication Grid

Class/ Subclass	Prototype/ Generic	Administration Considerations	Therapeutic Effects	Adverse/Side Effects
Antiar- rhythmic Class I	quinidine	Monitor blood pressure, heart rate, and QT with administration Avoid grapefruit juice Maintain consistent sodium intake Health care provider should review medications, as this medication may interact with many medications	Control supraven- tricular arrhythmias	Lengthen the QT interval, arrhyth- mia, dizziness, and headache Thrombocytopenia GI: Nausea, diarrhea, and vomiting

---

67   This work is a derivative of *Daily Med* by U.S. National Library of Medicine in the public domain.

68   uCentral from Unbound Medicine. https://www.unboundmedicine.com/ucentral.

69   This work is a derivative of *Daily Med* by U.S. National Library of Medicine in the public domain.

Class II – Beta Blockers

Class II medications are beta blockers that are used to decrease conduction velocity, automaticity, and the refractory period of the cardiac conduction cycle. Sotalol is a Beta-1 and Beta-2 blocker that also has Class III antiarrhythmic properties. Recall that other types of beta blockers, such as metoprolol, are also used to treat hypertension. See the "Antihypertensives" section later in this chapter for more information about the use of beta blockers to treat hypertension.

Mechanism of Action

Sotalol is a non-selective beta-adrenergic blocker that prolongs the cardiac action potential.

Indications for Use

Sotalol is given to patients for life-threatening arrhythmias, such as ventricular arrhythmias or supraventricular arrhythmias. It is not recommended for patients with less than severe arrhythmias.

Nursing Considerations Across the Life Span

Titration of this medication is done by evaluating renal function and monitoring QTc on the ECG 2-4 hours after each medication upon initiation. Patients with decreased renal function require dosage adjustment. Sotalol is contraindicated for patients with decreased serum potassium, bradycardia, 2nd or 3rd degree heart block, heart failure, and conditions leading to bronchospasm.

Adverse/Side Effects

Black Box Warning: This drug can cause arrhythmias. This medication lengthens a patient's QTc interval. Initiation of this medication requires a patient to be in a facility to determine baseline QT and intermittent QT interval checks. QT interval checks are done 2-4 hours after each dose. If the QT corrected interval is greater than 500 msec, the dosing must be changed. Common side effects for sotalol are arrhythmias, chest pain, palpitations, fatigue, dizziness, hypotension, bradycardia, heart failure, cardiac ischemia, bronchospasm, thyroid abnormalities, and hypoglycemia.[70]

Patient Teaching and Education

Patients should be instructed regarding the significance of compliance with therapeutic drug regimen and take medications as prescribed, even if not symptomatic. Patients or family members may need instruction on how to take pulse rate and blood pressure. They should receive parameters regarding reporting to their healthcare provider. They should report any pulse rate less than 50 bpm and significant changes in blood pressure.

Patients should also be advised that these medications may cause dizziness and visual changes. Patients may also notice orthostatic blood pressure decrease with position changes and should be advised to change positions slowly. If the patient notices irregular, fast heart rate or experiences any fainting episodes, they should notify their healthcare provider immediately.

---

70 This work is a derivative of *Daily Med* by U.S. National Library of Medicine in the public domain.

Additionally, these medications may also mask the signs of hypoglycemia, so diabetic patients must use extra caution to monitor for low blood sugar. They may also increase cold sensitivity.[71]

Now let's take a closer look at the medication grid for sotalol in Table 6.6b.[72]

Table 6.6b: Sotalol Medication Grid				
Class/ Subclass	Prototype/ Generic	Administration Considerations	Therapeutic Effects	Adverse/Side Effects
Antiar-rhythmic Class 2	sotalol	Black Box Warning: Drug induced arrhythmias Strict QTc monitoring with initiation of therapy Do not double dose Monitor blood pressure and heart rate	Treatment of life-threatening arrhythmias	Arrhythmias due to lengthening QTc Chest pain, palpitations, dizziness, fatigue, hypotension, heart failure, cardiac ischemia, and bradycardia Bronchospasm Thyroid abnormalities Hypoglycemia

Critical Thinking Activity 6.6a

1. What should a nurse assess before and after administration of sotalol?

Class III – Potassium Channel Blockers

Class III medications prolong repolarization by blocking the potassium channels in cardiac cells that are responsible for repolarization. They are used for emergency treatment of ventricular dysrhythmias. Amiodarone is an example of an antidysrhythmic that has predominantly Class III properties.

Mechanism of Action

Class III medications prolong repolarization by blocking the potassium channels in cardiac cells that are responsible for repolarization. Amiodarone also antagonizes alpha and beta receptors.

Indications for Use

Amiodarone is indicated only for the treatment of life-threatening recurrent ventricular arrhythmias when these have not responded to documented adequate doses of other available antiarrhythmics or when alternative agents could not be tolerated.

71   uCentral fromUnbound Medicine. https://www.unboundmedicine.com/ucentral.

72   This work is a derivative of *Daily Med* by U.S. National Library of Medicine in the public domain.

My Notes

Nursing Considerations Across the Life Span

Amiodarone can cause fetal injury when administered to a pregnant patient. Use cautiously with the geriatric population who may have decreased hepatic, cardiac, or renal function. Read drug label information carefully due to several potential drug interactions.

Adverse/Side Effects

Black Box Warnings: Amiodarone has several fatal toxicities such as pulmonary toxicity, exacerbation of arrhythmia, liver injury, and heart block. Patients who require initiation of this therapy should be hospitalized and monitored closely. Neurological impairments (such as fatigue, tremors, involuntary movements, poor coordination, and gait) and GI disturbances are common adverse effects. Vision changes/loss of vision and photosensitivity may also occur.

Patient Teaching and Education

Patients should be advised to closely follow the recommended dosing regimen. If one dose of medication is missed, the patient should follow the normal dosing schedule and resume with the next dose. If more than one dose of medication is missed, the patient should call the healthcare provider for guidance. Patients should be compliant with all follow-up appointments and monitoring.

Patients should avoid drinking grapefruit juice during medication therapy. Some patients may experience photosensitivity and protective measures should be taken.[73]

Now let's take a closer look at the medication grid for amiodarone in Table 6.6c.[74]

Table 6.6c: Amiodarone Medication Grid				
Class/ Subclass	**Prototype/ Generic**	**Administration Considerations**	**Therapeutic Effects**	**Adverse/Side Effects**
Antiar- rhythmic Class 3	amiodarone	Black Box Warning: Fatal toxicities Read drug label information due to several drug interactions Monitor blood pressure and heart rate for profound hypotension and bradycardia Initiation of therapy typically requires patients to be hospitalized to receive a loading dose	Treatment of life-threatening ventricular arrhythmia	Fatal toxicities Neurological impairments GI upset Worsening arrhythmia, bradycardia, hypotension Thyroid abnormalities Vision changes Photosensitivity

Class IV – Calcium Channel Blockers

Class IV medications include the calcium channel blockers verapamil and diltiazem. These medications increase the refractory period of the AV node by slowing the influx of calcium ions, thus decreasing the ventricular response and decreasing the heart rate. This medication may be used to control heart rate associated with supraventricular

---

73 uCentral from Unbound Medicine. https://www.unboundmedicine.com/ucentral.

74 This work is a derivative of *Daily Med* by U.S. National Library of Medicine in the public domain.

tachycardias. Calcium channel blockers are also used to treat hypertension because they relax smooth muscle and cause vasodilation. See the "Antihypertensives" section later in this chapter for more information about their use in treating hypertension.

Mechanism of Action

Diltiazem inhibits calcium during depolarization to decrease the workload of the heart and increase oxygen supply to the myocardium. This medication will relax smooth muscle and decrease peripheral resistance.

Indications for Use

Diltiazem is used to treat angina, hypertension, and supraventricular tachycardias.

Nursing Considerations Across the Life Span

This medication is not given to hypotensive patients, patients with acute myocardial infarction, or patients with 2nd or 3rd degree heart block or sick sinus syndrome.

Adverse/Side Effects

Diltiazem can potentially worsen signs and symptoms of heart failure due to the negative inotropic effect. Patients may experience bradycardia, worsening 1st degree AV block, syncope, edema, hypotension, headache, dizziness, or hepatic injury.[75]

Patient Teaching and Education

Patients should be advised to closely follow the recommended dosing regimen. Patients or family members may need instruction on how to take a pulse rate and should report any pulse less than 50 bpm. Patients should also be advised that this medication may cause dizziness and visual changes.

Patients may also notice orthostatic blood pressure decrease with position changes and should be advised to change positions slowly.

Patients should be advised to avoid grapefruit juice during medication therapy. They should also monitor for gingival sensitivity and be sure to maintain good oral hygiene. Patients may also notice increased photosensitivity and should take protective measures.[76]

Now let's take a closer look at the medication grid for diltiazem in Table 6.6.d.[77]

Table 6.6d: Diltiazem Medication Grid

Class/Subclass	Prototype/ Generic	Administration Considerations	Therapeutic Effects	Adverse/Side Effects
Antiarrhythmic Class 4	diltiazem	Monitor blood pressure and heart rate	Reduce workload of the heart, increase oxygen to myocardium, and control heart rate	Worsening heart failure, hypotension, bradycardia, lower extremity edema, syncope, and worsening 1st degree block Headache and dizziness Hepatic injury

Adenosine

Adenosine is a unique medication given to patients who are experiencing paroxysmal supraventricular tachycardia. It is given all at once as a bolus in either a 6 or 12 mg dose to slow electrical conduction to restore a normal sinus rhythm.

Mechanism of Action

Adenosine will slow conduction through the AV node to restore normal sinus rhythm.

Indications for Use

Adenosine is used to treat paroxysmal supraventricular tachycardia.

Nursing Considerations Across the Life Span

This medication is an emergent type of medication. Use cautiously with geriatric patients with decreased cardiac function.

This medication is contraindicated with patients who have 2nd or 3rd degree AV block, sinus node disease, or any known hypersensitivity.

At time of administration, a nurse may see no electrical activity on an ECG for a brief few seconds before normal sinus rhythm is restored. It is important to warn the patient about an extremely uncomfortable feeling during this short period of time.

77   This work is a derivative of *Daily Med* by U.S. National Library of Medicine in the public domain.

Adverse/Side Effects

Patients receiving adenosine may experience prolonged asystole, arrhythmias, palpitations, facial flushing, hypotension, bronchospasm, shortness of breath, dizziness, seizures, loss of consciousness, numbness and tingling to upper extremities, and nausea.[78]

Patient Teaching and Education

Patients should be advised to closely follow the recommended dosing regimen. Patients or family members may need instruction on how to take a pulse rate and should report any abnormalities. Patients should also be advised that this medication may cause dizziness and visual changes. Patients may also notice orthostatic blood pressure decrease with position changes and should be advised to change positions slowly.

Patients should be advised to avoid grapefruit juice during medication therapy. They should also monitor for gingival sensitivity and be sure to maintain good oral hygiene. Patients may also notice increased photosensitivity and should take protective measures.[79]

Now let's take a closer look at the medication grid for adenosine in Table 6.6e.[80]

Table 6.6e: Adenosine Medication Grid				
Class/ Subclass	**Prototype/ Generic**	**Administration Considerations**	**Therapeutic Effects**	**Adverse/Side Effects**
Antiarrhythmic	adenosine	Place the patient in a supine position and inject medication rapidly followed by saline flush	Restore normal sinus rhythm	Prolonged asystole, arrhythmias, palpitations, facial flushing, hypotension, bronchospasm, shortness of breath, and dizziness Seizures, loss of consciousness, numbness, and tingling to upper extremities Nausea

---

78 This work is a derivative of *Daily Med* by U.S. National Library of Medicine in the public domain.

79 uCentral from Unbound Medicine. https://www.unboundmedicine.com/ucentral.

80 This work is a derivative of *Daily Med* by U.S. National Library of Medicine in the public domain.

6.7   CARDIAC GLYCOSIDES

Digoxin

Digoxin is a cardiac glycoside medication that has been used for centuries to treat heart failure. It has three effects on heart muscle: positive inotropic action (increases contractility, stroke volume and, thus, cardiac output), negative chronotropic action (decreases heart rate), and negative dromotropic action (decrease conduction of cardiac cells).[81]

Mechanism of Action

Digoxin works by inhibiting the sodium and potassium pump, which results in an increase in intracellular sodium and an influx of calcium into cardiac cells, causing the cardiac muscle fibers to contract more efficiently and increase cardiac output.[82]

Indications for Use

This medication is used as second-line treatment for patients who have heart failure or atrial fibrillation. Due to the risk for digoxin toxicity, the clinical use of digoxin has decreased and alternative, safer medications are being used.

Nursing Considerations Across the Life Span

Apical pulse should be taken for a full minute before administration of this medication. If the apical pulse is less than 60, the dose should be withheld and the prescribing provider notified.

Serum digoxin levels should be monitored, with a normal therapeutic range from 0.8 to 2 ng/mL.

Serum potassium levels should also be closely monitored for patients on digoxin because hypokalemia increases the effect of digoxin and can result in digoxin toxicity. Normal potassium level is 3.5 to 5.0 mEq/L, and a result less than 3.5 should be immediately reported to the provider.

Nurses should closely monitor signs of digoxin toxicity. Geriatric patients have an increased risk for developing digoxin toxicity. Digibind is used to treat digoxin toxicity.

Adverse/Side Effects

Overdose or accumulation of digoxin causes digoxin toxicity. Signs and symptoms of digoxin toxicity are bradycardia (heart rate less than 60), nausea, vomiting, visual changes (halos), and arrhythmias. Cardiotoxicity is a serious adverse effect with ventricular dysrhythmias. Toxicity of this medication typically occurs at greater than 2 ng/mL, but some patients may have signs and symptoms at lower levels. Pediatric patients typically present with bradycardia or arrhythmias if toxicity is occuring.

Decreased renal function, hypokalemia, hypercalcemia, and hypomagnesemia may increase risk for digoxin toxicity.

---

81   McCuistion, L., Vuljoin-DiMaggio, K., Winton, M, and Yeager, J. (2018). *Pharmacology: A patient-centered nursing process approach*. pp. 443–454. Elsevier.

82   McCuistion, L., Vuljoin-DiMaggio, K., Winton, M, and Yeager, J. (2018). *Pharmacology: A patient-centered nursing process approach*. pp. 443–454. Elsevier.

Common side effects include GI symptoms, headache, weakness, dizziness, anxiety, depression, delirium, and hallucination.[83]

Patient Teaching and Education

The patient should be instructed to follow the prescribed dosing regimen and take medications at the same time each day. The patient should be cautious not to double up on medication doses. Additionally, the patient should consult the healthcare provider if two or more doses of medication are missed for follow-up instruction.

Patients should receive education regarding pulse rate monitoring and report any pulse rate less than 60. If the patient experiences signs of digoxin toxicity, this should be reported to the provider immediately. The medication should be stored in its original container and care should be taken not to mix the medication with other medications.[84]

Now let's take a closer look at the medication grid for digoxin in Table 6.7a.[85]

Table 6.7a: Digoxin Medication Grid				
Class/ Subclass	**Prototype-generic**	**Administration Considerations**	**Therapeutic Effects**	**Adverse/Side Effects**
Cardiac glycosides	digoxin	Assess apical heart rate Assess serum digoxin and potassium levels Assess for signs and symptoms of digoxin toxicity	Increased cardiac output	Digoxin toxicity; early signs include nausea, vomiting, and diarrhea Bradycardia and arrhythmias Headache, weakness, dizziness, and mental changes such as anxiety or hallucinations Gynecomastia (with prolonged use)

---

83 This work is a derivative of *Daily Med* by U.S. National Library of Medicine in the public domain.

84 uCentral from Unbound Medicine. https://www.unboundmedicine.com/ucentral.

85 This work is a derivative of *Daily Med* by U.S. National Library of Medicine in the public domain.

Digibind

Digibind is used to treat digoxin toxicity.

Mechanism of Action

Digibind binds to digoxin molecules, reducing free digoxin.

Indications for Use

This medication is the antidote for digoxin. Digibind will be administered when a patient is experiencing life-threatening digoxin toxicity.

Nursing Considerations Across the Life Span

There are no contraindications when using digibind.

Adverse/Side Effects

The most common effects a patient may experience are to have worsening heart failure, worsening atrial fibrillation, and hypokalemia.[86]

Patient Teaching and Education

The patient should report any signs of worsening heart failure, atrial fibrillation, or hypokalemia immediately to the healthcare provider.[87]

Now let's take a closer look at the medication grid for digibind in Table 6.7b.[88]

---

86   This work is a derivative of *Daily Med* by U.S. National Library of Medicine in the public domain.

87   uCentral from Unbound Medicine. https://www.unboundmedicine.com/ucentral.

88   This work is a derivative of *Daily Med* by U.S. National Library of Medicine in the public domain.

Table 6.7b: Medication Grid for Digibind

Class/ Subclass	Prototype- generic	Administration Considerations	Therapeutic Effects	Adverse/Side Effects
Antidote	digoxin immune fab (Digibind)	Give when patients are experiencing life-threatening digoxin toxicity	Reduce free digoxin	Worsening heart failure Worsening atrial fibrillation Hypokalemia

6.8   ANTIANGINAL - NITRATES

Antianginal medication is used to treat angina pectoris. Angina is chest pain caused by inadequate blood flow, resulting in hypoxia of the cardiac tissue. Angina can be chronic pain caused by atherosclerosis in coronary artery disease or acute pain caused by a myocardial infarction.

Antianginals increase blood flow to the heart or decrease oxygen demand by the heart. Nitrates promote vasodilation of coronary arteries and veins. Beta blockers and calcium channel blockers are also used to decrease workload of the heart and decrease oxygen demands.

Nitrates may come in a variety of routes, such as sublingual, extended-release tablets, creams, transdermal patches, and intravenously. The grid below focuses on administration via sublingual tablets. Sublingual tablets are prescribed PRN ("as needed") for patients who are experiencing chronic, stable angina due to coronary artery disease.

Mechanism of Action

Nitroglycerin relieves angina by relaxing vascular smooth muscle, resulting in vasodilation.

Indications for Use

Nitroglycerin is used to relieve angina due to coronary artery disease, during times of an acute attack, or prophylactically.

Nursing Considerations Across the Life Span

Patients taking sildenafil (Viagra) or similiar medications for erectile dysfunction in the previous 24 hours may not take nitroglycerin as this may result in a dangerous drop in blood pressure.

Nitroglycerin should not be used in pregnant women or those who are breastfeeding.

Nitroglycerin is contraindicated in patients who have severe anemia, increased intracranial pressure, hypersensitivity, or circulatory failure.

Adverse/Side Effects

Patients taking nitroglycerin may experience hypotension, palpitations, headache, weakness, sweating, flushing, nausea, vomiting, or dizziness.

Patients should allow medication to dissolve under their tongue. This route allows immediate absorption into the circulation and avoids first-pass metabolism by the liver. Patients may take up to one tablet every 5 minutes, up to 3 sublingual tablets within 15 minutes to relieve chest pain. If chest pain is not relieved after the first dose, 911 should be called. Nitroglycerin may also be used prophylactically 5 to 10 minutes prior to engaging in activities that might precipitate an acute attack.

Patient Teaching and Education

Instruct patients to avoid eating or smoking during administration as this may alter absorption. Patients should sit during administration to decrease the risk for injury due to the possibility of hypotension, dizziness, and weakness. Nitroglycerin decomposes when exposed to heat or light, so it should be stored in the original, airtight glass container. See Figure 6.24[89] for an image of nitroglycerin containers.[90]

Historically, patients have been taught to seek emergency help (call 911) if pain persists after the 3rd dose of medication. However, new guidelines from the American Heart Association urge patients to call 911 after the first dose if symptoms are not improved or become worse.[91]

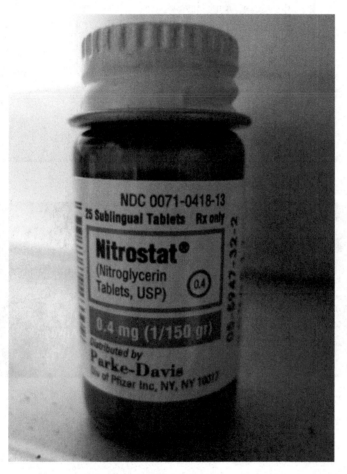

Figure 6.24 Sublingual nitroglycerin should be stored in its original, air tight glass container

---

89   "Nitroglycerin (1).JPG" by Intropin is licensed under CC BY 3.0.

90   This work is a derivative of *Daily Med* by U.S. National Library of Medicine in the public domain.

91   O'Gara, P., Kushner, F. , Ascheim, D. , Casey, D., Chung, M., de Lemos, J., Ettinger, S., Fang, J, Fesmire, F., Franklin, B., Granger, C., Krumholz, H., Linderbaum, J., Morrow, D., Newby, L., Ornato, J., Ou, N., Radford, M., Tamis-Holland, J., Tommaso, C., Tracy, C., Woo, Y., and Zhao, D. (2013). ACCF/AHA guideline for the management of ST-elevation myocardial infarction: a report of the American College of Cardiology Foundation/American Heart Association task force on practice guidelines. *Circulation, 127*(4). https://www.ahajournals.org/doi/full/ 10.1161/CIR.0b013e3182742cf6?url_ver=Z39 .88-2003&rfr_id=ori%3Arid%3Acrossref.org&rfr_dat=cr_pub%3Dpubmed.

My Notes

Now let's take a closer look at the medication grid for nitroglycerin in Table 6.8.[92]

Table 6.8: Nitroglycerine Medication Grid

Class/ Subclass	Prototype-generic	Administration Considerations	Therapeutic Effects	Adverse/Side Effects
Nitrate	nitroglycerin	Patients may take up to 3 sublingual tablets within 15 minutes (1 every 5 minutes) to relieve chest pain If symptoms are not improved after the first dose or become worse, or if the pain persists after the 3rd dose of medication, seek emergency help (call 911). Nurses should check BP after each dose No eating or smoking during administration of SL tablet Do not chew or crush SL tablet Advise patients to sit while taking this medication	Decrease chest pain	Hypotension and palpitations Headache, weakness, sweating, flushing, nausea, vomiting, and dizziness

Critical Thinking Activity 6.8

A patient was administered the first dose of nitroglycerin at 1305 for acute angina. What should the nurse evaluate after administration?

Note: Answers to the Critical Thinking activities can be found in the "Answer Key" sections at the end of the book.

---

92   This work is a derivative of *Daily Med* by U.S. National Library of Medicine in the public domain.

6.9   DIURETICS

Diuretics are used to decrease blood pressure and to decrease symptoms of fluid overload such as edema. There are many classifications of diuretics. We will discuss loop, thiazide, and potassium-sparing diuretics. Other diuretics, such as osmotic diuretics, are used to decrease fluid from cerebrospinal fluid and the brain.

Diuretics cause diuresis (increased urine flow) by inhibiting sodium and water reabsorption from the kidney tubules. By eliminating excess water, blood volume and blood pressure, as well as preload, are decreased.

Diuretics are often used in combination with other antihypertensive agents to reduce a patient's blood pressure.

Furosemide

Mechanism of Action

Loop diuretics inhibit absorption of sodium and chloride in the loop of henle and proximal and distal tubules, thus causing fluid loss, along with sodium, potassium, calcium, and magnesium losses. Loop diuretics are very potent diuretics and are used when a patient has an exacerbation of fluid overload.

Indications for Use

Furosemide is used to treat patients with edema and is also used to treat hypertension. IV furosemide is used to urgently treat pulmonary edema.

Nursing Considerations Across the Life Span

The onset of diuresis following oral administration is within 1 hour. The peak effect occurs within the first or second hour. The duration of diuretic effect is 6 to 8 hours. When possible, loop diuretics should be administered in the morning, and evening doses should be avoided (unless urgent) so that sleep is not disturbed.

Nurses should continually monitor for dehydration and electrolyte imbalances that can occur with excessive diuresis, such as dryness of mouth, thirst, weakness, lethargy, drowsiness, restlessness, muscle pains or cramps, muscular fatigue, hypotension, oliguria, tachycardia, arrhythmia, or gastrointestinal disturbances such as nausea and vomiting.

Use cautiously in the geriatric population who have decreased renal function. Kidney function should be monitored closely for all patients because this is a potent medication that works within the kidney tubules.

Monitor the patient closely for hypokalemia if furosemide is used concomitantly with digoxin. Hypokalemia may increase the risk of digoxin toxicity.

Adverse/Side Effects

Adverse effects include dehydration, hypotension, and electrolyte imbalances such as hypokalemia. Health care providers may add potassium to a patient's scheduled medication list to decrease risk of hypokalemia. If using IV route, the administration must be given slowly to reduce the risk of the patient developing ototoxicity.[93]

---

93   This work is a derivative of *Daily Med* by U.S. National Library of Medicine in the public domain.

Patient Teaching and Education

Advise patients to change position slowly as they may experience orthostatic changes. Patients should also report weight gain of more than three pounds in a day to their healthcare provider. Patients should also be encouraged to enjoy potassium-rich foods during loop diuretic drug therapy.[94] Now let's take a closer look at the medication grid for furosemide in Table 6.9a.[95]

Table 6.9a: Furosemide Medication Grid

Class/ Subclass	Prototype-generic	Administration Considerations	Therapeutic Effects	Adverse/Side Effects
Loop diuretic	furosemide	Assess blood pressure Monitor electrolytes (potassium) Promote potassium-rich diet Assess renal function Assess for dehydration, intake and output Monitor weight	Based on indication; decreased blood pressure or edem	Dehydration Electrolyte depletion (especially potassium) Ototoxicity with rapid IV infusion Renal impairment

Critical Thinking Activity 6.9

Mrs. Smith is a 79-year-old widow who has lived alone for the past 5 years. Three years ago she was hospitalized for an MI, which resulted in heart failure. She is compliant with her medications, which include digoxin (Lanoxin) 0.125 mg daily, furosemide (Lasix) 40 mg daily, and potassium (K-Dur) 20 mEq daily.

Recently Mrs. Smith ran out of her potassium and thought that because it was "just a supplement," it would be OK to go without it until the next time she went to town to fill the prescription. She has not taken her potassium for a week.

Today she comes into the clinic with generalized weakness, fatigue, nausea, and diarrhea. Her BP is 104/62, pulse 98 bpm and slightly irregular, RR 20, and temp 97.2 F. Blood is drawn and shows serum sodium level of 150 mEq/L, digoxin level of 2.6ng/ml and potassium level of 3.2 mEq/L.

1. What assessments should a nurse do before and after administering a diuretic?

2. What are the signs and symptoms of digoxin toxicity? What can happen to a patient who has toxic levels of digoxin?

3. What is the normal range for serum potassium level?

4. What classification of medication is furosemide (Lasix)?

5. Is dehydration a risk for patients on furosemide (Lasix)? Why or why not?

---

94   uCentral from Unbound Medicine. https://www.unboundmedicine.com/ucentral.

95   This work is a derivative of *Daily Med* by U.S. National Library of Medicine in the public domain.

6. How would you assess for dehydration?

7. What electrolyte imbalance(s) can occur in patients taking furosemide (Lasix)?

8. What relationship exists between this patient's furosemide, digoxin, and potassium levels?

Note: Answers to the Critical Thinking activities can be found in the "Answer Key" sections at the end of the book.

Hydrochlorothiazide

Mechanism of Action

Thiazide diuretics work near the distal tubule to promote the excretion of sodium and water, thus causing diuresis. They are not effective for immediate diuresis.

Indications for Use

Hydrochlorothiazide diuretics are used to manage hypertension and edema.

Nursing Considerations Across the Life Span

Thiazide diuretics are contraindicated for patients who have anuria or hypersensitivity.

After oral use, diuresis begins within 2 hours, peaks in about 4 hours, and lasts about 6 to 12 hours.

Use with caution in severe renal disease.

Adverse/Side Effects

Patients who are taking thiazide diuretics should be monitored for electrolyte depletion, dehydration, weakness, hypotension, renal impairment, and hypersensitivities.[96]

Patient Teaching and Education

Patients should be instructed to take these medications at the same time each day and notify their healthcare provider if they experience significant changes in weight. Thiazide diuretics may cause orthostatic changes so individuals should change positions slowly. Additionally, some patients may note increased photosensitivity so protective measures should be taken. Patients should monitor their blood pressure and comply with interventions to reduce hypertension.[97]

Now let's take a closer look at the medication grid for hydrochlorothiazide in Table 6.9b.[98]

---

96   This work is a derivative of *Daily Med* by U.S. National Library of Medicine in the public domain.

97   uCentral from Unbound Medicine. https://www.unboundmedicine.com/ucentral.

98   This work is a derivative of *Daily Med* by U.S. National Library of Medicine in the public domain.

Table 6.9b: Hydrochlorothiazide Medication Grid				
Class/ Subclass	Prototype-generic	Administration Considerations	Therapeutic Effects	Adverse/Side Effects
Thiazide diuretics	hydrochlorothiazide	Assess blood pressure Monitor electrolytes (potassium) Promote potassium-rich diet Assess renal function Assess for dehydration, intake and output Monitor weight	Decrease blood pressure Decrease edema	Electrolyte depletion Dehydration and weakness Hypotension Renal impairment Hypersensitivity (vasculitis, respiratory distress, photosensitivity, rash)

Spironolactone

Spironolactone is a potassium-sparing diuretic that is used as a mild diuretic or in combination with another diuretic.

Mechanism of Action

Spironolactone acts primarily through competitive binding of receptors at the aldosterone-dependent sodium-potassium exchange site in the distal convoluted renal tubule. Spironolactone causes increased amounts of sodium and water to be excreted, while potassium is retained.

Indications for Use

Spironolactone is used to treat hypertension and to control edema for patients with heart failure or liver dysfunction.

Nursing Considerations Across the Life Span

This medication may cause hyperkalemia. Monitor urine output and report if less than 30 ml/hour. Use cautiously with patients who have renal impairment due to increased risk for hyperkalemia. Use cautiously in patients with liver impairment. Administer in the morning to avoid nocturia.

Adverse/Side Effects

Hyperkalemia, hyperglycemia, hyperuricemia, dehydration, hypotension, renal impairment, hypersensitivity, and gynecomastia. This medication may increase risk for lithium toxicity.[99]

Patient Teaching and Education

Patients should be instructed to take these medications at the same time each day and notify their healthcare provider if they experience significant changes in weight. Diuretics may cause orthostatic changes so individuals should change positions slowly. Patients should be advised to avoid salt substitutes and foods that contain high levels of potassium.[100]

---

99   This work is a derivative of *Daily Med* by U.S. National Library of Medicine in the public domain.

100   uCentral from Unbound Medicine. https://www.unboundmedicine.com/ucentral.

Now let's take a closer look at the medication grid for spironolactone in Table 6.9c[101]

Table 6.9c: Spironolactone Medication Grid

Class/ Subclass	Prototype-generic	Administration Considerations	Therapeutic Effects	Adverse/Side Effects
Potassium Sparing diuretics	spironolactone	Assess blood pressure Monitor electrolytes (potassium) Assess renal function Assess for dehydration, intake and output Monitor weight	Decrease blood pressure Decrease edema	Hyperkalemia, hyperglycemia, hyperuricemia Dehydration Hypotension Renal impairment Hypersensitivity (vasculitis, fever, anaphylactic reactions, rash) Gynecomastia

---

101   This work is a derivative of *Daily Med* by U.S. National Library of Medicine in the public domain.

6.10 ANTIHYPERTENSIVES

Many different medication classifications are used to treat **hypertension**. It is important to understand the different mechanisms of action for different classes of antihypertensives because patients are often on a combination of medications that work synergistically to manage blood pressure. These medications are also discussed in the "Autonomic Nervous System" chapter, with more information provided regarding the specific receptors they affect.

Alpha-2 Agonist

Clonidine is an Alpha-2 agonist. You can read more information about Alpha-2 agonists in the "Autonomic Nervous System" chapter.

Mechanism of Action

Clonidine stimulates the alpha-adrenergic receptors, resulting in vasodilation and decreased blood pressure, thus decreasing peripheral resistance, increased blood flow to the kidneys, and decreased afterload.

Indications for Use

Clonidine is used to treat hypertension and ADHD.

Nursing Considerations Across the Life Span

Monitor BP and pulse rate. Dosage is usually adjusted to patient's blood pressure because it can cause hypotension, bradycardia, and sedation. Rebound hypertension may occur if stopped abruptly.[102]

Patient Teaching and Education

Patients should be compliant with medication therapy and take the medication at the same time each day. They should be careful not to take more than the prescribed dose within a 24-hour period. Do not abruptly cease medication as rebound hypertension might occur. Medications may cause orthostatic changes so individuals should change positions slowly. Additionally, medications may cause dry mouth and dry eyes. Individuals should also avoid the use of alcohol and other CNS depressants while taking these medications.[103]

---

102   This work is a derivative of *Daily Med* by U.S. National Library of Medicine in the public domain.

103   uCentral from Unbound Medicine. https://www.unboundmedicine.com/ucentral.

Now let's take a closer look at the medication grid for clonidine in Table 6.10a.[104]

Table 6.10a: Clonidine Medication Grid

Class	Prototype	Administration Considerations	Therapeutic Effects	Adverse/Side Effects
Alpha-2 Agonist	clonidine	Monitor blood pressure and pulse rate frequently Dosage is usually adjusted to patient's BP and tolerance	Treat hypertension or ADHD	Hypotension Bradycardia Sedation Rebound HTN if stopped abruptly

Beta-1 Antagonist

Metoprolol is a selective Beta-1 blocker. You can read more information about Beta-1 antagonists in the "Autonomic Nervous System" chapter.

Mechanism of Action

Metoprolol primarily blocks Beta-1 receptors in the heart, causing decreased heart rate and decreased blood pressure. However, higher doses can also block Beta-2 receptors in the lungs, causing bronchoconstriction.

Indications for Use

Metoprolol is commonly used to treat high blood pressure, chest pain due to poor blood flow to the heart, and several heart conditions involving an abnormally fast heart rate. It is used as an early intervention during myocardial infarction (MI) to reduce workload of the heart.

Nursing Considerations Across the Life Span

ER formulations should not be crushed. Assess patient's apical pulse rate before administering; if it is less than 60 beats/minute, withhold the drug and call the prescriber immediately, unless other parameters are provided. In diabetic patients, monitor glucose level closely because the drug masks common signs and symptoms of hypoglycemia.

Adverse Effects

The most serious potential adverse effects are shortness of breath, bradycardia, and worsening heart failure. Other adverse effects include fatigue, dizziness, depression, insomnia, nightmares, GI upset, erectile dysfunction, dyspnea, and wheezing. Black Box Warning: When stopping therapy, taper dosage over 1 to 2 weeks because abrupt discontinuation may cause chest pain or MI.[105]

---

104   This work is a derivative of *Daily Med* by U.S. National Library of Medicine in the public domain.

105   This work is a derivative of *Daily Med* by U.S. National Library of Medicine in the public domain.

My Notes

Patient Teaching and Education

Patients should be compliant with medication therapy and take the medication at the same time each day. Do not abruptly cease medication as arrhythmias, hypertension, or ischemia may develop. Patients and families should be instructed to check pulse and blood pressure and report abnormalities to the healthcare provider. Additionally, these medications may cause side effects of dizziness and cold sensitivity.[106]

Now let's take a closer look at the medication grid for metoprolol in Table 6.10b.[107]

Table 6.10b: Medication Grid for Metoprolol				
Class	**Prototype–generic**	**Administration Considerations**	**Therapeutic Effects**	**Adverse/Side Effects**
Beta-1 Antagonist	Selective B blocker: **metoprolol**	Do not crush ER formulations Always assess apical HR and if less than 60, do not administer and call the prescriber unless other parameters are provided Monitor blood sugar in diabetic patients because drug can mask symptoms of hypoglycemia	Decreases blood pressure or controls rapid heart rate	Most serious: hypotension, bradycardia, and worsening HF Other: CNS: fatigue, dizziness, depression, insomnia, nightmares GI upset GU: erectile dysfunction Respiratory: dyspnea and wheezing

ACE Inhibitor (Angiotensin Converting Enzyme)

Captopril is an example of an ACE (angiotensin converting enzyme) inhibitor.

Mechanism of Action

This medication blocks the conversion of Angiotensin I to Angiotensin II in the renin-angiotensin-aldosterone system. This will lead to vasodilation and sodium and water excretion by blocking aldosterone. See more information about the renin-angiotensin-aldosterone system in the "Review of Basic Concepts" section of this chapter.

Indications for Use

Captopril is used to treat hypertension and heart failure. This medication also helps reduce diabetic nephropathy.

Nursing Considerations Across the Life Span

Do not administer to patients who are pregnant. Use with caution with patients who have diabetes.

Avoid use with other medications that increase potassium. This medication may increase risk for lithium toxicity.

---

106   uCentral from Unbound Medicine. https://www.unboundmedicine.com/ucentral.

107   This work is a derivative of *Daily Med* by U.S. National Library of Medicine in the public domain.

Adverse/Side Effects

Black Box Warning: Patients who become pregnant should discontinue this medication due to the risk of fetal harm or fetal death.

Patients taking this medication may experience hypotension, cough, hyperkalemia, increased risk for infection, angioedema, anaphylactoid reactions, or proteinuria. Patients who experience increased facial swelling or difficulty swallowing or breathing should seek emergency medical attention. Report a persistent cough or angioedema to the health care provider.[108]

Patient Teaching and Education

Medications should be taken as directed. Patients taking ACE inhibitors should be cautioned to avoid salt substitutes or foods high in potassium. Additionally, the medication may alter the sense of taste, but this generally resolves within 2-3 months of medication therapy.

Patients taking ACE inhibitors may also experience a persistent cough throughout the duration of medication therapy.[109]

Now let's take a closer look at the medication grid for captopril in Table 6.10c.[110]

Table 6.10c: Captopril Medication Grid				
Class/ Subclass	**Prototype- generic**	**Administration Considerations**	**Therapeutic Effects**	**Adverse/Side Effects**
ACE Inhibitor	captopril	Black Box Warning: Do not use while pregnant Monitor blood pressure Report cough Assess for facial swelling or difficulty breathing	Decrease blood pressure Decrease fluid volume status	Hypotension Cough Hyperkalemia Neutropenia or agranulocytosis Angioedema Anaphylactoid reactions Proteinuria

Angiotensin II Receptor Blocker (ARB)

Losartan is an example of an Angiotensin II receptor blocker, also referred to as an ARB. ARBs are similar to ACE inhibitors in that they act on the renin-angiotensin-aldosterone system (RAAS). However, the difference is that they block Angiotensin II and cause vasodilation and decreased peripheral resistance, but are not likely to cause the cough that ACE inhibitors can.

---

108   This work is a derivative of *Daily Med* by U.S. National Library of Medicine in the public domain.

109   uCentral from Unbound Medicine. https://www.unboundmedicine.com/ucentral.

110   This work is a derivative of *Daily Med* by U.S. National Library of Medicine in the public domain.

Mechanism of Action

Losartan blocks Angiotensin II in the renin-angiotensin-aldosterone system to produce vasodilation.

Indications for Use

ARB is used for treatment of hypertension and to prevent nephropathy in diabetic patients.

Nursing Considerations Across the Life Span

Do not administer to patients who are pregnant. It is not recommended for children under 6. Anticipate dosage adjustment with hepatic impairment. This drug can cause renal impairment and hyperkalemia.

Adverse/Side Effects

Black Box Warning: Patients who become pregnant should discontinue this medication due to the risk of fetal harm or fetal death.

Patients taking this medication may experience hypotension, dizziness, increased risk for infection, angioedema, or proteinuria. Patients who experience increased facial swelling or difficulty swallowing or breathing should seek emergency medical attention.

Patient Teaching and Education

Medications should be taken as directed at the same time each day. Patients should not discontinue therapy unless directed to by their healthcare provider. Patients should be careful to avoid salt substitutes and foods with high levels of potassium. ARBs may cause orthostatic changes and patients should be cautioned to change positions slowly.[111]

---

111   uCentral from Unbound Medicine. https://www.unboundmedicine.com/ucentral.

Now let's take a closer look at the medication grid for losartan in Table 6.10d.[112]

Table 6.10d: Medication Grid for Losartan

Class/ Subclass	Prototype- generic	Administration Considerations	Therapeutic Effects	Adverse/Side Effects
ARB	losartan (Cozaar)	Black Box Warning: Do not use while pregnant Monitor blood pressure	Decrease blood pressure	Hypotension and dizziness Hyperkalemia Proteinuria

Critical Thinking Activity 6.10

A male 65-year-old patient has the following medications ordered: metoprolol succinate 100 mg daily, lisinopril 5 mg daily, verapamil ER 100 mg daily, and hydrochlorothiazide 25 mg daily. He has a history of hyperlipidemia, hypertension, and coronary artery disease. The patient asks the nurse, "Why do I have to take so many medications?"

1. What is the class and mechanism of action of each of these medications?

2. What is the nurse's best response to the patient's question?

Note: Answers to the Critical Thinking activities can be found in the "Answer Key" sections at the end of the book.

Vasodilator

Hydralazine is an example of a direct vasodilator.

Mechanism of Action

Hydralazine's direct mechanism of action is unknown, but it causes vasodilation via direct relaxation of vascular smooth muscle. Peripheral vasodilation results in a reduction of blood pressure and decreased vascular resistance, resulting in increased cardiac output.

Indications for Use

Vasodilators are used to treat hypertension.

---

112   This work is a derivative of *Daily Med* by U.S. National Library of Medicine in the public domain.

Nursing Considerations Across the Life Span

Use with caution in patients with coronary artery disease, mitral valve rheumatic heart disease, and cerebral vascular accidents.

This medication should only be used in pregnancy if the benefits outweigh the risks due to lack of safety studies.

Adverse/Side Effects

Patients should be monitored for infection and are at risk of developing systemic lupus erythematosus (SLE). SLE is a chronic disease that causes inflammation in connective tissues. The signs and symptoms of SLE vary among affected individuals and can involve many organs and systems, including the skin, joints, kidneys, lungs, central nervous system, and blood-forming (hematopoietic) system. A characteristic sign of SLE is a flat, red rash across the cheeks and bridge of the nose. This rash is called a "butterfly rash" because of its shape.

Hypotension, palpitations, angina, tremors, numbness, tingling, disorientation, nasal congestion, headache, nausea, vomiting, and diarrhea are effects associated with hydralazine.[113]

Patient Teaching and Education

Patients should remain compliant with the therapeutic dosing regimen, even if symptoms resolve. The patient should be cautious not to double up on medication doses. Additionally, the patient should consult the healthcare provider if two or more doses of medication are missed for follow-up instruction. Patients should be instructed to monitor their weight and assess for fluid retention in the feet and ankles. Additionally, the medication can cause side effects of orthostatic hypotension and drowsiness.[114]

Now let's take a closer look at the medication grid on hydralazine in Table 6.10e.[115]

Table 6.10e: Medication Grid for Hydralazine				
Class/ Subclass	Prototype- generic	Administration Considerations	Therapeutic Effects	Adverse/Side Effects
Vasodilator	hydralazine (Apresoline)	Monitor blood pressure Obtain complete blood count (CBC) and antibody titers prior to beginning this medication Report signs and symptoms of infection	Reduce blood pressure	Systemic lupus erythematosus (SLE) Hypotension, palpitations, and angina Tremors, numbness, tingling, and disorientation Nasal congestion Headache, nausea, vomiting, and diarrhea

113   This work is a derivative of *Daily Med* by U.S. National Library of Medicine in the public domain.

114   uCentral from Unbound Medicine. https://www.unboundmedicine.com/ucentral.

115   This work is a derivative of *Daily Med* by U.S. National Library of Medicine in the public domain.

6.11 ANTILIPEMICS

Antilipemic agents reduce hyperlipidemia that may lead to additional health problems such as stroke, myocardial infarction, angina, and heart failure. Medications should be used in adjunct with a healthy diet and exercise regime approved by the patient's health care provider.

Atorvastatin

Mechanism of Action

Atorvastatin inhibits HMG-CoA reductase and cholesterol synthesis, which reduces LDL (low density lipoprotein).

Indications for Use

This medication is used for hyperlipidemia and the prevention of cardiovascular disease.

Nursing Considerations Across the Life Span

Do not use with patients who have hepatic disease.

This medication is contraindicated with patients who are pregnant or breastfeeding. Do not give to patients under 10 years of age.

Use caution with geriatric patients due to increased risk for myopathy.

Adverse/Side Effects

Patients who are pregnant or breastfeeding should not take this medication. A health care provider will assess routine liver function for a patient taking atorvastatin. Nausea, diarrhea, dyspepsia, increase in blood glucose, rhabdomyolysis, myalgia, or muscle spasms may be produced by taking this medication. Rhabdomyolysis is a condition in which damaged skeletal muscle breaks down rapidly, causing muscle pain and weakness. Some of the muscle breakdown products are harmful to the kidneys and can cause kidney failure. There may be tea-colored urine or an irregular heartbeat with rhabdomyolysis.[116]

Patient Teaching and Education

Patients should take the prescribed medication as directed and avoid consuming grapefruit juice during drug therapy. The medication should be used with dietary modifications. If the patient experiences muscle pain, tenderness, or weakness, these should be reported to the healthcare provider.[117]

---

116   This work is a derivative of *Daily Med* by U.S. National Library of Medicine in the public domain.

117   uCentral from Unbound Medicine. https://www.unboundmedicine.com/ucentral.

My Notes

Now let's take a closer look at the medication grid on atrovastatin in Table 6.11a.[118]

Table 6.11a: Atorvastatin Medication Grid

Class/Subclass	Prototype-generic	Administration Considerations	Therapeutic Effects	Adverse/Side Effects
HMG-CoA Reductase Inhibitors	atorvastatin	Take at the same time each day, with or without food Report muscle weakness, feeling tired, abdominal pain, or yellowing of skin or eyes	Reduce LDL	Rhabdomyolysis, myalgia, and muscle spasms Abnormal liver enzymes May increase blood glucose Nausea, diarrhea, and dyspepsia

Ezetimibe

Mechanism of Action

Ezetimibe blocks the absorption of cholesterol in the small intestines to reduce LDL.

Indications for Use

This medication is used for treatment of hyperlipidemia and familial hypercholesterolemia.

Nursing Considerations Across the Life Span

If medication is combined with HMG-CoA reductase inhibitors, do not give to pregnant or breastfeeding patients.

Adverse/Side Effects

Use with caution when ezetimibe is combined with additional medication. Patients may experience arthralgia, rhabdomyolysis, hepatic impairment, dizziness, upper respiratory infections, or diarrhea if they are taking this medication. Minimal side effects were reported with monotherapy.[119]

Patient Teaching and Education

Patients should take the prescribed medication as directed and avoid consuming grapefruit juice during drug therapy. The medication should be used with dietary modifications. If the patient experiences muscle pain, tenderness, or weakness, this should be reported to the healthcare provider.[120]

Now let's take a closer look at the medication grid for ezetimibe in Table 6.11b.[121]

---

118   This work is a derivative of *Daily Med* by U.S. National Library of Medicine in the public domain.

119   This work is a derivative of *Daily Med* by U.S. National Library of Medicine in the public domain.

120   uCentral from Unbound Medicine. https://www.unboundmedicine.com/ucentral.

121   This work is a derivative of *Daily Med* by U.S. National Library of Medicine in the public domain.

Table 6.11b: Ezetimibe Medication Grid

Class/Subclass	Prototype-generic	Administration Considerations	Therapeutic Effects	Adverse/Side Effects
Cholesterol Absorption Inhibitor	ezetimibe	Take at the same time each day, with or without food Report muscle weakness, feeling tired, abdominal pain, or yellowing of skin or eyes	Reduce LDL	Arthralgia, rhabdomyolysis Hepatic impairment Dizziness Upper respiratory infection Diarrhea

6.12 BLOOD COAGULATION MODIFIERS

This section will discuss medications that affect blood coagulation and includes several types of medications including anticoagulants, antiplatelets, and thrombolytics, as well as their associated reversal agents.

Anticoagulants prevent the formation of a clot by inhibiting certain types of clotting factors. Anticoagulants include the following drug classes: heparins or unfractionated heparin and low molecular weight heparin (LMWH), warfarin (Coumadin), selective factor Xa inhibitors (rivaroxaban), and direct thrombin inhibitors (dabigatran). Antiplatelets include aspirin and other aggregation inhibitors such as clopidogrel, and thrombolytics include alteplase (tPA). All these types of medications are included on the List of High Alert Medications (HAMs) by the Institute for Safe Medication Practices (ISMP) that require special safeguards to reduce the risk of errors or adverse effects.[122]

The most common anticoagulant errors in acute hospital settings are administration mistakes, including incorrect dosage calculation and infusion rates. The Health Research and Educational Trust focuses on reducing harm related to HAMs by 50% and recommends the following interventions to achieve this goal:

- Educate staff based on evidence and best practices.
- Use standardized order sets and protocols.
- Perform medication reconciliation at all transitions.

Specific interventions regarding anticoagulant therapy include standardization of protocols for withholding and restarting warfarin perioperatively, including pharmacists on rounds to provide decision support for staff administering HAMs and to reduce prescribing errors, pharmacist monitoring of anticoagulants, and pharmacist notification when rescue medications are given.[123]

According to the *Institute for Safe Medication Practices (ISMP) 2016 Annual Report*, there is also a high risk of acute injuries for patients taking anticoagulants outside of the hospital setting. Anticoagulants are commonly used by the elderly to reduce the risk of ischemic stroke, with an estimated 3.8 million people taking oral anticoagulants in 2016. CDC data show that adverse effects of oral anticoagulants account for more emergency department visits than any other class of drugs. Adverse effects range from gastrointestinal bleeding to cerebral hemorrhages, resulting in over 3,000 deaths in 2016.[124]

Since 1954, warfarin has been a standard but hazardous treatment for preventing blood clots. Warfarin requires close laboratory monitoring and individual dose adjustments based on PT and INR lab results. When the pharmaceutical industry began marketing modern replacements for warfarin, including dabigatran (Pradaxa), rivaroxaban (Xarelto), and apixaban (Eliquis), they designed them to be easier to use than warfarin because no laboratory monitoring was required, but not necessarily safer. It is vital for nurses to provide thorough patient and caregiver education for patients prescribed anticoagulants at home. Suggested patient education topics are included for each type of medication below.

---

122   Institute for Safe Medication Practices (ISMP). (2018). *ISMP List of High-Alert Medications in Acute Care Settings*. https://www.ismp.org/sites/default/files/attachments/2018-08/highAlert2018-Acute-Final.pdf.

123   Anderson, P. and Townsend, T. (2015) Preventing high-alert medication errors in hospital patients. *Nurse Today, 10*(5). https://www.americannursetoday.com/wp-content/uploads/2015/05/ant5-CE-421.pdf.

124   Institute for Safe Medication Practices (ISMP). (2017). *QuarterWatch™ (2016 Annual Report) Part II: Oral Anticoagulants—The Nation's Top Risk of Acute Injury from Drugs*. https://www.ismp.org/resources/ quarterwatchtm-2016 -annual-report-part-ii-oral-anticoagulants-nations-top-risk-acute.

Heparin Sodium

Heparin sodium is an anticoagulant that can be injected or used intravenously and is formulated in several dosages. (See Figure 6.25.)[125] Due to heparin being a high-alert medication, hospitals use several processes for storing and labeling the medication to help prevent errors. It is also important to note that there is a type of heparin flush often referred to as "Hep-Lock" that is used to maintain the patency of central lines. The dosage of heparin in heparin IV flushes is much different than the heparin dose used as an intravenous medication to prevent or treat a blood clot.

Most hospitals have weight-based protocols for IV heparin administration that titrate a patient's dosage to be within a therapeutic range based on the results of a lab test called **Partial thromboplastin time (PTT)**. PTT is a blood test that looks at how long it takes for blood to clot. Patients receiving heparin subcutaneous injections to prevent DVTs (deep vein thrombosis) do not require PTT monitoring.

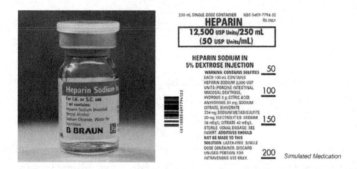

Figure 6.25 Heparin comes in many dosages, and overdose can be deadly, so it is important for the nurse to use safeguards to prevent potential medication errors

Mechanism of Action

Heparin inhibits the activated coagulation factors involved in the clotting sequence, particularly Xa and IIa. Heparin also prevents the formation of a stable fibrin clot by inhibiting the activation of the fibrin stabilizing factor. Heparin does not have fibrinolytic activity; therefore, it will not breakdown existing clots.

Indications for Use

IV heparin is commonly indicated for the treatment of deep venous thromboembolism (DVT) or pulmonary embolism. It is also indicated for use during an acute myocardial infarction. Subcutaneous heparin is commonly indicated to prevent DVT or embolization caused by atrial fibrillation. Heparin IV flushes ("Hep-Locks") are used to maintain the patency of central IV lines.

Nursing Considerations Across the Life Span

When bleeding requires the reversal of heparinization, protamine sulfate by slow infusion will neutralize heparin sodium.

A higher incidence of bleeding has been reported in patients over 60 years of age, especially women.

---

125   "Heparin Sodium sample.jpg" by LHcheM is licensed under CC BY-SA 3.0 and "Heparin in Dextrose Injection" by Chippewa Valley Technical College is licensed under CC BY 4.0.

My Notes

Fatal hemorrhages have occurred due to medication errors. Carefully examine all heparin products to confirm the correct dose prior to the administration of the drug.

IV heparin therapy requires close monitoring of frequent partial thromboplastin time (PTT) results to ensure dosage is in therapeutic range and to reduce the risk of overdose with associated bleeding. Dosage is considered adequate when the activated partial thromboplastin time (APTT) is 1.5 to 2 times the normal or when the whole blood clotting time is elevated approximately 2.5 to 3 times the control value.

This drug is contraindicated in patients with a history of Heparin-Induced Thrombocytopenia (HIT) and Heparin-Induced Thrombocytopenia and Thrombosis (HITT). HIT is a condition where platelets drop 30% or more below a patient's baseline after heparin is administered and can lead to HITT where thrombi are formed.

Use with caution with medication that affects the coagulation cascade due to additive effects that increase the risk of bleeding. When a patient is receiving IV heparin therapy to treat a blood clot, it may be overlapped with oral warfarin to establish anticoagulation therapy after discharge. See more information about this process under the "Warfarin" section.

Adverse/Side Effects

There is a high risk of bleeding that can lead to hemorrhaging. Notify prescribing provider immediately of new signs of bleeding or bruising or sudden changes in vital signs that indicate internal bleeding, such as decreasing blood pressure with an associated increase in heart rate.

Some patients may develop Heparin-Induced Thrombocytopenia (HIT) or Heparin-Induced Thrombocytopenia and Thrombosis (HITT); therefore, heparin should be immediately discontinued.

Patient Teaching and Education

Notify health care staff immediately of new signs of bleeding or bruising. Remind physicians and dentists that they are receiving heparin before any surgery or invasive procedure is scheduled.[126] Patients should avoid medications containing aspirin or NSAIDS. Bleeding precautions should be taken, including the avoidance of IM injections, use of a soft toothbrush, and elective razor.[127]

---

126 This work is a derivative of *Daily Med* by U.S. National Library of Medicine in the public domain.

127 uCentral from Unbound Medicine. https://www.unboundmedicine.com/ucentral.

Now let's take a closer look at the medication grid for heparin in Table 6.12a.[128]

Table 6.12a: Heparin Medication Grid

Class/Subclass	Prototype-generic	Administration Considerations	Therapeutic Effects	Adverse/Side Effects
Anticoagulant	heparin	Injection (subq) or IV Carefully examine all heparin products to confirm the correct choice prior to administration Closely monitor PTT levels in IV therapy to ensure in therapeutic range Protamine sulfate is the reversal agent	Prevention or treatment of DVT or PE	High risk of bleeding Risk of gastrointestinal or cerebral hemorrhage, especially in elderly Risk of Heparin-Induced Thrombocytopenia (HIT) and Heparin-Induced Thrombocytopenia and Thrombosis (HITT)

Low Molecular Weight Heparin (LMWH)

Enoxaparin (Lovenox) is a low molecular weight heparin (LMWH) that is supplied in a prefilled syringe (see Figure 6.26).[129] LMWH heparin formulations do not require lab monitoring.

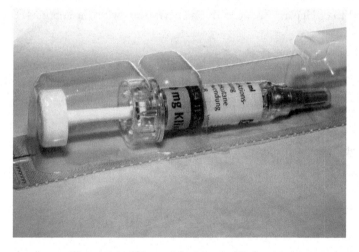

Figure 6.26 Enoxaparin in a prefilled syringe

Mechanism of Action

Enoxaparin is a low molecular weight heparin, which has antithrombotic properties with a higher ratio of anti-Factor Xa to anti-Factor IIa activity compared to heparin.

---

128 This work is a derivative of *Daily Med* by U.S. National Library of Medicine in the public domain.

129 "syringe-disposable-syringe-blister-103059" by stux is licensed under CC0.

My Notes

Indications for Use

It is indicated for the prevention and treatment of deep vein thrombosis (DVT), which may lead to pulmonary embolism (PE). It is also used in combination with aspirin for the treatment of acute myocardial infarction.

Nursing Considerations Across the Life Span

Enoxaparin is administered subcutaneously and preferably in the abdomen for best absorption.

Safety and effectiveness have not been established in pediatric patients. The risk of bleeding increases with age, especially if used concurrently with antiplatelet medications.

Use with caution in patients with renal impairment; risk of bleeding is increased. A dosage adjustment is recommended for patients with severe renal impairment.

Overdosage can be neutralized with a slow IV infusion of protamine sulfate.

Adverse/Side Effects

Black Box Warning: Epidural or spinal hematomas may occur in patients who are anticoagulated with low molecular weight heparins (LMWH) and are receiving neuraxial anesthesia or undergoing spinal puncture. These hematomas may result in long-term or permanent paralysis.

There is a risk of bleeding and hemorrhaging, especially following percutaneous coronary revascularization procedures or with concurrent medication conditions such as recent GI ulcer. It may cause Heparin-Induced Thrombocytopenia (HIT) or Heparin-Induced Thrombocytopenia with Thrombosis (HITT).[130]

Patient Teaching and Education

Notify health care staff immediately of new signs of bleeding or bruising. Remind physicians and dentists that they are receiving heparin before any surgery or invasive procedure is scheduled.[131] Patients should avoid medications containing aspirin or NSAIDS.[132]

Now let's take a closer look at the medication grid on enoxaparin in Table 6.12b.[133]

---

130   This work is a derivative of *Daily Med* by U.S. National Library of Medicine in the public domain.

131   This work is a derivative of *Daily Med* by U.S. National Library of Medicine in the public domain.

132   uCentral from Unbound Medicine. https://www.unboundmedicine.com/ucentral.

133   This work is a derivative of *Daily Med* by U.S. National Library of Medicine in the public domain.

Table 6.12b: Enoxaparin Medication Grid				
Class/Subclass	Prototype-generic	Administration Considerations	Therapeutic Effects	Adverse/Side Effects
Anticoagulant	enoxaparin	Use with caution in patients with kidney disease. If used for a patient undergoing neuraxial anesthesia or a spinal puncture, monitor frequently for neurological impairment. If neurological compromise is noted, urgent treatment is necessary	Prevention	Bleeding Risk of hemorrhage Thrombocytopenia, HIT, or HITT

Warfarin

Warfarin (Coumadin) is an oral anticoagulant formulated in various strengths in different colors to help prevent errors when patients self-administer different dosages at home (see Figure 6.27[134]). Close monitoring of **prothrombin time (PT)** or **international normalized ratio (INR)** is required.

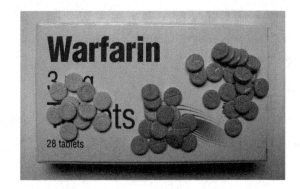

Figure 6.27 Warfarin is an oral pill with various strengths in different colors

Mechanism of Action

Warfarin acts by inhibiting the synthesis of vitamin K-dependent clotting factors, which include Factors II, VII, IX, and X and the anticoagulant proteins C and S.

Indications for Use

Warfarin is indicated for the following:

- Prophylaxis and treatment of venous thrombosis and its extension, pulmonary embolism (PE).

- Prophylaxis and treatment of thromboembolic complications associated with atrial fibrillation (AF) and/or cardiac valve replacement.

---

134   "Warfarintablets5-3-1.jpg" by Gonegonegone is licensed under CC BY-SA 3.0.

- Reduction in the risk of death, recurrent myocardial infarction (MI), and thromboembolic events such as stroke or systemic embolization after myocardial infarction.

Nursing Considerations Across the Life Span

Warfarin is contraindicated in pregnant women except for those with mechanical heart valves; it can cause fetal harm.

Vitamin K is the reversal agent. Fresh frozen plasma may be considered if the requirement to reverse the effects of warfarin sodium is urgent.

Close monitoring of prothrombin time (PT) or international normalized ratio (INR) is required. Therapeutic INR ranges from 2.0 to 3.5, depending on the indication.

In hospitalized patients receiving heparin therapy, there is often a period of overlap where the patient is prescribed both IV heparin and warfarin until the INR reaches therapeutic range. At that point, the IV heparin is discontinued.

Warfarin has significant interactions with many medications; read drug label information before administering.

Warfarin sodium is contraindicated in patients with many conditions, including, but not limited to:

- Hemorrhagic tendencies or blood dyscrasias
- Recent or contemplated surgery of the central nervous system or eye, or traumatic surgery resulting in large open surfaces

Bleeding tendencies associated with:

- Active ulceration or overt bleeding of the gastrointestinal, genitourinary, or respiratory tracts
- Central nervous system hemorrhage
- Cerebral aneurysms and dissecting aorta
- Pericarditis and pericardial effusions
- Bacterial endocarditis

Adverse/Side Effects

Black Box Warnings: Warfarin can cause major or fatal bleeding. Perform regular monitoring of INR in all treated patients. Drugs, dietary changes, and other factors affect INR levels achieved with warfarin therapy. Instruct patients about prevention measures to minimize risk of bleeding and to report signs and symptoms of bleeding. Warfarin can cause acute kidney injury and bleeding risks are increased in patients with liver disease.

Patient Education

Advise patients to:

- Avoid alcohol, cranberries, and grapefruit as they increase the effect of warfarin and the risk for bleeding.

- Strictly adhere to the prescribed dosage schedule.

- Follow INR monitoring guidelines as provided by the prescriber.

- Avoid any activity or sport that may result in traumatic injury.

- Tell their provider if they experience frequent falls because warfarin can increase their risk for bleeding in the brain.

- Eat a normal, balanced diet to maintain a consistent intake of vitamin K (such as green, leafy vegetables).

- Tell all health care professionals and dentists that they are taking warfarin, especially before surgery or dental procedures.

- Use electric razors instead of straight razors.

- Carry identification stating that they are taking warfarin.

- Notify their provider immediately if any unusual bleeding or symptoms occur, such as pain, swelling or discomfort, prolonged bleeding from cuts, increased menstrual flow or vaginal bleeding, nosebleeds, bleeding of gums from brushing, unusual bleeding or bruising, red or dark brown urine, red or tar black stools, headache, dizziness, or weakness. [135]

Now let's take a closer look at the medication grid on warfarin in Table 6.12c. [136]

Table 6.12c: Warfarin Medication Grid				
Class/Subclass	**Prototype-generic**	**Administration Considerations**	**Therapeutic Effects**	**Adverse/Side Effects**
Anticoagulant	warfarin	Oral route Vitamin K is the antidote Monitor INR results before administering medication Use with caution in patients with liver disease	Prevent DVT or PE	Bleeding Hemorrhage

135   This work is a derivative of *Daily Med* by U.S. National Library of Medicine in the public domain.

136   This work is a derivative of *Daily Med* by U.S. National Library of Medicine in the public domain.

Critical Thinking Activity 6.12

A patient who was treated in the hospital for DVT in his left leg has been prescribed warfarin.

1. The patient asks, "Will the warfarin dissolve the clot in my leg?" What is the nurse's best response?

The nurse plans to assess the patient's lab work before administering the warfarin.

2. What blood test(s) are important to monitor for patients taking warfarin, and what is the therapeutic range?

The nurse knows that the patient will need to monitor his diet when taking warfarin.

3. What dietary instructions should be provided to the patient?

The nurse plans to provide patient education regarding this newly prescribed medication.

4. Outline the topics to cover with this high-risk medication.

5. What is the reversal agent for warfarin?

Note: Answers to the Critical Thinking activities can be found in the "Answer Key" sections at the end of the book.

Rivaroxaban

Rivaroxaban (Xarelto) is a selective Xa inhibitor.

Mechanism of Action

Rivaroxaban is a selective inhibitor of factor Xa and indirectly inhibits platelet aggregation induced by thrombin.

Indications for Use

Rivaroxaban is indicated for prevention or treatment of DVT and PE. In combination with aspirin, it is indicated to reduce the risk of major cardiovascular events such as cardiovascular (CV) death, myocardial infarction (MI) and stroke and in patients with chronic coronary artery disease (CAD) or peripheral artery disease (PAD).

Nursing Considerations Across the Life Span

For overdose, activated charcoal can be used to reduce absorption and Andexxa is a reversal agent.

Avoid in patients with moderate to severe liver impairment. Report any unusual bleeding or bruising.

Adverse/Side Effects

Black Box Warning: Epidural or spinal hematomas may occur in patients who are anticoagulated with rivaroxaban and are receiving neuraxial anesthesia or undergoing spinal puncture. These hematomas may result in long-term or permanent paralysis.

Risk of bleeding can be fatal.[137]

Patient Teaching and Education

Patients should report any signs of unusual bleeding or bruising to the healthcare provider. The patient should also notify the provider of all prescriptions, OTC medications, vitamins, and herbal products.[138]

Now let's take a closer look at the medication grid on rivaroxaban in Table 6.12d.[139]

Table 6.12d: Rivaroxaban Medication Grid				
Class/Subclass	**Prototype-generic**	**Administration Considerations**	**Therapeutic Effects**	**Adverse/Side Effects**
Selective Xa Inhibitors	rivaroxaban	Activated charcoal or Andexxa can be used in overdose Avoid in patients with liver impairment	Prevent DVT and PE and and risk of severe cardiovascular events	Bleeding Epidural or spinal hematomas if neuraxial anesthesia or spinal puncture

Dabigatran

Dabigatran (Pradaxa) is a direct-acting thrombin inhibitor.

Mechanism of Action

Dabigatran is a competitive, direct thrombin inhibitor. Because thrombin enables the conversion of fibrinogen into fibrin during the coagulation cascade, its inhibition prevents the development of a thrombus.

Indications for Use

This drug is used to prevent or treat deep vein thromboses (DVT) or pulmonary emboli (PE).

Nursing Considerations Across the Life Span

Overdose: Idarucizumab, a specific reversal agent, is available.

Safety and effectiveness in pediatric patients have not been established.

Adverse/Side Effects

Black Box Warning: Epidural or spinal hematomas may occur in patients who are anticoagulated with dabigatran and are receiving neuraxial anesthesia or undergoing spinal puncture. These hematomas may result in long-term or permanent paralysis.

---

137 This work is a derivative of *Daily Med* by U.S. National Library of Medicine in the public domain.

138 uCentral from Unbound Medicine. https://www.unboundmedicine.com/ucentral.

139 This work is a derivative of *Daily Med* by U.S. National Library of Medicine in the public domain.

OPEN RN
OPEN RESOURCES FOR NURSING

My Notes

Risk of bleeding can be fatal.[140]

Patient Teaching and Education

Patients should report any signs of unusual bleeding or bruising to the healthcare provider. Additionally, dabigatran bottles should be disposed of four months after opening. The patient should also notify the provider of all prescriptions, OTC medications, vitamins, and herbal products.[141]

Now let's take a closer look at the medication grid for dabigatran in Table 6.12e.[142]

Table 6.12e: Dabigatran Medication Grid				
Class/ Subclass	Prototype- generic	Administration Considerations	Therapeutic Effects	Adverse/Side Effects
Direct-acting thrombin inhibitors	dabigatran	Idarucizumab is a specific reversal agent	Prevent or treat DVT or PE	Risk of bleeding that can be fatal Epidural or spinal hematomas if receiving neuraxial anesthesia or undergoing spinal puncture

Antiplatelets

Acetylsalicylic acid (aspirin) and clopidogrel (Plavix) are antiplatelet medications.

During an active myocardial infarction (heart attack), chewable aspirins are used due to their rapid absorption (see Figure 6.28[143]).

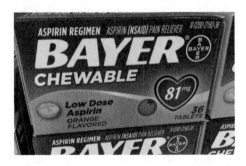

Figure 6.28 Chewable aspirin are used for patients experiencing a MI

Mechanism of Action

Aspirin inhibits platelet activation and aggregation.

---

140 This work is a derivative of *Daily Med* by U.S. National Library of Medicine in the public domain.

141 uCentral from Unbound Medicine. https://www.unboundmedicine.com/ucentral.

142 This work is a derivative of *Daily Med* by U.S. National Library of Medicine in the public domain.

143 "Bayer Aspirin Low Dose" by Mike Mozart is licensed under CC BY 2.0.

Indications for Use

Aspirin is indicated in patients with established peripheral arterial disease or a history of recent myocardial infarction (MI) or stroke to reduce the rate of MI and stroke. It is also indicated to reduce the rate of myocardial infarction (MI) and stroke in patients with ST-elevation and non–ST-segment elevation ACS.

Nursing Considerations Across the Life Span

It is important to remember that the effects of these medications last the life of the platelet (7-10 days), so aspirin will need to be withheld for several days before surgery or certain procedures to prevent excessive bleeding. In elderly patients, there is an increased risk of bleeding events with concurrent use of clopidogrel plus aspirin. Aspirin is contraindicated in children under the age of 12 with flu-like symptoms due to the risk of Reye's syndrome.

Overdose is irreversible.

Clopidogrel is metabolized to its active metabolite by CYP2C19.

Concomitant use of drugs that inhibit the activity of this enzyme results in reduced plasma concentrations of the active metabolite of clopidogrel and a reduction in platelet inhibition.

Adverse/Side Effects

Increased risk of bleeding.

Black Box Warning: Reduced effectiveness for patients referred to as "CYP2C19 poor metabolizers."

Patient Teaching and Education

Patients should report tinnitus, unusual bleeding of the gums, bruising, or blood in the stool to the healthcare provider immediately. While on antiplatelet therapy, patients should avoid alcohol to prevent gastric irritation. Additionally, patients should avoid NSAIDs while receiving antiplatelet therapy.[144]

Now let's take a closer look at the medication grid for acetylsalicylic acid and clopidogrel in Table 6.12f.[145]

Table 6.12f: Acetylsalicylic Acid and Clopidogrel Medication Grid				
Class/ Subclass	Prototype-generic	Administration Considerations	Therapeutic Effects	Adverse/Side Effects
Antiplatelets	acetylsalicylic acid (Aspirin) clopidogrel	Administer with food to reduce risk of GI upset and bleeding Monitor for bleeding Effects last for 7-10 days	Reduce risk of MI and stroke	Increased risk of bleeding

---

144   uCentral from Unbound Medicine. https://www.unboundmedicine.com/ucentral.

145   This work is a derivative of *Daily Med* by U.S. National Library of Medicine in the public domain.

Alteplase (tPA)

Alteplase (tPA) is a thrombolytic used to break up clots. It has a very short half-life of 5 minutes so it can open a clogged artery rapidly. It is often given with heparin to prevent reocclusion of the affected blood vessel. There is also a smaller dosage form that is used to flush clogged IV or arterial lines.[146]

Mechanism of Action

Alteplase binds to fibrin in a thrombus and converts the entrapped plasminogen to plasmin, thus breaking down the clot.

Indications for Use

Alteplase is indicated for the acute treatment of myocardial infarction (MI), stroke, or massive pulmonary embolism (PE). It is also used to clear central lines such as a peripherally inserted central line catheter (PICC).

Nursing Considerations Across the Life Span

The drug is contraindicated in situations in which the risk of significant bleeding is greater than the potential benefit such as:

- Active internal or intracranial bleeding
- History of recent stroke
- Recent (within 3 months) intracranial or intraspinal surgery or serious head trauma
- Presence of intracranial conditions that may increase the risk of bleeding (e.g., some neoplasms, arteriovenous malformations, or aneurysms)
- Current severe uncontrolled hypertension

Significant post-administration monitoring is performed due to the risk of life-threatening bleeding.

Adverse/Side Effects

This drug can cause significant, sometimes fatal, internal or external bleeding, especially at arterial and venous puncture sites. Avoid intramuscular injections and perform venipunctures carefully and only as required. It can increase the risk of thrombo-embolic events in patients with high likelihood of left heart thrombus, such as patients with atrial fibrillation.

Patient Teaching and Education

Patients must institute bleeding precautions to prevent complications of therapy.[147]

Now let's take a closer look at the medication grid for alteplase in Table 6.12g.[148]

---

146   McCuistion, L., Vuljoin-DiMaggio, K., Winton, M, and Yeager, J. (2018). *Pharmacology: A patient-centered nursing process approach*. pp. 443–454. Elsevier.

147   uCentral from Unbound Medicine. https://www.unboundmedicine.com/ucentral.

148   This work is a derivative of *Daily Med* by U.S. National Library of Medicine in the public domain.

Table 6.12g: Alteplase Medication Grid

Class/ Subclass	Prototype- generic	Administration Considerations	Therapeutic Effects	Adverse/Side Effects
Thrombolytic	alteplase (tPA)	Contraindicated in many conditions where the risk of bleeding outweighs the potential benefit	Break down a life-threatening clot in MI, stroke, or massive PE	Risk of severe bleeding that can be fatal

My Notes

6.13 ERECTILE AGENTS

Sildenafil (Viagra) is commonly known to treat erectile dysfunction. This medication was originally developed for improvement of pulmonary hypertension, but has been found to be useful for additional indications. However, patients taking this medication cannot take nitroglycerin due to severe hypotension.

Mechanism of Action

Sildenafil inhibits phosphodiesterase (PDE-5) in the pulmonary smooth muscle and corpus cavernosum. This allows for relaxation in the smooth muscle.

Indications for Use

Sildenafil is used in the treatment of pulmonary hypertension and erectile dysfunction.

Nursing Considerations Across the Life Span

Pediatric patients have shown to have an increase in mortality with sildenafil. Dose adjustments are needed for patients with hepatic and renal impairment. Use cautiously with geriatric patients with decreased hepatic, renal, and cardiac functions.

Adverse/Side Effects

Patients taking sildenafil may expect to experience hypotension, visual or hearing loss, priapism (male), headache, or vaso-occlusive crisis. If patients have priapism that lasts longer than 4 hours, they should seek medical attention.[149]

Patient Education and Teaching

Patients should be instructed to take medications as directed and should seek immediate medical attention if chest pain occurs. Patients need education regarding the need to report priapism lasting longer than 4 hours or if they notice any dizziness or decrease in hearing ability.[150]

---

149   This work is a derivative of *Daily Med* by U.S. National Library of Medicine in the public domain.

150   uCentral from Unbound Medicine. https://www.unboundmedicine.com/ucentral.

Now let's take a closer look at the medication grid on sildenafil in Table 6.13.[151]

Table 6.13: Sildenafil Medication Grid

Class/Subclass	Prototype-generic	Administration Considerations	Therapeutic Effect	Adverse/Side Effects
Phosphodiesterase inhibitor	sildenafil	Do not administer with organic nitrates If priapism persists longer than 4 hours, seek medical attention	Decrease pulmonary hypertension Improving erectile dysfunction symptoms	Hypotension Visual loss, hearing loss Priapism Headache Vaso-occlusive crisis due to sickle cell anemia

---

151   This work is a derivative of *Daily Med* by U.S. National Library of Medicine in the public domain.

6.14 MODULE LEARNING ACTIVITIES

Interactive Activities

 An interactive or media element has been excluded from this version of the text. You can view it online here: https://wtcs.pressbooks.pub/pharmacology/?p=2800

GLOSSARY

Afterload: The tension that the ventricles must develop to pump blood effectively against the resistance in the vascular system.

Anticoagulant: Any substance that opposes coagulation.

Arrhythmia: A deviation from the normal pattern of impulse conduction and contraction of the heart, which if serious and untreated, can lead to decreased cardiac output and death.

Arteriosclerosis: A condition when compliance in an artery is reduced and pressure and resistance within the vessel increase. This is a leading cause of hypertension and coronary heart disease, as it causes the heart to work harder to generate a pressure great enough to overcome the resistance.

Artery: A blood vessel that carries blood away from the heart (except for pulmonary arteries that carry oxygenated blood from the lungs back to the heart).

Atherosclerosis: A buildup, called plaque, that can narrow arteries enough to impair blood flow.

Blood pressure: A type of hydrostatic pressure, or the force exerted by blood on the walls of the blood vessels or the chambers of the heart.

Capillaries: Smallest arteries where nutrients and wastes are exchanged at the cellular level.

Cardiac Output (CO): To calculate this value, multiply stroke volume (SV), the amount of blood pumped by each ventricle, by heart rate (HR), in contractions per minute (or beats per minute, bpm). It can be represented mathematically by the following equation: CO = HR × SV.

Cerebrovascular Accident (CVA): Lack of blood flow to the brain that can cause irreversible brain damage, often referred to as a "stroke."

Coagulation: The formation of a blood clot.

Compliance: The ability of any compartment to expand to accommodate increased content. The greater the compliance of an artery, the more effectively it is able to expand to accommodate surges in blood flow without increased resistance or blood pressure. Veins are more compliant than arteries and can expand to hold more blood. When vascular disease causes stiffening of arteries, compliance is reduced and resistance to blood flow is increased.

Contractility: The force of contraction of the heart.

Diastole: The period of relaxation that occurs as the chambers fill with blood.

Edema: The presence of excess tissue fluid around the cells.

Embolus: When a portion of a thrombus breaks free from the vessel wall and enters the circulation. An embolus that is carried through the bloodstream can be large enough to block a vessel critical to a major organ. When it becomes trapped, an embolus is called an embolism. In the heart, brain, or lungs, an embolism may accordingly cause a heart attack, a stroke, or a pulmonary embolism.

Fibrillation: An uncoordinated beating of the heart, which if serious and untreated, can lead to decreased cardiac output and death.

Fibrinolysis: The gradual degradation of a clot.

Hemostasis: The process by which the body temporarily seals a ruptured blood vessel and prevents further loss of blood.

Hyperlipidemia: Elevated cholesterol levels in the blood that increase a patient's risk for heart attack and stroke.

Hypertension: Chronically elevated blood pressure.

Hypervolemia: Excessive fluid volume caused by retention of water and sodium, as seen in patients with heart failure, liver cirrhosis, and some forms of kidney disease.

Hypovolemia: Decreased blood volume that may be caused by bleeding, dehydration, vomiting, severe burns, or by diuretics used to treat hypertension. Treatment typically includes intravenous fluid replacement.

My Notes

International Normalized Ratio (INR): A blood test used to monitor the effects of warfarin and to achieve therapeutic range, generally between 2.0 and 3.5 based on the indication.

Ischemia: Reduced blood flow to the tissue region "downstream" of the narrowed vessel.

Loop of Henle: A component of the nephron where loop diuretics act to eliminate sodium and water.

Myocardial Infarction (MI): Commonly referred to as a heart attack, resulting from a lack of blood flow (ischemia) and oxygen to a region of the heart, resulting in death of the cardiac muscle cells.

Negative Inotropic factors: Factors that decrease contractility.

Partial Thromboplastin Time (PTT): A blood test used to monitor how long it takes for a patient's blood to clot. PTT is used for patients receiving IV heparin therapy to achieve therapeutic range. Dosage is considered adequate when the activated partial thromboplastin time (APTT) is 1.5 to 2 times the normal or when the whole blood clotting time is elevated approximately 2.5 to 3 times the control value.

Positive inotropic factors: Factors that increase contractility.

Preload: The amount of blood in the atria just prior to atrial contraction.

Prothrombin Time (PT): A blood test that measures how long it takes for a patient's blood to clot. PT is used to monitor the effects of warfarin in preventing clot formation.

Renin-Angiotensin-Aldosterone System (RAAS): Renin converts the plasma protein angiotensinogen into its active form—Angiotensin I. Angiotensin I circulates in the blood and is then converted into angiotensin II in the lungs. This reaction is catalyzed by the angiotensin-converting enzyme (ACE). Angiotensin II is a powerful vasoconstrictor, greatly increasing blood pressure. It also stimulates the release of ADH and aldosterone, a hormone produced by the adrenal cortex. Aldosterone increases the reabsorption of sodium into the blood by the kidneys, causing reabsorption of water and increasing blood volume and raising blood pressure.

Sinoatrial (SA) node: Normal cardiac rhythm is established by the sinoatrial (SA) node. The SA node has the highest inherent rate of depolarization and is known as the pacemaker of the heart.

Sinus rhythm: Normal electrical pattern followed by contraction of the heart.

Stroke Volume (SV): The amount of blood that both ventricles pump during each contraction, normally in the range of 70–80 mL.

Systole: The period of contraction that the heart undergoes while it pumps blood into circulation.

Thrombus: An aggregation of platelets, erythrocytes, and WBCs trapped within a mass of fibrin strands that adhere to the vessel wall and decrease the flow of blood or totally block the flow of blood.

Transient Ischemic Attack (TIA): Occurs when blood flow is interrupted to the brain, even for just a few seconds, resulting in loss of consciousness or temporary loss of neurological function.

Veins: Blood vessels that conduct blood toward the heart (except for pulmonary veins that carry deoxygenated blood from the heart to the lungs).

Venous reserve: Volume of blood located in venous networks within the liver, bone marrow, and integument.

Chapter VII

Gastrointestinal

7.1   GASTROINTESTINAL INTRODUCTION

Learning Objectives

- Cite the classifications and actions of gastrointestinal system drugs
- Give examples of when, how, and to whom gastrointestinal system drugs may be administered
- Identify the side effects and special considerations associated with gastrointestinal system drug therapy
- Identify considerations and implications of using gastrointestinal system medications across the life span
- Apply evidence-based concepts when using the nursing process
- Identify indications and adverse/side effects associated with the use of herbal supplements
- Identify and interpret related laboratory tests

Gastrointestinal complaints are a commonplace occurrence. How many times have you heard someone complaining of an upset stomach, heartburn, nausea, constipation, or diarrhea? Occasionally, these ailments will go away on their own . . . but if they do not, there are a variety of medications that can be used to treat the disease or symptom. Treatment can involve both the use of prescription and nonprescription drug therapy, in addition to nonpharmacological interventions. In this chapter, you will learn about medications used to treat common disorders within the gastrointestinal system.

Prior to the examination of specific medication classes, it is important to have a clear understanding of the various components that make up the gastrointestinal system. Use the following "Basics" section to review selected anatomy and physiology of the gastrointestinal system.

7.2 BASICS: GASTROINTESTINAL SYSTEM REVIEW

Overview of Gastrointestinal System and Processes

There are several supplementary sources you can use to review anatomy and physiology information that is important to know to understand how GI medications work. Figure 7.1[1] illustrates the anatomical components of the gastrointestinal system. Links are provided below to the OpenStax *Anatomy and Physiology* book for further details regarding the following selected areas: overview of the digestive system, digestive system processes and regulation, the stomach, the small and large intestines, and chemical digestion and absorption. Box 7.2 contains links to supplementary videos further explaining the gastrointestinal system and digestive system. Medications related to hyperacidity, bowel disorders, and nausea and vomiting will be discussed in this chapter with reference to how they target pathophysiological concepts related to these organs and processes.

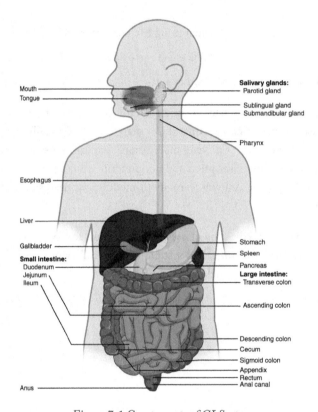

Figure 7.1 Components of GI System

Links to Open Stax A&P detailed content related to this module:[2]

🔗 **Overview of the Digestive System**

🔗 **Digestive System Processes and Regulation**

---

1 "Components of the Digestive System" by CNX OpenStax is licensed under CC BY 4.0 Access for free at https://openstax.org/books/anatomy-and-physiology/pages/23-1-overview-of-the-digestive-system.

2 This work is a derivative of *Anatomy and Physiology* by OpenStax licensed under CC BY 4.0. Access for free at https://openstax.org/books/anatomy-and-physiology/pages/1-introduction.

🔗 **The Stomach**

🔗 **The Small and Large Intestines**

🔗 **Chemical Digestion and Absorption: A Closer Look**

Box 7.2 – Video links reviewing the gastrointestinal system and digestive processes

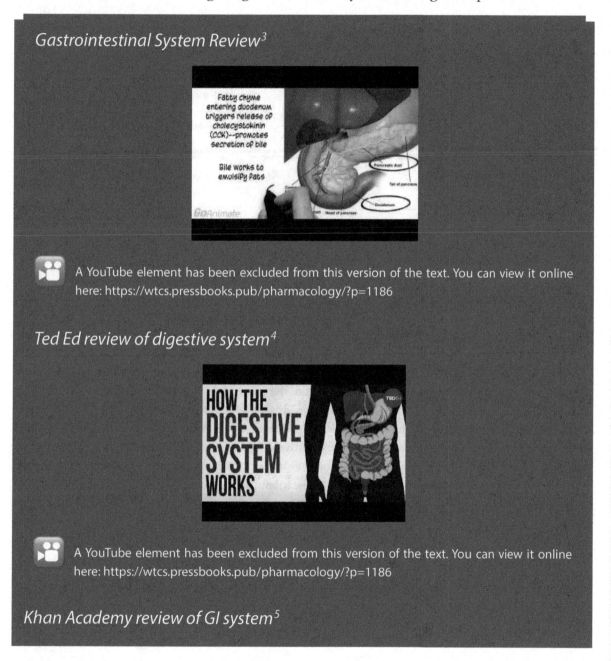

Gastrointestinal System Review[3]

A YouTube element has been excluded from this version of the text. You can view it online here: https://wtcs.pressbooks.pub/pharmacology/?p=1186

Ted Ed review of digestive system[4]

A YouTube element has been excluded from this version of the text. You can view it online here: https://wtcs.pressbooks.pub/pharmacology/?p=1186

Khan Academy review of GI system[5]

---

3   Forciea, B. (2015, March 18). *Anatomy and Physiology of the Digestive System* [Video]. YouTube. All rights reserved. Video used with permission. https://youtu.be/1ssJV-EpfiQ.

4   Bryce, E. (2017, December 14). *How Your Digestive System Works.* [YouTube]. https://youtu.be/Og5xAdC8EUI.

5   Meet the Gastrointestinal Tract! by Raja Narayan is licensed under CC BY-NC-SA 3.0.

7.3 ANTI-ULCER MEDICATIONS

Pathophysiology

The stomach contains cells that secrete different substances as part of the digestive process: parietal cells, chief cells, and surface epithelium cells. See an image of the stomach and these cells in Figure 7.2.[6]

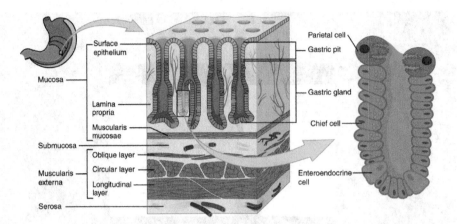

Figure 7.2 An image of the stomach with surface epithelium cells in the mucosa, and an enlarged image of the gastric gland showing chief cells and parietal cells

Surface epithelium cells are found within the lining of the stomach and secrete mucus as a protective coating. Parietal cells and chief cells are found within the gastric glands. **Parietal cells** produce and secrete hydrochloric acid (HCl) to maintain the acidity of the environment of a pH of 1 to 4. Parietal cells also secrete a substance called **intrinsic factor**, which is necessary for the absorption of vitamin B12 in the small intestine. Parietal cells are the primary site of action for many drugs that treat acid-related disorders. Chief cells secrete pepsinogen that becomes **pepsin**, a digestive enzyme, when exposed to acid. The stomach also contains enteroendocrine cells (ECL or enterochromaffin-like cells) located in the gastric glands that secrete substances including serotonin, histamine, and somatostatin. G cells in the stomach secrete gastrin that promotes secretions of digestive substances. Although these cells play an important role in the digestive system, acid-related diseases can occur when there is an imbalance of secretions. The most common mild to moderate hyperacidic condition is **gastroesophageal reflux disease (GERD)**, often referred to by patients as heartburn, indigestion, or sour stomach. GERD is caused by excessive hydrochloric acid that tends to back up, or reflux, into the lower esophagus. See Figure 7.3 for an illustration of GERD.[7]

6 "2415 Histology of StomachN.jpg" by CNX OpenStax is licensed under CC BY 3.0 Access for free at https://cnx.org /contents/FPtK1zmh@16.7:O9dvCxUQ@8/23-4-The-Stomach.

7 "GERD.png" by BruceBlaus is licensed under CC BY-SA 4.0.

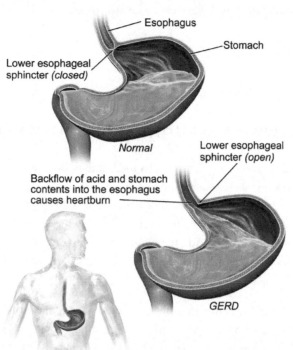

Gastroesophageal Reflux Disease (GERD)

Figure 7.3 Illustration of GERD

Peptic ulcer disease (PUD) occurs when gastric or duodenal ulcers are caused by the breakdown of GI mucosa by pepsin, in combination with the caustic effects of hydrochloric acid. PUD is the most harmful disease related to hyperacidity because it can result in bleeding ulcers, a life-threatening condition.

Stress-related mucosal damage is another common condition that can occur in hospitalized patients leading to PUD. Thus, many post-operative or critically ill patients receive medication to prevent the formation of a stress ulcer, which is also called **prophylaxis**.[8] See an image of a duodenal ulcer in Figure 7.4.[9]

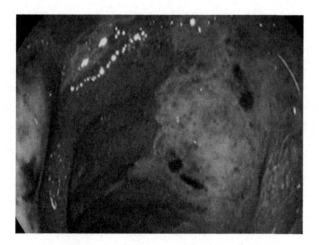

Figure 7.4 Image of a duodenal ulcer

---

8   Lilley, L., Collins, S., and Snyder, J. (2014). *Pharmacology and the Nursing Process*. pp. 782–862. Elsevier.

9   ""Duodenal ulcer01.jpg" by melvil is licensed under CC BY-SA 4.0.

Links to supplementary videos illustrating heartburn and gastric ulcers:

🔗 **Heartburn**[10]

🔗 **Gastric ulcer**[11]

Overall Nursing Considerations for Hyperacidity Medications

Assessments: Whenever a nurse administers hyperacidity medications, there are common assessments that should be documented, such as an abdominal assessment and documentation of bowel patterns. During therapy, the nurse should continue to assess for potential medication interactions and side effects and be aware that vitamin B12 malabsorption may occur whenever stomach acidity levels are altered. Based on the category of medication, renal and liver function may require monitoring. Additionally, if a patient complains of chest pain, the nurse should perform a complete focused cardiac assessment and not assume it is GI-related because patients may erroneously attribute many cardiac conditions to "heartburn."

Implementation: The nurse should read the drug label information and follow the recommendations for administering hyperacidity medications with other medications or the intake of food. Cultural preferences should also be accommodated when safe and feasible because the patient may believe in alternative methods for treating GI discomfort. A written plan of care with modifications for safe use of medications with these alternative methods may be required.

Evaluation: Patients should experience improvement of symptoms within the defined time period; if not, the provider should be notified. Increased pain or new symptoms of coughing/vomiting of blood should be immediately reported because these symptoms can be signs of a life-threatening bleeding ulcer.

Hyperacidity Medication Classes

There are four major classes of medications used to treat hyperacidity conditions: antacids, H2-receptor antagonists, proton pump inhibitors, and mucosal protectants. Each class of medication is further described below.

Antacids

Antacids (see Figure 7.5[12]) are used to neutralize stomach acid and reduce the symptoms of heartburn. There are many OTC medications available for this purpose, such as calcium carbonate, aluminum hydroxide, and magnesium hydroxide. Calcium carbonate is the prototype discussed as an example. Be sure to read drug label information regarding antacids as you administer them because each type has its own specific side effects. Many antacids also contain simethicone, an antiflatulent used for gas relief. Simethicone is further described in the medication grid below.

---

10   MedlinePlus. Bethesda (MD): National Library of Medicine (US); [updated 2019 October 23]. Heartburn; [updated 2019 October 2; cited 2019 October 27] https://medlineplus.gov/ency/anatomyvideos/000068.htm.

11   Blausen Medical. (2015, November 17). *Gastric Ulcers* [Video].https://blausen.com/en/video/gastric-ulcers/#.

12   "Antacid-L478.jpg" by Midnightcomm is licensed under CC BY-SA 3.0.

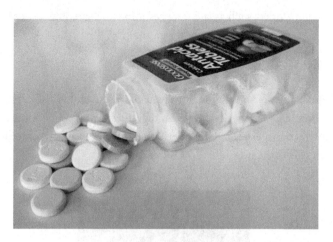

Figure 7.5 Antacids

Indications

Antacids are used to relieve heartburn, acid indigestion, and upset stomach.

Mechanism of Action

Antacids neutralize gastric acidity and elevate the pH of the stomach. Elevated pH also inactivates pepsin, a digestive enzyme.

Specific Administration Considerations

Calcium carbonate comes in various formations such as a tablet, a chewable tablet, a capsule, or liquid to take by mouth. It is usually taken three or four times a day. Chewable tablets should be chewed thoroughly before being swallowed; do not swallow them whole. The patient should drink a full glass of water after taking either the regular or chewable tablets or capsules. Some liquid forms of calcium carbonate must be shaken well before use. Do not administer calcium carbonate within 1-2 hours of other medicines because calcium may decrease the effectiveness of the other medicine. Calcium carbonate may be contraindicated in patients with preexisting kidney disease because it may cause **hypercalcemia**. Common side effects of calcium carbonate include constipation and **rebound hyperacidity** when it is discontinued.[13]

Patient Teaching and Education

In addition to the information under "Specific Administration Considerations," patients should be reminded to take OTC meds appropriately as prescribed and to not exceed the maximum dose. Other interventions to prevent

---

13   A.D.A.M. Medical Encyclopedia [Internet]. Atlanta (GA): A.D.A.M., Inc.; ©2019. Heartburn; [reviewed 2019 May 10; cited 2019 October 27]. https://medlineplus.gov/ency/anatomyvideos/000068.htm.

hyperacidity can also be recommended, such as smoking cessation and avoiding food and beverages that can cause increased acidity (alcohol, high-fat or spicy foods, and caffeine).[14, 15, 16, 17]

H2-Receptor Antagonist

A common H2-receptor antagonist is famotidine. It is available OTC and is also often prescribed orally or as an IV injection in the hospital setting. Other H2-receptor antagonists include cimetidine and ranitidine. Cimetidine has a high risk of drug interactions, especially in elderly patients because of its binding to **cytochrome P-450 enzymes** in the liver, which affects the metabolism of other drugs.

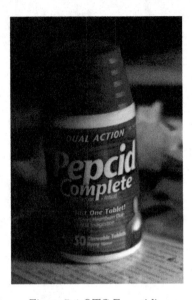

Figure 7.6 OTC Famotidine

Indications

Famotidine (see Figure 7.6[18]) is used to treat GERD, peptic ulcer disease, erosive esophagitis, and hypersecretory conditions, or as adjunct treatment for the control of upper GI bleeding. OTC famotidine is also used to treat heartburn or sour stomach.

Mechanism of Action

H2-receptor antagonists block histamine's action at the H2 receptor of the parietal cell, thus reducing the production of hydrochloric acid.

---

14   Lilley, L., Collins, S., and Snyder, J. (2014). *Pharmacology and the Nursing Process. pp. 782–862. Elsevier.*

15   McCuistion, L., Vuljoin-DiMaggio, K., Winton, M, and Yeager, J. (2018). *Pharmacology: A patient-centered nursing process approach.* pp. 443–454. Elsevier.

16   This work is a derivative of *Daily Med* by U.S. National Library of Medicine in the public domain.

17   A.D.A.M. Medical Encyclopedia [Internet]. Atlanta (GA): A.D.A.M., Inc.; ©2019. Heartburn; [reviewed 2019 May 10; cited 2019 October 27]. https://medlineplus.gov/ency/anatomyvideos/000068.htm.

18   "My Still LIfe" by Bast Productions is licensed under CC BY-NC-ND 2.0.

Specific Administration Considerations

To prevent symptoms, oral famotidine is taken 15 to 60 minutes before eating foods or drinking drinks that may cause heartburn. Preexisting liver and kidney disease may require dosage adjustment. Famotidine is supported by evidence as safe for use in pediatric patients younger than 1 year old, as well as in geriatric patients.

Patient Teaching and Education

Patients taking the oral suspension should be instructed to shake it vigorously for 5 to 10 seconds prior to each use.[19, 20] The medication may cause constipation so fluids and high-fiber diet should be encouraged. Additionally, smoking interferes with histamine antagonists and should be discouraged.[21, 22]

Proton Pump Inhibitors

A common proton pump inhibitor (PPI) is pantoprazole (see Figure 7.7[23]). It may be prescribed in various routes including orally, with an NG tube, or as an IV injection in the hospital setting. Other PPIs include esomeprazole, lansoprazole, and omeprazole. PPIs are more powerful than antacids and H2-receptor antagonists.

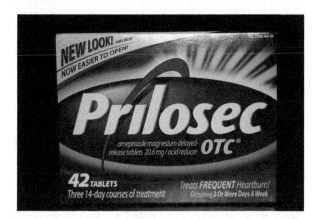

Figure 7.7 OTC Omeprazole

Indications

Pantoprazole is used to treat damage from gastroesophageal reflux disease (GERD) in adults and children five years of age and older by allowing the esophagus to heal and prevent further damage. It is also used to treat conditions where the stomach produces too much acid, such as Zollinger-Ellison syndrome in adults. PPIs may also be given in combination with antibiotics to treat *H. Pylori* infections, a common cause of duodenal ulcers.

---

19   Lilley, L., Collins, S., Snyder, J. (2014). *Pharmacology and the Nursing Process*. pp. 782–862. Elsevier.

20   McCuistion, L., Vuljoin-DiMaggio, K., Winton, M, and Yeager, J. (2018). *Pharmacology: A patient-centered nursing process approach*. pp. 443–454. Elsevier.

21   This work is a derivative of *Daily Med* by U.S. National Library of Medicine in the public domain.

22   A.D.A.M. Medical Encyclopedia [Internet]. Atlanta (GA): A.D.A.M., Inc.; ©2019. Heartburn; [reviewed 2019 May 10; cited 2019 October 27]. https://medlineplus.gov/ency/anatomyvideos/000068.htm.

23   "Prilosec Box 001" by cygnus921 is licensed under CC BY 2.0.

Mechanism of Action

PPIs bind to the hydrogen-potassium ATPase enzyme system of the parietal cell, also referred to as the "proton pump" because it pumps hydrogen ions into the stomach. PPIs inhibit the secretion of hydrochloric acid, and the antisecretory effect lasts longer than 24 hours.

Specific Administration Considerations

Packets of delayed-release granules must be mixed with applesauce or apple juice and taken by mouth or given through a feeding tube. Consult the labeling of concomitantly used drugs to obtain further information about interactions because PPIs can interfere with the liver metabolism of other drugs. IV pantoprazole can potentially exacerbate zinc deficiency, and long-term therapy can cause hypomagnesemia, so the nurse should monitor for these deficiencies.

Patient Teaching and Education

In addition to the considerations above, instruct patients to call their provider if their condition does not improve or gets worse, especially if bleeding occurs.[24, 25] Use of alcohol, NSAIDS, or foods that cause GI irritation should be discouraged.[26, 27]

Mucosal Protectants

Sucralfate is a mucosal protectant used to cover and protect gastrointestinal ulcers.

Indications

Sucralfate is used in the treatment of ulcers.

Mechanism of Action

Sucralfate locally covers the ulcer site in the GI tract and protects it against further attack by acid, pepsin, and bile salts. It is minimally absorbed by the gastrointestinal tract.

Specific Administration Considerations

Administer sucralfate on an empty stomach, 2 hours after or 1 hour before meals. Constipation may occur. Sucralfate should be cautiously used with patients with chronic renal failure or those receiving dialysis due to impaired excretion of small amounts of absorbed aluminum that can occur with sucralfate.

24   Lilley, L., Collins, S., Snyder, J. (2014). *Pharmacology and the Nursing Process.* pp. 782–862. Elsevier.

25   McCuistion, L., Vuljoin-DiMaggio, K., Winton, M, Yeager, J. (2018). *Pharmacology: A patient-centered nursing process approach.* pp. 443–454. Elsevier.

26   This work is a derivative of *Daily Med* by U.S. National Library of Medicine in the public domain.

27   A.D.A.M. Medical Encyclopedia [Internet]. Atlanta (GA): A.D.A.M., Inc.; ©2019. Heartburn; [reviewed 2019 May 10; cited 2019 October 27; https://medlineplus.gov/ency/anatomyvideos/000068.htm.

Patient Teaching and Education

In addition to the considerations above, instruct patients to call their provider if their condition does not improve or gets worse. [28, 29, 30, 31]

Antiflatulent

Simethicone is an antiflatulent that is commonly found in other OTC antacids (see Figure 7.8[32]). It is also safe for use in infants. Gas commonly occurs in the GI tract due to digestive processes and the swallowing of air. Gaseous distension can also occur postoperatively.

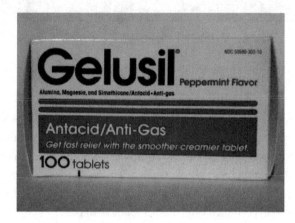

Figure 7.8 OTC Simethicone

Indications

Simethicone is used to treat the symptoms of gas such as uncomfortable or painful pressure, fullness, and bloating.

Mechanism of Action

Simethicone works by altering the elasticity of the mucous-coated gas bubbles, which cause them to break into smaller bubbles, thus reducing pain and facilitating expulsion.

Specific Administration Considerations

Simethicone is usually taken four times a day, after meals and at bedtime. For liquid form, shake drops before administering.

28   Lilley, L., Collins, S., Snyder, J. (2014). *Pharmacology and the Nursing Process.* pp. 782–862. Elsevier.

29   McCuistion, L., Vuljoin-DiMaggio, K., Winton, M, and Yeager, J. (2018). *Pharmacology: A Patient-Centered Nursing Process Approach.* p.188–194 and 604–633. Elsevier.

30   This work is a derivative of *Daily Med* by U.S. National Library of Medicine in the public domain.

31   A.D.A.M. Medical Encyclopedia [Internet]. Atlanta (GA): A.D.A.M., Inc.; ©2019. Heartburn; [reviewed 2019 May 10; cited 2019 October 27]. https://medlineplus.gov/ency/anatomyvideos/000068.htm.

32   "Gelusil Antacid and Anti-Gas" by Wellspring Pharmaceutical is licensed under CC BY 2.0.

Patient Teaching and Education

Patients can be instructed about other measures to assist with gas expulsion such as changing position, ambulation, avoiding the use of straws, and tapering intake of beans and cruciferous vegetables. [33, 34, 35, 36]

Interactive Activity

 An interactive or media element has been excluded from this version of the text. You can view it online here: https://wtcs.pressbooks.pub/pharmacology/?p=1194

Now let's take a closer look at the medication grids comparing medications used to treat hyperacidity in Table 7.3. [37, 38, 39, 40]

Medication grids are intended to assist students to learn key points about each medication. Because information about medication is constantly changing, nurses should always consult evidence-based resources to review current recommendations before administering specific medication. Basic information related to each class of medication is outlined below. Detailed information on a specific medication can be found for free at *Daily Med*. On the home page, enter the drug name in the search bar to read more about the medication. Prototype/generic medications listed in the grids below are also hyperlinked directly to a *Daily Med* page.

---

33   Lilley, L., Collins, S., Snyder, J. (2014). *Pharmacology and the Nursing Process.* pp. 782–862. Elsevier.

34   McCuistion, L., Vuljoin-DiMaggio, K., Winton, M, and Yeager, J. (2018). *Pharmacology: A patient-centered nursing process approach.* pp. 443–454. Elsevier.

35   This work is a derivative of *Daily Med* by U.S. National Library of Medicine in the public domain.

36   A.D.A.M. Medical Encyclopedia [Internet]. Atlanta (GA): A.D.A.M., Inc.; ©2019. Heartburn; [reviewed 2019 May 10; cited 2019 October 27]. https://medlineplus.gov/ency/anatomyvideos/000068.htm.

37   Lilley, L., Collins, S., and Snyder, J. (2014). *Pharmacology and the Nursing Process.* pp. 782–862. Elsevier.

38   McCuistion, L., Vuljoin-DiMaggio, K., Winton, M, and Yeager, J. (2018). *Pharmacology: A patient-centered nursing process approach.* pp. 443–454. Elsevier.

39   This work is a derivative of *Daily Med* by U.S. National Library of Medicine in the public domain.

40   A.D.A.M. Medical Encyclopedia [Internet]. Atlanta (GA): A.D.A.M., Inc.; ©2019. Heartburn; [reviewed 2019 May 10; cited 2019 October 27]. https://medlineplus.gov/ency/anatomyvideos/000068.htm.

Table 7.3: Medication Grid Comparing Hyperacidity Medications

Class	Prototype	Administration Considerations	Therapeutic Effects	Adverse/Side Effects
Antacid	calcium carbonate	Do not administer within 1-2 hours of other medications Drink a full glass of water after administration Use cautiously with renal disease	Decreased symptoms of heartburn or sour stomach	Constipation Hypercalcemia Rebound hyperacidity when discontinued
H2 blocker	famotidine	Administer 15 to 60 minutes before eating foods or drinking drinks that may cause heartburn Preexisting liver and kidney disease may require dosage adjustment	Decreased symptoms of heartburn or sour stomach Decreased pain if ulcers are present	Side effects: headache, dizziness, constipation, and diarrhea Immediately report increased pain or other signs of bleeding ulcers such as coughing/vomiting of blood
Proton Pump Inhibitor	pantoprazole	Delayed release can be taken with or without food Administer granules with apple juice or applesauce	Decreased symptoms of heartburn and pain	Hypersensitivity; anaphylaxis and serious skin reactions Potential zinc, magnesium, or B12 deficiency Headache, abdominal pain, diarrhea, constipation Acute renal dysfunction Osteoporosis-related bone fracture Acute lupus erythematosus Immediately report increased pain or other signs of bleeding ulcers such as coughing/vomiting of blood
Mucosal protectants	sucralfate	Administer sucralfate on an empty stomach, 2 hours after or 1 hour before meals Use cautiously used patients with chronic renal failure	Healing of ulcer	Constipation
Antiflatulant	simethicone	Shake drops before administering	Relief of gas discomfort	None

Critical Thinking Activity 7.3

A patient who recently underwent surgery has a medication order for daily pantoprazole. The nurse reviews the patient's medical history and finds no history of GERD or peptic ulcer disease. The patient does not report any symptoms of heartburn, stomach pain, or sour stomach. The nurse reviews the physician orders for an indication for this medication before calling the provider to clarify.

What is the likely indication for this drug therapy for this patient?

Note: Answers to the Critical Thinking activities can be found in the "Answer Key" sections at the end of the book.

7.4   ANTIDIARRHEAL MEDICATIONS AND LAXATIVES

The digestive system is continually at work, but unless something goes amiss, you don't notice your digestive system working. This section will focus on bowel disorders that occur in the lower intestine during the final step of digestion called **defecation**, when undigested materials are removed from the body as feces. During this final step, the large intestine absorbs water and changes the waste from liquid into stool; then peristalsis helps move the stool into the rectum. Diarrhea and constipation occur when conditions occur that affect this final step of defection.

The process of defecation begins when mass movements force feces from the colon into the rectum, stretching the rectal wall and provoking the defecation reflex, which eliminates feces from the rectum. This parasympathetic reflex is mediated by the spinal cord. It contracts the sigmoid colon and rectum, relaxes the internal anal sphincter, and initially contracts the external anal sphincter. Figure 7.9[41] reviews the anatomy of the rectum and its external and internal sphincters. The presence of feces in the anal canal sends a signal to the brain, which gives the person the choice of voluntarily opening the external anal sphincter (defecating) or keeping it temporarily closed. If defecation is delayed until a more convenient time, it takes a few seconds for the reflex contractions to stop and the rectal walls to relax. The next mass movement will trigger additional defecation reflexes until defecate occurs.[42]

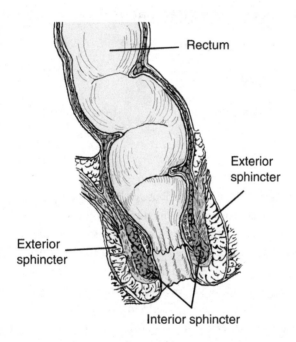

Figure 7.9 Anatomy of the Rectum

If defecation is delayed for an extended time, additional water is absorbed, making the feces firmer and potentially leading to constipation. Alternatively, if the waste matter moves too quickly through the intestines, not enough water is absorbed, and diarrhea can result. Figure 7.10[43] demonstrates the Bristol Stool Chart that is used to assess stool characteristics ranging from very constipated to diarrhea.

41   "Anorectum.gif" by U.S. Government National Institutes of Health is licensed under CC0.

42   This work is a derivative of *Anatomy and Physiology* by OpenStax licensed under CC BY 4.0. Access for free at https://openstax.org/books/anatomy-and-physiology/pages/1-introduction.

43   "BristolStoolChart.png" by Cabot Health, Bristol Stool Chart is licensed under CC BY-SA 3.0.

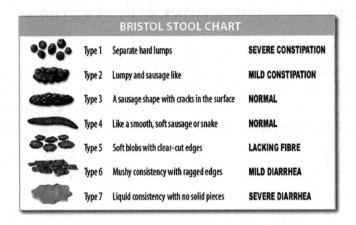

Figure 7.10 Bristol Stool Chart

You can further review how the digestive system works at the following links:

🔗 **Digestive System Processes and Regulation**[44]

🔗 **Your Digestive System and How it Works**[45]

🔗 **Video on Digesting Food**[46]

7.4a Antidiarrheals

Pathophysiology

Diarrhea is defined as the passage of three or more loose or liquid stools per day (or more frequent passage than is normal for the individual). Frequent passing of formed stools is not considered diarrhea. Diarrhea has multiple causes such as bacteria from contaminated food or water; viruses such as influenza, norovirus, or rotavirus; parasites found in contaminated food or water; medicines such as antibiotics, cancer drugs, and antacids that contain magnesium; food intolerances and sensitivities; and diseases that affect the colon, such as Crohn's disease or irritable bowel syndrome.[47] The most severe threat posed by diarrhea is dehydration caused by the loss of water and electrolytes. Diarrheal disease is a leading cause of child mortality and morbidity throughout the world due to dehydration; frail elderly are also at risk. When severe diarrhea occurs, assessment for dehydration and electrolyte imbalances receive top priority and rehydration with oral rehydration solutions or IV fluids may be required.[48] Common medications used to manage the symptoms of diarrhea are discussed below.

---

44 https://openstax.org/books/anatomy-and-physiology/pages/23-2-digestive-system-processes-and-regulation.

45 National Institute of Diabetes and Digestive and Kidney Diseases, National Institute of Health. (2018). *Treatment for constipation*.https://www.niddk.nih.gov/health-information/digestive-diseases/constipation/ treatment.

46 *Digesting Food* by Stanford School of Medicine and Khan Academy is licensed under CC BY-NC-SA 3.0.

47 A.D.A.M. Medical Encyclopedia [Internet]. Atlanta (GA): A.D.A.M., Inc.; ©2019. Heartburn; [reviewed 2019 May 10; cited 2019 October 27]. https://medlineplus.gov/ency/anatomyvideos/000068.htm.

48 World Health Organization. (2017, May 2). *Diarrhoeal disease*.https://www.who.int/en/news-room/fact-sheets/ detail/diarrhoeal-disease.

Nursing Considerations

Assessment

When administering antidiarrheals, the nurse should document an abdominal assessment, frequency of bowel movements and stool characteristics, and if there is skin breakdown in the anal area. Dehydration is a serious risk in patients with severe diarrhea, so priority assessments and documentation relate to monitoring for dehydration, especially in vulnerable populations of infants, children, and elderly. If signs of dehydration occur, the provider should be immediately notified and treatment initiated for dehydration.

Implementation

Teach the patient to not exceed dosages of OTC medications because life-threatening adverse effects may occur. Probiotics have been found to be likely safe in all populations, and the nurse can advocate for the use of probiotics in patients with diarrhea or those at risk for diarrhea because of other medications prescribed. In addition to teaching about medication therapy, nurses can also teach patients with diarrhea other nonpharmacological interventions, such as replacing fluid and electrolytes by drinking water, sports drinks, or sodas without caffeine; and eating soft, bland food like bananas, rice, and toast. Children with severe diarrhea may also require oral rehydration solutions to replace lost fluids and electrolytes. The nurse should also keep in mind that antidiarrheals should be used very cautiously with children because some categories are contraindicated.

Evaluation

Because antidiarrheals treat the symptoms of diarrhea but do not eliminate the cause of it, if symptoms do not resolve within 48 hours, the provider should be notified and other potential causes of diarrhea investigated. Monitor for serious adverse effects such as increased bleeding in patients taking salicylates and for abnormal heart rhythms in patients taking loperamide and notify the provider immediately. Evaluation for dehydration should continuously occur until the condition resolves.

Antidiarrheal Medication Classes

There are three common mechanisms of action of **antidiarrheal** medications: adsorbents, which help eliminate the toxin or bacteria from the GI tract; **antimotility** agents, which slow peristalsis; and probiotics, which help to restore the normal bacteria found in the lower intestine. Oral rehydration agents may also be used in patients with diarrhea to replace fluid and electrolyte loss, but they do not treat the diarrhea. Antibacterial agents may also be used to treat diarrhea caused by specific infections, such as campylobacter or giardia, but they are not routinely needed.[49]

Adsorbents

Adsorption is the adhesion of molecules to a surface. This process differs from absorption, where a substance is dissolved or penetrates into a surface. Bismuth subsalicylate (brand name Pepto Bismol) is an example of an adsorbent (see Figure 7.11[50]).

---

49   World Health Organization. (2017, May 2). *Diarrhoeal disease*.https://www.who.int/en/news-room/fact-sheets/detail/diarrhoeal-disease.

50   "PeptoBismol Bottle.JPG" by ParentingPatch is licensed under CC BY-SA 3.0.

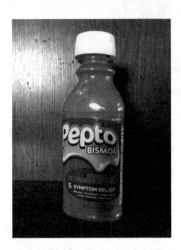

Figure 7.11 Bismuth Subsalicylate

Mechanism of Action

Adsorbent medications work by coating the walls of the GI tract and binding the causative bacteria or toxin for elimination from the GI tract through the stool.[51] Bismuth subsalicylate also decreases the flow of fluids and electrolytes into the bowel, reducing inflammation within the intestine.[52]

Specific Administration Considerations

Bismuth subsalicylate contains salicylate. It should be avoided if the patient has an allergy to salicylates (including aspirin) or if the patient is taking other salicylate products such as aspirin. It should not be used if the patient has an ulcer, a bleeding problem, or bloody or black stool. Children and teenagers who have or are recovering from chicken pox or flu-like symptoms should not use this product. When using this product, if changes in behavior with nausea and vomiting occur, consult a doctor because these symptoms could be an early sign of Reye's syndrome, a rare but serious illness. Liquid products should be shaken well before use. Tablets should be swallowed whole and not chewed unless they are a chewable tablet. Medication can cause a black or darkened tongue. If symptoms worsen, a fever, or ringing in the ears occurs, or if diarrhea lasts longer than 48 hours, contact the provider.[53, 54]

Patient Teaching and Education

Patients should be advised to take medication as directed. They should be aware of potential color changes to stool that may occur and that the medication contains aspirin. They should discontinue the medication if tinnitus occurs.[55]

---

51   Lilley, L., Collins, S., and Snyder, J. (2014). *Pharmacology and the Nursing Process.* pp. 782–862. Elsevier.

52   A.D.A.M. Medical Encyclopedia [Internet]. Atlanta (GA): A.D.A.M., Inc.; ©2019. Heartburn; [reviewed 2019 May 10; cited 2019 October 27]. https://medlineplus.gov/ency/anatomyvideos/000068.htm.

53   This work is a derivative of *Daily Med* by U.S. National Library of Medicine in the public domain.

54   A.D.A.M. Medical Encyclopedia [Internet]. A.D.A.M. Medical Encyclopedia [Internet]. Atlanta (GA): A.D.A.M., Inc.; ©2019. Heartburn; [reviewed 2019 May 10; cited 2019 October 27]. https://medlineplus.gov/ency/anatomyvideos/000068.htm.

55   uCentral from Unbound Medicine. https://www.unboundmedicine.com/ucentral.

Antimotility

Antimotility medications help to treat diarrhea by slowing peristalsis. There are two categories of antimotility medication: anticholinergics and opiate-like medication.

Anticholinergics

Mechanism of Action

Hyoscyamine is an anticholinergic that works on the smooth muscle of the GI tract to inhibit propulsive motility and decreases gastric acid secretion.

Specific Administration Considerations

Read drug label information for all contraindications, including but not limited to, glaucoma, myasthenia gravis, and paralytic ileus. Diarrhea may be an early symptom of incomplete intestinal obstruction, and the use of this drug would be inappropriate and possibly harmful. CNS symptoms and other adverse effects may occur that are common with anticholinergic medications.[56, 57]

Patient Teaching and Education

Patients should receive instruction that these medications may cause dizziness and drowsiness. If patients experience dry mouth, frequent oral hygiene may alleviate discomfort.[58]

Opioid-Like Medication

Mechanism of Action

Loperamide has an opioid-like chemical structure but causes fewer CNS effects. It works by decreasing the flow of fluids and electrolytes into the bowel and by slowing down the movement of the bowel to decrease the number of bowel movements (see Figure 7.12[59]).

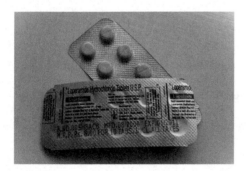

Figure 7.12 Loperamide

---

56   This work is a derivative of *Daily Med* by U.S. National Library of Medicine in the public domain.

57   A.D.A.M. Medical Encyclopedia [Internet]. Atlanta (GA): A.D.A.M., Inc.; ©2019. Heartburn; [reviewed 2019 May 10; cited 2019 October 27]. https://medlineplus.gov/ency/anatomyvideos/000068.htm.

58   uCentral from Unbound Medicine. https://www.unboundmedicine.com/ucentral.

59   "Loperamide2mg.JPG" by Kristoferb is licensed under CC BY-SA 3.0.

My Notes

Specific Administration Considerations

Loperamide should not be given to a child younger than two years of age because of the risk of serious breathing and heart problems. Taking more than the prescribed dose can cause a serious abnormal heart rhythm that can lead to death. Read the drug label carefully for information about interaction with other medications, especially antidysrhythmics and antipsychotics.[60, 61]

Patient Teaching and Education

Patients should take medications as directed. They should also avoid alcohol and other CNS depressants. The medications may cause drowsiness.[62]

Probiotics

Probiotics are used for the prevention and treatment of diarrhea. They are often used concomitantly with antibiotics to prevent the common associated side effects of diarrhea (see Figure 7.13[63]). An example of a probiotic is lactobacillus.

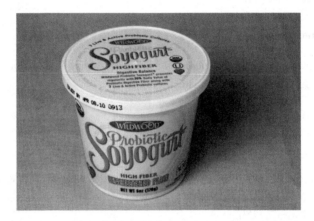

Figure 7.13 Probiotics come in several forms

Mechanism of Action

Probiotics help replenish normal bacterial flora in the gastrointestinal tract.

Specific Administration Considerations/Patient Teaching and Education

Side effects of probiotics are mild such as gas and bloating. Probiotics are safe for use in children.[64, 65]

---

60   This work is a derivative of *Daily Med* by U.S. National Library of Medicine in the public domain.

61   A.D.A.M. Medical Encyclopedia [Internet]. Atlanta (GA): A.D.A.M., Inc.; ©2019. Heartburn; [reviewed 2019 May 10; cited 2019 October 27]. https://medlineplus.gov/ency/anatomyvideos/000068.htm.

62   uCentral from Unbound Medicine. https://www.unboundmedicine.com/ucentral.

63   "WildWood Probiotic Soyogurt" by Veganbaking.net is licensed under CC BY-SA 2.0.

64   This work is a derivative of *Daily Med* by U.S. National Library of Medicine in the public domain.

65   A.D.A.M. Medical Encyclopedia [Internet]. Atlanta (GA): A.D.A.M., Inc.; ©2019. Heartburn; [reviewed 2019 May 10; cited 2019 October 27]. https://medlineplus.gov/ency/anatomyvideos/000068.htm.

Now let's take a closer look at medication grids comparing medications used to treat diarrhea. (See Table 7.4a[66,67].)

Medication grids are intended to assist students to learn key points about each medication. Because information about medication is constantly changing, nurses should always consult evidence-based resources to review current recommendations before administering specific medication. Basic information related to each class of medication is outlined below. Detailed information on a specific medication can be found for free at *Daily Med*. On the home page, enter the drug name in the search bar to read more about the medication. Prototype/generic medications listed in the grids below are also hyperlinked directly to a *Daily Med* page.

Table 7.4a: Comparison of Medications Used to Treat Diarrhea

Class	Prototype/ Generic	Administration Considerations	Therapeutic Effects	Adverse/Side Effects
Adsorbents	bismuth subsalicy- late (Pepto Bismol)	Avoid if taking other salicylates Do not use in children or teenagers recovering from chicken pox or flu-like symptoms as may cause Reye's syndrome Do not use if patient has an ulcer, bleeding problem, or bloody or black stool	Decreased diarrhea symptoms	May cause black or darkened tongue Contact provider if symptoms worsen, a fever, or ringing in the ears occurs, or if diarrhea lasts longer than 48 hours
Anticholin-ergic	hyoscyamine	Contraindicated in glaucoma, myas-thenia gravis, or paralytic ileus	Decreased diarrhea symptoms	May cause CNS and other adverse effects associated with anticholinergic medication
Opiate-like medication	loperamide (Imodium)	Contraindicated in children younger than 2 and with several other medications; read drug label infor-mation before administering	Decreased diarrhea symptoms	Black Box Warning: May cause abnormal heart rhythm
Probiotics	lactobacillus	Pediatric dosing is age based and varies by product	Prevention of diarrhea or decreased symptoms of diarrhea	Mild such as gas and bloating

66   This work is a derivative of *Daily Med* by U.S. National Library of Medicine in the public domain.

67   A.D.A.M. Medical Encyclopedia [Internet]. Atlanta (GA): A.D.A.M., Inc.; ©2019. Heartburn; [reviewed 2019 May 10; cited 2019 October 27]. https://medlineplus.gov/ency/anatomyvideos/000068.htm.

My Notes

> ## Critical Thinking Activity 7.4a
>
> 1. A patient has been prescribed loperamide for diarrhea associated with gastroenteritis. The patient begins to complain of "heart palpitations." What is the nurse's next best response?
>
> 2. A child, aged 6, has diarrhea. The mother asks the nurse what OTC medications she can provide to her child to help resolve the diarrhea. What is the nurse's best response?
>
> *Note:* Answers to the Critical Thinking activities can be found in the "Answer Key" sections at the end of the book.

7.4.b Constipation

Pathophysiology

Constipation is defined as "three or fewer bowel movements in a week; stools that are hard, dry or lumpy; stools that are difficult or painful to pass; or the feeling that not all stool has passed."[68] If defecation is delayed for an extended time, additional water is absorbed, thus making the feces firmer and potentially leading to constipation. There are several causes of constipation, such as lack of proper fluids or fiber in the diet, lack of ambulation, various disease processes, recovery from surgical anesthesia and opiates, and side effects of many medications. A list of these potential causes can be found in Figure 7.6.[69] Because there are several potential causes of constipation, treatment should always be individualized to the patient. Many times, constipation can be treated with simple changes in diet, exercise, or routine. However, when medications are also needed to resolve constipation, there are several categories of laxative medications that work in different ways. Classes of laxative medications are described below.

Figure 7.6 Common Causes of Constipation

Medications	Antacids that contain aluminum and calcium
	Anticholinergics and antispasmodics
	Anticonvulsants—used to prevent seizures
	Calcium channel blockers
	Diuretics
	Iron supplements
	Medicines used to treat Parkinson's disease
	Narcotic pain medicines
	Some medicines used to treat depression

---

68   National Institute of Diabetes and Digestive and Kidney Diseases, National Institute of Health. (2018). *Symptoms and causes of constipation.*https://www.niddk.nih.gov/health-information/digestive-diseases/ constipation/symptoms-causes.

69   National Institute of Diabetes and Digestive and Kidney Diseases, National Institute of Health. (2018). *Symptoms and causes of constipation.*https://www.niddk.nih.gov/health-information/digestive-diseases/ constipation/symptoms-causes.

Health and Nutrition Problems	Not eating enough fiber
	Not drinking enough liquids or dehydration
	Not getting enough physical activity
	Celiac disease
	Disorders that affect the brain and spine, such as Parkinson's disease
	Spinal cord or brain injuries
	Diabetes
	Hypothyroidism
	Inflammation linked to diverticular disease or proctitis
	Intestinal obstructions, including anorectal blockage and tumors
Daily Routine Changes	Pregnancy
	Aging
	Traveling
	Ignoring the urge to have a bowel movement
	Medication changes
	Change in diet

Figure 7.6 Common Causes of Constipation

Nursing Considerations

Assessment

The nurse should assess for the potential cause of the patient's constipation and appropriately individualize the treatment and patient education. The nurse should document an abdominal assessment that includes discomfort, distention, and decreased bowel sounds. The date of the last bowel movement should also be documented. The patient may be asked additional history questions such as the appearance of the stool to determine if it is hard and dry, if passing the stool is difficult or painful, or if there is a feeling of incomplete emptying.

Implementation

Many facilities have a bowel medication protocol with progressive treatment of constipation ranging from stool softeners to stimulants to enemas, depending on the length of time since the last bowel movement. Medications should be administered according to label instructions, and the patient should be instructed when to expect a bowel movement will occur. Measures to prevent constipation should also be discussed with the patient.

Patient teaching for all classes of laxative medications should be individualized based on the cause of constipation. Measures to prevent constipation should be reviewed with the patient, such as:

- Getting enough fiber in the diet
- Drinking plenty of water and other liquids
- Getting regular physical activity
- Trying to have a bowel movement at the same time every day[70]

---

70   National Institute of Diabetes and Digestive and Kidney Diseases, National Institute of Health. (2018). *Treatment for constipation*. https://www.niddk.nih.gov/health-information/digestive-diseases/constipation/treatment.

My Notes

Evaluation

If a bowel movement does not occur within the expected timeframe, the provider should be notified and other causes investigated for individualized treatment. It is imperative that good documentation of bowel movements and communication among staff occur when constipation is being treated with various medications. If there is a complete absence of bowel sounds, worsening distension or abdominal pain, a smearing of stool, or other findings indicating that a paralytic ileus or blockage may be occurring, the provider should be immediately notified.

Laxative Classes

There are five categories of laxative medications commonly used to treat constipation: fiber supplements, **stool softeners**, **osmotic agent**, lubricants, and **stimulants** (see Table 7.4b.1). Fiber supplements and stool softeners are often used daily to prevent constipation, whereas the other laxative categories are used to treat constipation. Table 7.4b1 compares the mechanism of action for each laxative category and includes common prototype and OTC brand names[71, 72, 73]

Table 7.4b1: Categories of Laxatives Used to Treat Constipation

Category	Prototypes	Mechanism of Action
Fiber supplements	psyllium (Metamucil)	Bulk forming to facilitate passage of stool through rectum
Stool softeners	Docusate (Colace)	Facilitates movement of water and fats into stool
Osmotic agents	Milk of Magnesia; polyethylene glycol (PEG) 3350 (Miralax)	Causes water to be retained with the stool, increasing the number of bowel movements and softening the stool so it is easier to pass
Lubricants	mineral oil enema (Fleet)	Coats the stool to help seal in water
Stimulants	Bisacodyl (Dulcolax)	Causes the intestines to contract, inducing stool to move through the colon

Fiber Supplements

Psyllium (brand name Metamucil) is an example of a common OTC fiber supplement (see Figure 7.14[74]).

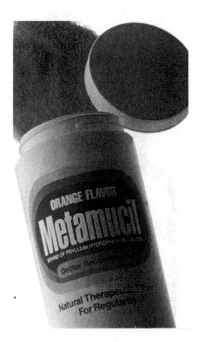

Figure 7.14 Psyllium in powder form

Mechanism of Action

Psyllium adds bulk to the stool to facilitate passage through the rectum.

Specific Administration Considerations

When administering, put one dose into an empty glass and mix with at least 8 ounces of water or other fluid. Taking this product without enough liquid may cause choking. Stir briskly and drink promptly. If mixture thickens, add more liquid and stir. Administer at least 2 hours before or 2 hours after other medications as it can affect absorption. Psyllium usually produces a bowel movement within 12 to 72 hours. It may cause bloating and cramping.

Patient Teaching and Education

When teaching patients how to take psyllium at home, in addition to the above considerations, advise them to start with 1 dose per day but may gradually increase to 3 doses per day as necessary to maintain soft stools.

Stool Softeners

Docusate is a common OTC stool softener that is also used frequently in health care settings.

Mechanism of Action

Docusate facilitates movement of water and fats into stool to make it soft and improve regularity of bowel movements.

Specific Administration Considerations

Docusate usually produces a bowel movement in 12 to 72 hours. It may cause stomach cramping.

My Notes

Osmotic Agents

Milk of Magnesia and polyethylene glycol 3350 (brand name Miralax) are examples of common osmotic agents used to promote a bowel movement (see figure 7.15[75].

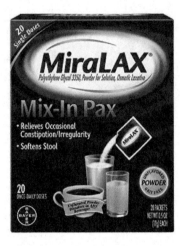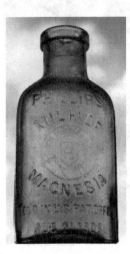

Figure 7.15 Miralax & Milk of Magnesia

Mechanism of Action

Osmotic agents cause water to be retained with the stool, increasing the number of bowel movements and softening the stool so it is easier to pass.

Specific Administration Considerations

Polyethylene glycol 3350 has a bottle top that can be used as a measuring cap to contain 17 grams of powder when filled to the indicated line. Fill to top of clear section in cap, which is marked to indicate the correct dose (17 g); stir and dissolve in any 4 to 8 ounces of beverage (cold, hot or room temperature), and then administer.

Patient Teaching and Education

In addition to the administration considerations above, teach patients that polyethylene glycol usually produces a bowel movement in 1-3 days. It may cause loose, watery stools.

Lubricants

A mineral oil enema (brand name Fleet enema) is an example of a lubricant laxative (see Figure 7.16[76]).

---

75   "MiraLax Mix-In Pax, Unflavored, 20 Little Packets" by Ava Williams is licensed under CC0 and "Phillips' Milk of Magnesia, 1910's" by Roadsidepictures is licensed under CC BY-NC 2.0.

76   "fleet_enema" by Logesh79 is licensed under CC BY-NC 2.0.

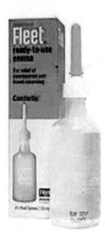

Figure 7.16 Mineral oil enema

Mechanism of Action

Mineral oil coats the stool to help seal in water.

Specific Administration Considerations

Read drug label for children as some brands can be used in children aged 2 or older, whereas others are not intended for children.

Patient Teaching and Education

A mineral oil enema generally produces a bowel movement in 2 to 15 minutes. It may cause stomach cramps, bloating, upset stomach, or diarrhea.

Stimulants

Bisacodyl is an example of a stimulant laxative.

Mechanism of Action

Bisacodyl causes the intestines to contract, inducing the stool to move through the colon.

Specific Administration Considerations

Oral dosage or rectal suppositories are available. See instructions for how to insert a rectal suppository. Instruct patient to retain suppository for about 15 to 20 minutes (see Figure 7.17[77]).

---

77   "Administering-med-rectally-2.png" by British Columbia Institute of Technology (BCIT) is licensed under CC BY 4.0.

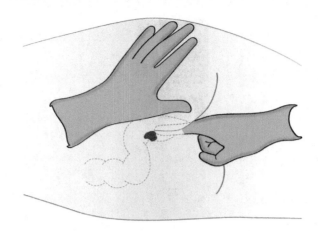

Figure 7.17 Administering a rectal suppository

Patient Teaching and Education

A bowel movement is generally produced in 15 minutes. Bisacodyl may cause stomach cramps, dizziness, or rectal burning.

Now let's take a closer look at the medication grids comparing medications used to treat constipation. (See Table 7.4b2).[78,79]

Medication grids are intended to assist students to learn key points about each medication. Because information about medication is constantly changing, nurses should always consult evidence-based resources to review current recommendations before administering specific medication. Basic information related to each class of medication is outlined below. Detailed information on a specific medication can be found for free at *Daily Med*. On the home page, enter the drug name in the search bar to read more about the medication. Prototype/generic medications listed in the grids below are also hyperlinked directly to a *Daily Med* page.

Table 7.4b2: Medication Grid Comparing Laxatives Used to Treat Constipation			
Prototype/ Generic	**Administration Considerations**	**Therapeutic Effects**	**Adverse/Side Effects**
psyllium (Metamucil)	Put one dose into an empty glass and mix with at least 8 ounces of water or other fluid. Taking this product without enough liquid may cause choking. Stir briskly and drink promptly. If mixture thickens, add more liquid and stir Usually produces a bowel movement within 12 to 72 hours Administer at least 2 hours before or 2 hours after other medications as it can affect absorption Start with 1 dose per day; may gradually increase to 3 doses per day as necessary	Improves regularity of bowel movements	May cause bloating and cramping

---

78   This work is a derivative of *Daily Med* by U.S. National Library of Medicine in the public domain.

79   Drugs.com [Internet]. *Metamucil*; © 2000–2019 [reviewed 20 November 2017; updated 1 October 2019; cited 27 October 2019]. https://www.drugs.com/mtm/metamucil.html.

docusate	Usually produces bowel movement in 12 to 72 hours	Softens stool and improves regular-ity of bowel movements	May cause abdominal cramping
polyethylene glycol 3350 (Miralax)	Usually produces a bowel movement in 1-3 days The bottle top is a measuring cap marked to contain 17 grams of powder when filled to the indicated line For adults and children 17 years of age and older: fill to top of clear section in cap, which is marked to indicate the correct dose (17 g) stir and dissolve in any 4 to 8 ounces of beverage (cold, hot or room temperature) and then drink use once a day use no more than 7 days	Softens stool and improves regular-ity of bowel movements	May cause loose, watery stools
Mineral oil enema	Read drug label for children as some brands can be used in children aged 2 or older, whereas others are not intended for children Generally produces bowel movement in 2 to 15 minutes	Bowel move-ment within 15 minutes	Stomach cramps, bloating, upset stomach, or diarrhea
bisacodyl	Oral dosage or rectal suppositories are available To administer a rectal suppository: Position patient on left side with the right knee up towards the chest. In the presence of anal fissures or hemorrhoids, suppositories should be coated at the tip with petroleum jelly. Remove foil and insert supposi-tory well into rectum touching the bowel wall. Instruct patient to retain suppository for about 15 to 20 minutes. A bowel movement is generally produced in 15 minutes to one hour. For children, read drug label for dosage	Bowel move-ment within one hour	Stomach cramps, dizziness, or rectal burning

Interactive Activity

 An interactive or media element has been excluded from this version of the text. You can view it online here: https://wtcs.pressbooks.pub/pharmacology/?p=1200

Critical Thinking Activity 7.4b

A patient who underwent hip surgery two days ago has not had a bowel movement since before admission. The patient is receiving oxycontin ER 10 mg every 12 hours and oxycodone 5 mg every 4 hours for pain. The patient describes abdominal discomfort and the nurse finds decreased bowel sounds in all quadrants. The nurse notifies the physician, follows the bowel protocol, and administers docusate sodium to the patient.

1. What are the potential causes of constipation that should be addressed for this patient?

2. What is the mechanism of action for docusate?

3. The patient asks how quickly the medication will work. What is the nurse's best response?

4. What other preventative measures for constipation should the nurse teach the patient?

5. If docusate is not effective within 24 hours, what other medications can the nurse anticipate to be ordered?

Note: Answers to the Critical Thinking activities can be found in the "Answer Key" sections at the end of the book.

7.5   ANTIEMETICS

Nausea and vomiting are common conditions. Nausea is the unpleasant sensation of having the urge to vomit, and vomiting (emesis) is the forceful expulsion of gastric contents.[80] There are many potential causes of nausea and vomiting, such as:

- Morning sickness during pregnancy
- **Gastroenteritis** and other infections
- Migraines
- Motion sickness
- Food poisoning
- Side effects of medicines, including those for cancer chemotherapy
- GERD and ulcers
- Intestinal obstruction
- Poisoning or exposure to a toxic substance
- Diseases of other organs (cardiac, renal, or liver)

Nausea and vomiting are common and are usually not serious. However, the health care provider should be contacted immediately if the following conditions occur:

- Vomiting for longer than 24 hours
- Blood in the vomit (also called **hematemesis**)
- Severe abdominal pain
- Severe headache and stiff neck
- Signs of dehydration, such as dry mouth, infrequent urination, or dark urine

Treatment of nausea and vomiting should be tailored to the cause. There are several medications that work on different neuroreceptors that when used can treat nausea and vomiting. For severe cases of vomiting, intravenous fluids may also be needed to treat the accompanying dehydration.[81, 82]

80   Bashashati, M. and McCallum, R. (2014). Neurochemical mechanisms and pharmacologic strategies in managing nausea and vomiting related to cyclic vomiting syndrome and other gastrointestinal disorders. *European Journal of Pharmacology*, 772, p 79.

81   MedlinePlus [Internet]. Bethesda (MD): National Library of Medicine (US); [updated 2019 October 23]. *Nausea and vomiting;* [updated 2019 February 7; reviewed 2016 March 17; cited 2019 October 27]. https://medlineplus.gov /nauseaandvomiting.html.

82   Bashashati, M. and McCallum, R. (2014). Neurochemical mechanisms and pharmacologic strategies in managing nausea and vomiting related to cyclic vomiting syndrome and other gastrointestinal disorders. *European Journal of Pharmacology*, 772, p 79.

Pathophysiology

The vomiting center can be activated directly by irritants or indirectly following input from four principal areas: gastrointestinal tract, cerebral cortex and thalamus, vestibular region, and chemoreceptor trigger zone (CRTZ). See Figure 7.14 for an illustration of the pathophysiology of nausea and vomiting.[83]

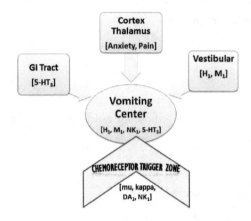

Figure 7.14 Pathophysiology of nausea and vomiting

An important part of the emesis circuit is the **chemoreceptor trigger zone (CTZ)**, located in the **area postrema** in the brain. The CTZ is not restricted by the blood–brain barrier, which allows it to respond directly to toxins in the bloodstream such as anesthesia and opioids. The CTZ also receives stimuli from several other locations in the body including the vestibular center; visceral organs such as the GI tract, kidneys, and liver; the thalamus; and the cerebral cortex.

The vestibular center and cerebral cortex can stimulate the vomiting center directly or indirectly through the CTZ. The **vestibular system** is located within the inner ear and gives a sense of balance and spatial orientation for the purpose of coordinating movement with balance. The feeling of nausea associated with motion sickness often arises from stimuli from the vestibular center. The gastrointestinal tract sends stimuli to the CTZ via cranial nerves IX and X related to obstruction, distension, inflammation, and infection. The cerebral cortex and other parts of the brain can also stimulate a sense of nausea related to odors, tastes, and images and send these stimuli to the CTZ. The CTZ forwards these signals to the vomiting center in the brain. Pain can also directly stimulate the vomiting center.

The **vomiting center** (VC) is located in the medulla in the brain. In response to these stimuli, the vomiting center initiates vomiting by inhibiting peristalsis and producing retro-peristaltic contractions beginning in the small bowel and ascending into the stomach. It also produces simultaneous contractions in the abdominal muscles and diaphragm that generate high pressures to propel the stomach contents upwards. Additionally, autonomic stimulation of the heart, airways, salivary glands, and skin cause other symptoms associated with vomiting such as salivation, palor, sweating, and tachycardia. Several neurotransmitters are involved in the nausea and vomiting process, and antiemetic medications are targeted to specific neuroreceptors.[84]

83 Becker D. E. (2010). Nausea, vomiting, and hiccups: a review of mechanisms and treatment. *Anesthesia progress*, 57(4), 150–157. doi:10.2344/0003-3006-57.4.150.

84 Becker D. E. (2010). Nausea, vomiting, and hiccups: a review of mechanisms and treatment. *Anesthesia progress*, 57(4), 150–157. https://www.ncbi.nlm.nih.gov/pmc/articles/PMC3006663/.

Table 7.5a compares the neurotransmitters involved in the nausea and vomiting process, classes of antiemetic medication targeting these neurotrasmitters, prototype antiemetic medications, and associated mechanisms of action.[85] Each medication class is also discussed in more detail later in this section.

Table 7.5a: Neurotransmitters and Associated Medications Used to Treat Nausea and Vomiting

Neurotransmitter	Medication Class	Antiemetic Drug	Mechanism of Action
Acetylcholine (M1)	Anticholinergics	scopolamine	Blocks ACh receptors in vestibular system
Histamine (H1)	Antihistamines	meclizine	Blocks H1 receptors and thus blocks ACh in vestibular system
Dopamine (DA2)	Dopamine antagonists	prochlorperazine	Blocks dopamine in CTZ and may block ACh
Dopamine and ACh (DA2 and M1)	Prokinetics	metoclopramide	Blocks dopamine in CTZ and stimulates ACh in GI tract
Serotonin (5HT)	Serotonin antagonists	ondansetron	Blocks serotonin in GI tract, CTZ, and VC
Substance P (NK1)	Neurokinin antagonists	aprepitant	Inhibits substance P neurokinin receptors
Cannabinoid (CB1)	Tetrahydrocannabinols (THC)	dronabinol or medical marijuana	Activated CB1 receptor leading to inhibitory effects on cerebral cortex

Nursing Considerations

Assessment

When administering antiemetics, identify factors contributing to the symptoms of nausea and vomiting so that treatment can correctly target the cause. Document the frequency and amount of emesis and effects on the patient's appetite and fluid intake. Assess for symptoms of dehydration, such as decreased blood pressure associated with tachycardia, decreased skin turgor, and decreased urine output or dark concentrated urine. If lab tests are ordered, monitor hemoglobin, hematocrit, and serum sodium levels for additional signs of dehydration.

Implementation

Advocate for the most effective route of administration if the patient is vomiting. Consider timing of administration of antiemetics in advance of meals when appetite is affected. Follow drug label administration information and monitor the patient closely for potential side effects associated with that category of medication. For example,

---

85   Bashashati, M. and McCallum, R. (2014). Neurochemical mechanisms and pharmacologic strategies in managing nausea and vomiting related to cyclic vomiting syndrome and other gastrointestinal disorders. *European Journal of Pharmacology, 772*, p 79.

when administering anticholinergics and antihistamines, monitor for anticholinergic side effects, especially in elderly patients.

Evaluation

Monitor for improvement of nausea and vomiting and notify the provider if expected improvement does not occur so that other treatment can be initiated. Continue to monitor for dehydration. Teach the patient nonpharmacological interventions for nausea such as:

- Drink enough fluids to avoid dehydration. If you are having trouble keeping liquids down, drink sips of clear liquids every few minutes.

- Eat bland foods; stay away from spicy, fatty, or salty foods.

- Eat smaller meals more often.

- Avoid strong smells because they can sometimes trigger nausea and vomiting.

- If you are pregnant and have morning sickness, eat crackers before you get out of bed in the morning.[86]

Antiemetic Medication Classes

Anticholinergics

Scopolamine is an example of an anticholinergic medication that is often used to treat motion sickness or nausea and vomiting associated with surgical recovery from anesthesia and/or opiate analgesia.

Mechanism of Action

Anticholinergics block ACh receptors in the vestibular center and within the brain to prevent nausea-inducing stimuli to the Chemoreceptor Trigger Zone (CTZ) and the Vomiting Center (VC). They also dry GI secretions and reduce smooth muscle spasms.

Specific Administration Considerations

The scopolamine transdermal patch (see Figure 7.15)[87] is designed for continuous release of scopolamine following application to an area of intact skin on the head, behind the ear. The system is formulated to deliver approximately 1 mg of scopolamine to the systemic circulation over 3 days. It is contraindicated in patients with glaucoma. It has been reported to exacerbate psychosis, induce seizures, and cause drowsiness, confusion, and sedation. Due to its anticholinergic properties, scopolamine can decrease gastrointestinal motility and cause urinary retention. Nurses should perform more frequent monitoring during treatment with Transderm Scōp and discontinue Transderm Scōp in patients who develop difficulty in urination. Transderm Scōp contains an aluminized membrane; skin burns have been reported at the application site in patients wearing an aluminized transdermal system during an MRI scan. Remove Transderm Scōp before undergoing an MRI.

86   MedlinePlus [Internet]. Bethesda (MD): National Library of Medicine (US); [updated 2019 October 23]. *Nausea and vomiting*; [updated 2019 February 7; reviewed 2016 March 17; cited 2019 October 27]. https://medlineplus.gov/nauseaandvomiting.html.

87   "Scopoderm 278:365" by Andreas Nilsson is licensed under CC BY-NC-ND 2.0.

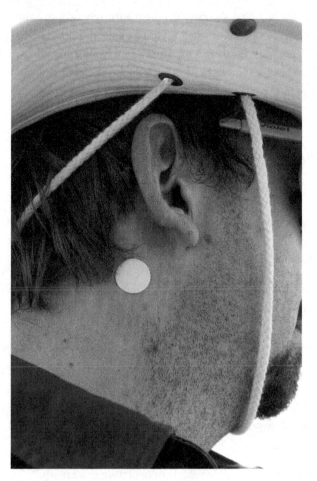

Figure 7.15 Scopolamine Transdermal Patch

Application instructions:

- Only wear one transdermal system at any time.

- Do not cut the transdermal system.

- Apply the transdermal system to the skin in the postauricular area (hairless area behind one ear).

- After the transdermal system is applied on the dry skin behind the ear, wash hands thoroughly with soap and water and dry hands.

- If the transdermal system becomes displaced, discard the transdermal system, and apply a new transdermal system on the hairless area behind the other ear.

- For surgeries other than cesarean section, apply one Transderm Scōp transdermal system the evening before scheduled surgery. Remove the transdermal system 24 hours following surgery.

Patient Teaching and Education

Transderm Scōp may impair the mental and/or physical abilities required for the performance of hazardous tasks such as driving a motor vehicle, operating machinery, or participating in underwater sports. Concomitant use of other drugs (e.g., alcohol, sedatives, hypnotics, opiates, and anxiolytics) that cause central nervous system (CNS) adverse reactions, or that have anticholinergic properties, may increase this impairment. Inform patients not to operate motor vehicles or other dangerous machinery or participate in underwater sports until they are

My Notes

reasonably certain that Transderm Scōp does not affect them adversely. Scopolamine can cause temporary dilation of the pupils resulting in blurred vision if it comes in contact with the eyes. Advise patients to wash their hands thoroughly with soap and water and dry their hands immediately after handling the transdermal system. Upon removal, fold the used transdermal system in half with the sticky side together, and discard in household trash in a manner that prevents accidental contact or ingestion by children, pets, or others.[88]

Antihistamines

Meclizine is an example of an antihistamine that is often used to treat motion sickness.

Mechanism of Action

Antihistamines block H1 receptors in the vestibular center and may also block acetylcholine (ACh).

Specific Administration Considerations

Antihistamines are contraindicated in patients with glaucoma or an enlarged prostate gland. Dosage should be started one hour before travel begins.

Patient Teaching and Education

- Do not exceed recommended dosage.
- Be advised that drowsiness may occur.
- Avoid alcohol, sedatives, and tranquilizers, which may increase drowsiness.
- Avoid alcoholic drinks.
- Be careful when driving a motor vehicle or operating machinery.[89]

Dopamine Antagonists

Prochlorperazine is an example of a dopamine antagonist used to treat nausea and vomiting. It can also be used as an antipsychotic medication.

Mechanism of Action

Prochlorperazine blocks dopamine in the Chemoreceptor Trigger Zone (CTZ). It also calms the central nervous system and may also block acetylcholine.

Specific Administration Considerations

Prochlorperazine can be administered orally, intramuscularly, rectally or intravenously. It is contraindicated in children under age 2 or under 20 pounds. Severe side effects have occurred when used to treat psychosis.

---

88   This work is a derivative of *Daily Med* by U.S. National Library of Medicine in the public domain.

89   This work is a derivative of *Daily Med* by U.S. National Library of Medicine in the public domain.

Patient Teaching and Education

Patients should be instructed to take medications as prescribed. They should avoid alcohol and other CNS depressants. Patients may experience increased photosensitivity and extreme temperatures should be avoided. Patients should be advised that urine may turn pinkish to reddish-brown.[90]

Prokinetics

Metoclopramide is an example of a prokinetic medication (see Figure 7.16).[91]

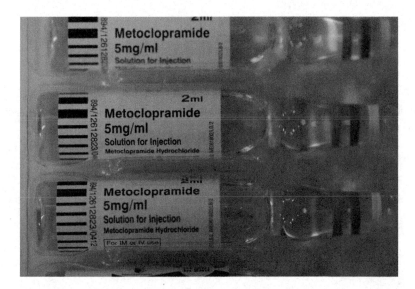

Figure 7.16 Prokinetics

Mechanism of Action

Metoclopramide blocks dopamine and may also sensitize tissues to acetylcholine. It is used to promote peristalsis to empty the gastrointestinal tract and thus reduce nausea.

Specific Administration Considerations

Metoclopramide can be administered orally, intramuscularly, and intravenously. The onset of pharmacological action of metoclopramide is 1 to 3 minutes following an intravenous dose, 10 to 15 minutes following intramuscular administration, and 30 to 60 minutes following an oral dose. Pharmacological effects persist for 1 to 2 hours.

Metoclopramide should not be used whenever stimulation of gastrointestinal motility might be dangerous (e.g., in the presence of gastrointestinal hemorrhage, mechanical obstruction, or perforation). Metoclopramide is contraindicated in patients with pheochromocytoma because the drug may cause a hypertensive crisis. Metoclopramide should not be used in epileptics or patients receiving other drugs that are likely to cause extrapyramidal reactions because the frequency and severity of seizures or extrapyramidal reactions may be increased. Rare reports of neuromalignant syndrome have occured.

---

90   uCentral from Unbound Medicine. https://www.unboundmedicine.com/ucentral.

91   "Metoclopramide" by John Campbell is licensed under CC0.

Patient Teaching and Education

Teach patients to immediately inform the healthcare provider if they experience new feelings of depression or abnormal muscle movements they cannot control such as:

- lip smacking, chewing, or puckering of the mouth
- frowning or scowling
- sticking out the tongue
- blinking and moving the eyes
- shaking of the arms and legs[92]

Serotonin Antagonists

Ondansetron is an example of a serotonin (5HT) antagonist often used to treat severe nausea and vomiting associated with chemotherapy, postoperative nausea and vomiting, and hyperemesis during pregnancy. (See Figure 7.17 for an image of odansetron blocking the 5-HT3 receptor.[93])

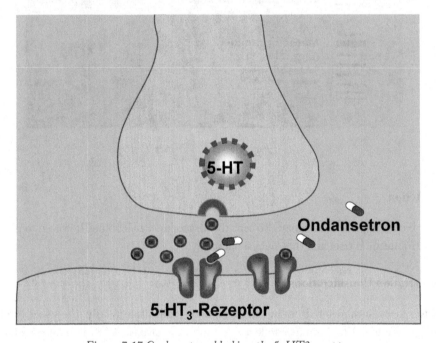

Figure 7.17 Ondansetron blocking the 5-HT3 receptor

---

92 This work is a derivative of *Daily Med* by U.S. National Library of Medicine in the public domain.

93 "Eichelbaum2.jpg" by Michel Eichelbaum is licensed under CC BY-SA 3.0 DE.

Mechanism of Action

Ondansetron blocks serotonin receptors in the GI tract, the chemoreceptor trigger zone (CTZ), and the vomiting center (VC). See Figures 7.18 and 7.19 for images of the injectable and oral formulations of ondansetron.[94, 95]

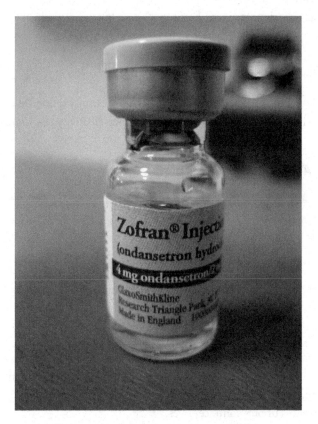

Figure 7.18 Ondansetron in injectable form

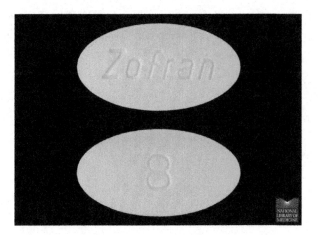

Figure 7.19 Ondansetron in tablet form

94   "000817lg Zofran 8 MG Oral Tablet.jpg" by NLM is licensed under CC0.

95   "Ondansetron (1)" by M is licensed under CC BY-NC 2.0.

Specific Administration Considerations

Ondansetron is available as an orally disintegrating tablet and as an injectable for those patients too nauseated to tolerate oral medication. It is contraindicated with apomorphine. **Serotonin syndrome** can occur if administered concurrently with other serotonin antagonists or selective serotonin reuptake inhibitors. Ondansetron can cause headaches, drowsiness, constipation, fever, and diarrhea. A rare but serious adverse effect of ondansetron is QT prolongation that can cause an abnormal cardiac rhythm.

Patient Teaching and Education

Teach patients to immediately inform their healthcare provider if they experience a change in heart rate, light-headedness, or feel faint or have any signs and symptoms of hypersensitivity reactions such as fever, chills, rash, or breathing problems.[96]

Neurokinin Receptor Antagonists

Aprepitant is an example of a neurokinin antagonist used to prevent nausea and vomiting associated with chemotherapy and surgery.

Mechanism of Action

Aprepitant inhibits substance-P neurokinin receptors in the brainstem.

Nursing Considerations

Aprepitant is usually administered concurrently with dexamethasone (a corticosteroid) and ondansetron. It can be administered orally or intravenously. It has clinically significant CYP3A4 drug interactions with medications such as pimozide, diltiazem, and rifampin, and can decrease INR levels when taken concurrently with warfarin. It can also reduce the effectiveness of oral contraceptives.

Patient Teaching and Education

Teach patients taking warfarin that they will need to monitor their INR levels more closely, which may require adjustment of the warfarin dosage, while taking aprepitant. Teach patients using an oral contraceptive to use backup birth control.[97]

Tetrahydrocannabinoids (THC)

Dronabinol or medical marijuana is an example of a **THC** medication used to treat nausea in patients with cancer or AIDS (see Figures 7.20 and 7.21).[98]

---

96   This work is a derivative of *Daily Med* by U.S. National Library of Medicine in the public domain.

97   This work is a derivative of *Daily Med* by U.S. National Library of Medicine in the public domain.

98   "Marinol - Dronabinol" by Steffen Geyer is licensed under CC BY-NC 2.0 and 7.21"Medical Marijuana" by Circe Denyer is licensed under CC0.

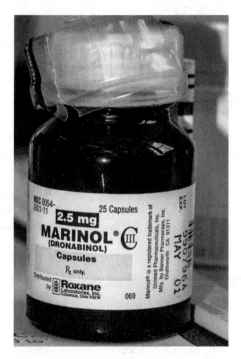

Figure 7.20 Dronabinol, a THC medication

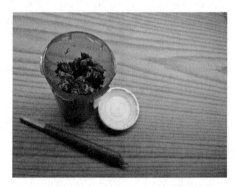

Figure 7.21 Medical Marijuana

Mechanism of Action

THC has inhibitory effects in the cerebral cortex causing an alteration in mood and the body's perception of its surroundings, which may relieve nausea and vomiting, as well as stimulate the appetite.

Specific Administration Considerations

THC will cause a dose-related "high" (easy laughing, elation, and heightened awareness). It is abusable and, thus, is a controlled substance and scheduled medication. THC should be used cautiously in elderly patients because they may be more sensitive to the neurological, psychoactive, and postural hypotensive effects of the drug. In general, dose selection for an elderly patient should be cautious, usually starting at the low end of the dosing range.

My Notes

Patient Teaching and Education

Teach patients to not drive, operate machinery, or engage in any hazardous activity when using THC. Keep out of reach of children and pets.[99]

Herbal and Vitamin Supplements

Ginger has been used in traditional Indian and Chinese medicine as an antiemetic. Although its mechanism of action is not completely understood, ginger is thought to antagonize the 5HT and cholinergic receptors and may have direct activity on the gastrointestinal tract. Although ginger can cause reflux and heartburn and may potentially cause bleeding because of its anticoagulant effects, dosages of up to 2 g per day in divided doses of 250 mg are considered safe even in pregnant women. Pyridoxine (vitamin B6) has also been recommended for treating nausea and vomiting in pregnancy. Typical dosages of pyridoxine 10 to 25 mg every eight hours cause minimal adverse effects.[100]

Antiemetics Medication Grid

Now let's take a closer look at the medication grid comparing medications used to treat nausea. See Table 7.5b.[101]

Medication grids are intended to assist students to learn key points about each medication. Because information about medication is constantly changing, nurses should always consult evidence-based resources to review current recommendations before administering specific medication. Basic information related to each class of medication is outlined below. Detailed information on a specific medication can be found for free at *Daily Med*. On the home page, enter the drug name in the search bar to read more about the medication. Prototype/generic medications listed in the grids below are also hyperlinked directly to a *Daily Med* page.

Table 7.5b: Medication Grid Comparing Antiemetics

Class	Prototype/ Generic	Administration Considerations	Therapeutic Effects	Adverse/Side Effects
Anticholin-ergic	scopolamine	Apply patch to hairless skin behind ear for 3 days or apply the night before surgery and remove 24 hours later Do not cut patch After application, thoroughly wash and dry hands Remove before an MRI Contraindicated in patients with glaucoma	Prevent or reduce nausea and vomiting associated with motion sickness or surgery	Monitor for anticholinergic effects such as decreased GI motility and urinary retention Discontinue if it exacerbates psychosis or causes seizures or cognitive impairment

99   This work is a derivative of *Daily Med* by U.S. National Library of Medicine in the public domain.

100   Flake, Z., Linn, B., and Hornecker, J. (2015). Practical selection of antiemetics in the ambulatory setting. *American Family Physician*, 91(5): pp 293–296.

101   This work is a derivative of *Daily Med* by U.S. National Library of Medicine in the public domain.

Antihista-mine	meclizine	Contraindicated in patients with glaucoma or an enlarged prostate gland Dosage should be started one hour before travel begins	Prevent or reduce nausea and vomiting associated with motion sickness	May cause drowsiness
Dopamine antagonist	prochlorpera-zine	Can be administered PO, IM, PR, or IV	To control nausea and vomiting associated with surgery	Drowsiness, dizziness, amenorrhea, blurred vision, skin reactions, and hypotension may occur
Prokinetic	metoclo-pramide	Can be administered PO, IM, and IV Onset of action is 1 to 3 minutes following an IV dose, 10 to 15 minutes following IM administration, and 30 to 60 minutes following an oral dose Pharmacological effects persist for 1 to 2 hours	To prevent or treat nausea and vomiting associated with surgery or chemotherapy	Restlessness, drowsiness, fatigue, depression, and suicide ideation Should be immediately discontinued if symptoms of tardive dyskinesia (abnormal muscle movements) or neuromalignant syndrome occur (hyperthermia, muscle rigidity, altered consciousness, irregular pulse or blood pressure, tachycardia, diaphoresis, and cardiac arrhythmias)
Serotonin antagonist	ondansetron	Can be administered as oral disintegrating tablet, PO, or IV	Prevention or treatment of severe nausea and vomiting associated with surgery, chemotherapy, or hyperemesis in pregnancy	Hypersensitivity reactions, including fever, chills, rash, or breathing problems Headache, drowsiness, constipation, fever, and diarrhea May cause QT prolongation Can cause serotonin syndrome if given concurrently with other serotonin antagonists or SSRIs
Neurokinin receptor antagonist	aprepitant	Can be administered PO or IV	Prevention of nausea and vomiting associated with chemotherapy and surgery	Hypersensitivity reaction, such as hives, rash. and itching; skin peeling or sores; or difficulty in breathing or swallowing If taking warfarin, increase monitoring of INR levels If taking oral contraceptives, use a backup method of birth control
THC	dronabinol or medical marijuana	Administered PO Most patients respond to 5 mg three or four times daily Dosage may be escalated during a chemotherapy cycle or at subsequent cycles, based on initial results	For treatment of nausea and vomiting associated with cancer chemotherapy when other treatment fails	Use cautiously in elderly patients because they may be more sensitive to the neurological, psychoactive, and postural hypotensive effects of the drug. In general, dose selection for an elderly patient should be cautious, usually starting at the low end of the dosing range

Critical Thinking Activity 7.5

A nurse is caring for a patient who underwent surgery earlier today and is experiencing nausea and vomiting. The original post-op orders included prochlorperazine, but the patient continues to experience vomiting despite receiving this medication. The nurse calls the provider and receives a new order for ondansetron orally dissolving tablets 8 mg three times daily as needed.

1. How will the nurse assess for symptoms of dehydration?

2. When administering the medication, the patient states, "This tastes terrible! Why can't I have a normal pill to swallow?" What is the nurse's best response?

3. What other measures should the nurse teach the patient to reduce feelings of nausea and avoid dehydration?

Note: Answers to the Critical Thinking activities can be found in the "Answer Key" sections at the end of the book.

7.6   MODULE LEARNING ACTIVITIES

> *Interactive Activity*
>
> An interactive or media element has been excluded from this version of the text. You can view it online here: https://wtcs.pressbooks.pub/pharmacology/?p=1444

GLOSSARY

Adsorption: The adhesion of molecules to a surface. For example, bismuth salicylate coats the walls of the GI tract and binds the causative bacteria or toxin for elimination from the GI tract through the stool.

Antacids: Used to neutralize stomach acid and reduce the symptoms of heartburn.

Antidiarrheals: Relieve the symptoms of diarrhea, such as an increased frequency and urgency when passing stools, but do not eliminate the cause of it.

Antimotility medications: Medications that help to treat diarrhea by slowing peristalsis.

Area Postrema: A structure in the medulla oblongata in the brainstem that controls vomiting. Its location in the brain also allows it to play a vital role in the control of autonomic functions by the central nervous system.

Chemoreceptor Trigger Zone (CTZ): Area in the brain that responds directly to toxins in the bloodstream and also receives stimuli from several other locations in the body that stimulate the vomiting center.

Cytochrome P-450 enzymes: Enzymes produced from the cytochrome P450 genes involved in the formation (synthesis) and breakdown (metabolism) of various molecules, chemicals, and medications within cells.

Defecation: The digestive process where undigested materials are removed from the body as feces.

Diarrhea: The passage of three or more loose or liquid stools per day (or more frequent passage than is normal for the individual).

Gastroenteritis: Infection of the intestines.

Gastroesophageal reflux disease (GERD): Caused by excessive hydrochloric acid that tends to back up, or reflux, into the lower esophagus.

Hematemesis: Blood in the vomit.

Hypercalcemia: Elevated levels of calcium in the bloodstream.

Intrinsic factor: Necessary for the absorption of vitamin B12 in the small intestine.

Osmotic agents: Cause water to be retained with the stool, increasing the number of bowel movements and softening the stool so it is easier to pass.

Parietal cells: Cells in the gastric glands that produce and secrete hydrochloric acid (HCl) and intrinsic factor.

Pepsin: A digestive enzyme.

Peptic ulcer disease (PUD): Occurs when gastric or duodenal ulcers are caused by the breakdown of GI mucosa by pepsin in combination with the caustic effects of hydrochloric acid.

Probiotics: Used for the prevention and treatment of diarrhea by restoring normal bacteria flora in the gastrointestinal tract.

Prokinetic: Medications used to promote peristalsis to empty the gastrointestinal tract and reduce nausea.

Proton pump inhibitors (PPIs): Bind to the hydrogen-potassium ATPase enzyme system of the parietal cell and inhibit the release of hydrogen ions into the stomach.

Rebound hyperacidity: A side effect of medication causing elevated levels of hydrochloric acid in the stomach after the medication is discontinued.

Serotonin Syndrome: Symptoms associated with serotonin syndrome may include the following: mental status changes (e.g., agitation, hallucinations, delirium, and coma), autonomic instability (e.g., tachycardia, labile blood pressure, dizziness, diaphoresis, flushing, hyperthermia), neuromuscular symptoms (e.g., tremor, rigidity, myoclonus, hyperreflexia, incoordination), seizures, with or without gastrointestinal symptoms (e.g., nausea, vomiting, diarrhea).

Stimulants: Laxatives that cause the intestines to contract, inducing stool to move through the colon.

Stool softeners: Laxatives that facilitate movement of water and fats into stool to make it soft and improve regularity of bowel movements.

Stress-related mucosal damage: A common condition in hospitalized patients that can lead to PUD.

Stress Ulcer Prophylaxis: Medication to prevent the formation of stress ulcers.

Surface epithelium cells: Cells found within the lining of the stomach that secrete mucus as a protective coating.

THC: Tetrahydrocannabinoids found in marijuana.

Vestibular system: An area located within the inner ear that gives a sense of balance and spatial orientation for the purpose of coordinating movement with balance.

Vomiting Center (VC): An area in the brain that initiates vomiting by inhibiting peristalsis and producing retro-peristaltic contractions beginning in the small bowel and ascending into the stomach. It also produces simultaneous contractions in the abdominal muscles and diaphragm that generate high pressures to propel the stomach contents upwards.

Chapter VIII

Central Nervous System

8.1   CENTRAL NERVOUS SYSTEM INTRODUCTION

Learning Objectives

- Cite the classifications and actions of central nervous system drugs
- Cite the classifications and actions of drugs used to treat psychiatric disorders
- Give examples of when, how, and to whom central nervous system drugs may be administered
- Identify the side effects and special considerations associated with central nervous system drug therapy
- Identify considerations and implications of using central nervous system medications across the life span
- Apply evidence-based concepts when using the nursing process
- Identify indications, side effects, and potential drug interactions associated with the use of herbal supplements
- Identify and interpret related laboratory tests

The nervous system is a very complex organ system. Even though progress has continued at an amazing rate within the scientific disciplines of neuroscience, our understanding of the intricacies within this science are limited. The nervous system may be just too complex for us to completely understand, and you may notice evidence of this within some of the "Mechanisms of Action" statements later in this chapter where exact understanding is unknown. The complexity of the nervous system and understanding of the brain can make treating and preventing diseases that affect this system complicated.[1]

---

1   This work is a derivative of *Anatomy and Physiology* by OpenStax licensed under CC BY 4.0. Access for free at https://openstax.org/books/anatomy-and-physiology/pages/1-introduction.

8.2   REVIEW OF BASIC CONCEPTS OF THE CENTRAL NERVOUS SYSTEM

Before we can begin to understand how different medications influence the brain, we need to review the central nervous system. The nervous system can be divided into two major regions: the central and peripheral nervous systems. The **central nervous system (CNS)** is the brain and spinal cord, and the **peripheral nervous system (PNS)** is everything else. The brain is contained within the cranial cavity of the skull, and the spinal cord is contained within the vertebral cavity of the vertebral column. It is a bit of an oversimplification to say that the CNS is what is inside these two cavities and the peripheral nervous system is outside of them, but that is one way to start to think about it. In actuality, there are some elements of the peripheral nervous system that are within the cranial or vertebral cavities. The peripheral nervous system is so named because it is on the periphery—meaning beyond the brain and spinal cord. Depending on different aspects of the nervous system, the dividing line between central and peripheral is not necessarily universal. The peripheral nervous system is further divided into the autonomic nervous system and the somatic nervous system, which are further discussed in the "Autonomic Nervous System" chapter.[2] (See Figures 8.1[3] and 8.2[4] for illustrations of the central and peripheral nervous systems.)

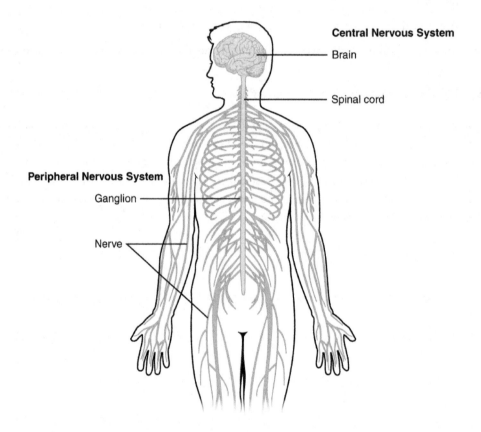

Figure 8.1 The Central and Peripheral Nervous System

---

2   This work is a derivative of *Anatomy and Physiology* by OpenStax licensed under CC BY 4.0. Access for free at https://openstax.org/books/anatomy-and-physiology/pages/1-introduction.

3   "1201 Overview of Nervous System.jpg" by OpenStax is licensed under CC BY 4.0. Access for free at https://openstax.org/books/anatomy-and-physiology/pages/12-1-basic-structure-and-function-of-the-nervous- system.

4   "1205 Somatic Autonomic Enteric StructuresN.jpg" by OpenStax is licensed under CC BY 4.0. Access for free at https://openstax.org/books/anatomy-and-physiology/pages/12-1-basic-structure-and-function-of-the-nervous- system.

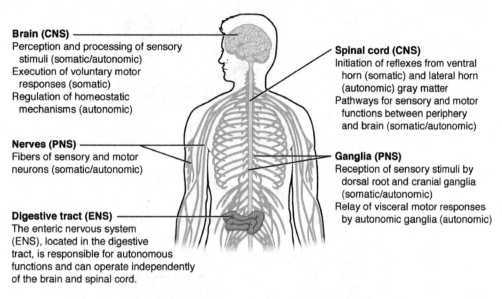

Brain (CNS)
Perception and processing of sensory
  stimuli (somatic/autonomic)
Execution of voluntary motor
  responses (somatic)
Regulation of homeostatic
  mechanisms (autonomic)

Nerves (PNS)
Fibers of sensory and motor
neurons (somatic/autonomic)

Digestive tract (ENS)
The enteric nervous system
(ENS), located in the digestive
tract, is responsible for autonomous
functions and can operate independently
of the brain and spinal cord.

Spinal cord (CNS)
Initiation of reflexes from ventral
  horn (somatic) and lateral horn
  (autonomic) gray matter
Pathways for sensory and motor
  functions between periphery
  and brain (somatic/autonomic)

Ganglia (PNS)
Reception of sensory stimuli by
  dorsal root and cranial ganglia
  (somatic/autonomic)
Relay of visceral motor responses
  by autonomic ganglia (autonomic)

Figure 8.2 Somatic, Autonomic, and Enteric Structures of the Nervous System

Review more detailed information about the nervous system function using this OpenStax link:

🔗 **Basic structure and function of the nervous system**

Communication in the Nervous System

Your brain communicates with electrical impulses that signal a release of a **neurotransmitter**, which then binds to the targeted cell. Understanding this communication will help you put the pieces together when you are trying to understand the mechanism of action of medication that works by influencing neurotransmitters. See Figure 8.3 for an illustration of the major elements in **neuron** communication.[5]

---

5 "Chemical synapse schema cropped.jpg" by Looie496 is licensed under public domain. Access for free at https://med
.libretexts.org/Bookshelves/Anatomy_and_Physiology/Book%3A_Anatomy_and_Physiology_(Boundless)/10%3A
_Overview_of_the_Nervous_System/10.1%3A_Introduction_to_the_Nervous_System/10.1A%3A_Organization_of
_the_Nervous_System.

My Notes

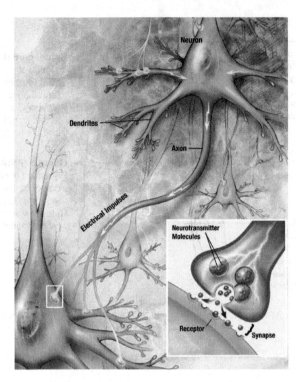

Figure 8.3 Major Elements in Neuron Communication

There are two types of connections between electrically active cells: chemical synapses and electrical synapses. In a **chemical synapse**, a chemical signal—namely, a neurotransmitter—is released from one cell and affects another cell. In comparison, in an **electrical synapse**, there is a direct connection between the two cells so that ions can pass directly from one cell to the next. In this unit we will be focusing on the communication of a neurotransmitter in a chemical synapse. Once in the synaptic cleft, the neurotransmitter diffuses the short distance to the postsynaptic membrane and can interact with neurotransmitter receptors. Receptors are specific for the neurotransmitter, and the two fit together like a key and lock. One neurotransmitter binds to its receptor and will not bind to receptors for other neurotransmitters, making the binding a specific chemical event.[6] (See Figure 8.4 for an illustration of a synapse.[7])

---

6   This work is a derivative of *Anatomy and Physiology* by OpenStax licensed under CC BY 4.0. Access for free at https://openstax.org/books/anatomy-and-physiology/pages/1-introduction.

7   "1225 Chemical Synapse.jpg" by Young, KA., Wise, JA., DeSaix, P., Kruse, DH., Poe, B., Johnson, E., Johnson, JE., Korol, O., Betts, JG., and Womble, M. is licensed under CC BY 4.0 Access for free at https://openstax.org/books/anatomy-and-physiology/pages/12-5-communication-between-neurons.

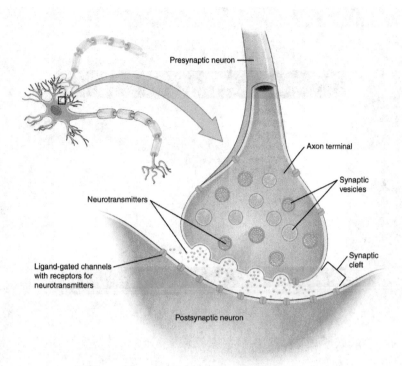

Figure 8.4 Major Elements in Neuron Communication

When the neurotransmitter binds to the receptor, the cell membrane of the target neuron changes its electrical state and a new graded potential begins. If that graded potential is strong enough to reach **threshold**, the second neuron generates an **action potential**. The target of this neuron is another neuron in the **thalamus** of the brain, the part of the CNS that acts as a relay for sensory information. The thalamus then sends the sensory information to the cerebral cortex, the outermost layer of gray matter in the brain, where conscious perception of that stimulus begins.[8]

A supplementary video explaining neuron communication via action potentials is provided below.

---

8   This work is a derivative of *Anatomy and Physiology* by OpenStax licensed under CC BY 4.0. Access for free at https://openstax.org/books/anatomy-and-physiology/pages/1-introduction.

Neuron communication via Action Potentials[9]

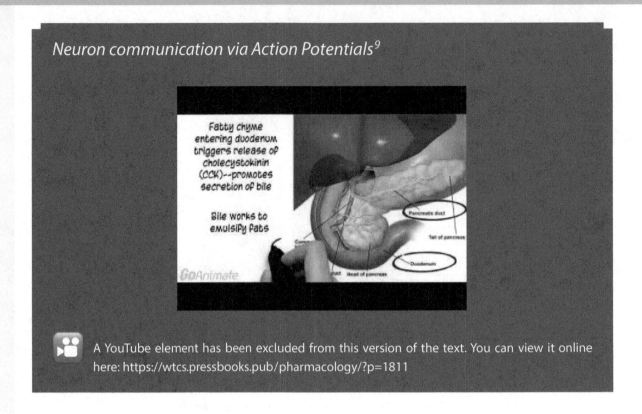

A YouTube element has been excluded from this version of the text. You can view it online here: https://wtcs.pressbooks.pub/pharmacology/?p=1811

Types of Neurotransmitters

Amino Acids

One group of neurotransmitters are amino acids. GABA (gamma-aminobutyric acid) is an example of an amino acid neurotransmitter. They each have their own receptors and do not interact with each other. Amino acid neurotransmitters are eliminated from the synapse by reuptake. A pump in the cell membrane of the presynaptic element, or sometimes a neighboring glial cell, will clear the amino acid from the synaptic cleft so that it can be recycled, repackaged in vesicles, and released again.

Biogenic Amine

Another class of neurotransmitter is the biogenic amine, a group of neurotransmitters that are enzymatically made from amino acids. For example, serotonin is made from tryptophan. It is the basis of the serotonergic system, which has its own specific receptors. Serotonin is transported back into the presynaptic cell for repackaging.

Other biogenic amines are made from tyrosine and include dopamine, norepinephrine, and epinephrine. Dopamine is part of its own system, the dopaminergic system, which has dopamine receptors. Norepinephrine and epinephrine belong to the adrenergic neurotransmitter system. The two molecules are very similar and bind to the same receptors, which are referred to as alpha- and beta-receptors. The biogenic amines have mixed effects. For example, dopamine receptors that are classified as D1 receptors are excitatory, whereas D2-type receptors are inhibitory.

---

9   Forciea, B. (2015, May 12). *Anatomy and Physiology: Nervous System: Action Potential Generation V2.0.* [Video]. YouTube. All rights reserved. Video used with permission. https://youtu.be/- xFliVq3MKg.

The important thing to remember about neurotransmitters and signaling chemicals is that the effect is entirely dependent on the receptor.[10]

Functions of Neurotransmitters

An alteration in CNS function is related to abnormal impulse transmission and can result in an imbalance of a neurotransmitter. A person with an imbalance of neurotransmitters may have signs and symptoms of a CNS disorder. The medications that are used to treat CNS disorders mimic or block the neurotransmitter based on the imbalance caused by the condition. Medications are used to either stimulate or depress the effect of the neurotransmitter. For example, CNS depressants alter the brain by decreasing excitability of neurotransmitters, blocking their receptor site, or increasing the inhibitory neurotransmitter. On the other hand, CNS stimulants increase brain activity by increasing excitability of neurotransmitters, decreasing the inhibitory neurotransmitters, or blocking their receptor sites.[11]

Norepinephrine is often associated with the fight-or-flight response. Abnormal levels of this neurotransmitter are also associated with depression, decreased alertness and interest, along with possible palpitations, anxiety, and panic attacks. Dopamine is strongly linked to motor and cognition. This neurotransmitter influences movement and can be associated with ADHD, paranoia, and schizophrenia. Serotonin is heavily involved in many bodily processes. Abnormal levels of serotonin can affect sleep, libido, mood, and temperature regulation. Alterations of this neurotransmitter have been linked to many mental health issues such as depression, bipolar disorder, anxiety, and body disorders. GABA (gamma-aminobutyric acid) can act as an inhibitory neurotransmitter. GABA assists with communication in the brain, and if this neurotransmitter is low, it has been linked to issues such as anxiety, seizures, mania, and impulse control. The neurotransmitter glutamate works as an excitatory neurotransmitter and works with GABA to control other functions of the brain.[12]

---

10   This work is a derivative of *Anatomy and Physiology* by OpenStax licensed under CC BY 4.0. Access for free at https://openstax.org/books/anatomy-and-physiology/pages/1-introduction.

11   This work is a derivative of *Pharmacology Notes: Nursing Implications for Clinical Practice* by Gloria Velarde licensed under CC BY-NC-SA 4.0.

12   This work is a derivative of *Pharmacology Notes: Nursing Implications for Clinical Practice* by Gloria Velarde licensed under CC BY-NC-SA 4.0.

8.3   DISORDERS OF THE CNS SYSTEM

Now that we have reviewed basic concepts of neurotransmitters and their function, let's review common CNS disorders.

Additional supplementary videos about mental disorders are available at:

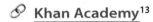 **Khan Academy**[13]

Anxiety

Anxiety disorders are a group of conditions marked by pathological or extreme anxiety or dread. People with anxiety experience disturbances of mood, behavior, and most systems in the body, making them unable to continue with everyday activities. Many feel anxious most of the time for no apparent reason.[14]

Anxiety is different from fear. Fear is a person's response to an event or object. The psychiatric disorder of anxiety occurs when the intensity and duration of anxiety does not match the potential for harm or threat to the affected person. Anxiety can be expressed with physical symptoms or behaviorally.[15]

Signs and Symptoms of Anxiety

- Aches
- Pains
- Stomach aches
- Headaches
- Heart racing or pounding
- Trembling
- Sweating
- Difficulty concentrating (see Figure 8.5)[16]
- Increased agitation
- Crying[17, 18]

---

13   Introduction to Mental Disorders by Khan Academy is licensed under CC BY-NC-SA 3.0.

14   This work is a derivative of *Supporting Individuals with Intellectual Disability and Mental Illness* by Sheri Melrose is licensed under CC BY 4.0.

15   This work is a derivative of *Supporting Individuals with Intellectual Disability and Mental Illness* by Sheri Melrose is licensed under CC BY 4.0.

16   "stress-2902537_960_720.jpg" by TheDigitalArtist is licensed under CC0 1.0.

17   This work is a derivative of *Supporting Individuals with Intellectual Disability and Mental Illness* by Sheri Melrose is licensed under CC BY 4.0.

18   Mayo Clinic Staff. (2018, May 4). *Anxiety disorders.* https://www.mayoclinic.org/diseases-conditions/anxiety/symptoms-causes/syc-20350961.

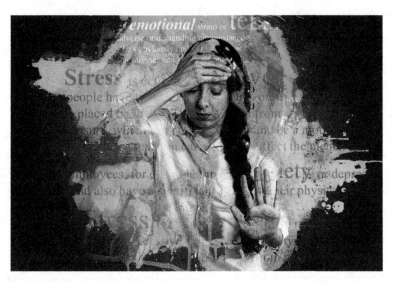

Figure 8.5 Many patients with anxiety experience difficulty concentrating

Treatment can include non-pharmacological interventions as well as medications. Non-pharmacological interventions to decrease anxiety include relaxation techniques such as deep breathing, exercise, psychotherapy, support groups, or cognitive behavioral therapy. Anti-anxiety medications can also be used to help both verbal and non-verbal clients feel a much-needed sense of peace.[19, 20]

Learn more about anxiety from the National Institute of Mental Health's website.

Depression

Depression is a frequent problem, affecting up to 5% of the population. To be diagnosed with depression, five of the following symptoms must be present during the same two-week period and represent a change from previous functioning. The symptoms cause clinically significant distress or impairment in social, occupational, or other important areas of functioning. The symptoms of depression cannot be due to effects of a substance or from bereavement.[21]

Signs and Symptoms of Depression

- Depressed mood
- Diminished interest
- Weight loss when not dieting or weight gain
- Insomnia or hypersomnia
- Agitation
- Fatigue or loss of energy

---

19 This work is a derivative of *Supporting Individuals with Intellectual Disability and Mental Illness* by Sheri Melrose is licensed under CC BY 4.0.

20 McCuistion, L., Vuljoin-DiMaggio, K., Winton, M, and Yeager, J. (2018). *Pharmacology: A patient-centered nursing process approach.* pp. 227–305).

21 This work is a derivative of *Principles of Pharmacology* by LibreTexts licensed under CC BY-NC-SA 4.0.

My Notes

- Feeling of worthlessness
- Inappropriate guilt
- Diminished ability to concentrate
- Recurrent thoughts of death, suicidal ideation, or suicide attempt[22, 23]

Treatment of depression may include medication, psychotherapy, cognitive therapy, electroconvulsive therapy (ECT), and group therapy. Patients who are depressed may not report symptoms unless specifically asked, and they may be suicidal. Using assessment techniques to gather information about the history of each patient's depression, support system, specific triggering events, psychosocial assessment, and risk for harm to self or others is imperative. Each patient's response to medication is unpredictable, and often medications will need to be adjusted based on reported symptoms.[24, 25]

Learn more about depression from the National Institute of Mental Health's website.

Bipolar

Bipolar affective disorder is marked by serious mood swings. Typically, patients experience extreme highs (called mania or hypomania) alternating with extreme lows (depression). See the "Depression" section for signs and symptoms of depression. People feel normal only in the periods between the highs and lows. For some people, the cycles occur so rapidly that they hardly ever feel a sense of control over their mood swings.[26]

Signs and Symptoms of a Manic Episode

- Rapid speech
- Hyperactivity
- Reduced need for sleep
- Flight of ideas
- Grandiosity
- Poor judgement
- Aggression/hostility
- Risky sexual behavior

---

22   This work is a derivative of *Daily Med* by U.S. National Library of Medicine in the public domain.

23   Mayo Clinic Staff. (2018, February 3). *Depression*. https://www.mayoclinic.org/diseases-conditions/depression/symptoms-causes/syc-20356007.

24   This work is a derivative of *Principles of Pharmacology by LibreTexts* licensed under CC BY-NC-SA 4.0.

25   Varcarolis, E. M. (2017). *Essentials of psychiatric mental health nursing: a communication approach to evidence-based care.* pp. 255–324. Elsevier.

26   This work is a derivative of *Supporting Individuals with Intellectual Disability and Mental Illness* by Sheri Melrose is licensed under CC BY 4.0.

- Neglect basic self-care
- Decreased impulse control[27, 28]

Treatment for a patient diagnosed with bipolar may include medication, safety initiatives during acute mania, ECT, psychotherapy, and support groups. The severity of manic and depressive episodes varies for each patient. Assessing if a patient is a danger to others or themselves is the priority. People with bipolar may need assistance with impulse control during times when they are in a manic state.[29]

Learn more about bipolar disorder from the National Institute of Mental Health's website.

Schizophrenia

Schizophrenia affects people from all walks of life and usually first appears between the ages of 15 and 30. Not everyone will experience the same symptoms, but many symptoms are common such as withdrawing, hearing voices, talking to oneself, seeing things that are not there, neglecting personal hygiene, and showing low energy.[30]

Schizophrenia refers to a group of severe, disabling psychiatric disorders marked by withdrawal from reality, illogical thinking, delusions (fixed false beliefs that cannot be changed through reasoning), hallucinations (hearing, seeing, smelling, tasting, or feeling touched by things that are not there), and flat affect (lack of observable expressions of emotions, monotone voice, expressionless face, immobile body).[31]

Signs and Symptoms of Schizophrenia

There are three types of symptoms related to schizophrenia: positive, negative, and cognitive.

Positive Symptoms

Note that in this context, the word *positive* is not the same as good. Rather, positive symptoms are psychotic and demonstrate how the individual has lost touch with reality. Positive symptoms include:

- Delusions
- Hallucinations
- Disorganized thinking and behavior

Delusions fall into several categories. Individuals with a persecutory delusion may believe they are being tormented, followed, tricked, or spied on. Individuals with a grandiose delusion may believe they have special powers. Individuals with a reference delusion may believe that passages in books, newspapers, television shows, song lyrics,

---

27   This work is a derivative of *Supporting Individuals with Intellectual Disability and Mental Illness* by Sheri Melrose is licensed under CC BY 4.0.

28   Mayo Clinic Staff. (2018, January 31)) *Bipolar disorder*. https://www.mayoclinic.org/diseases-conditions /bipolar- disorder/symptoms-causes/syc-20355955.

29   Varcarolis, E. M. (2017). *Essentials of psychiatric mental health nursing: a communication approach to evidence-based care.* pp. 255–324. Elsevier.

30   This work is a derivative of *Supporting Individuals with Intellectual Disability and Mental Illness* by Sheri Melrose is licensed under CC BY 4.0.

31   This work is a derivative of *Supporting Individuals with Intellectual Disability and Mental Illness* by Sheri Melrose is licensed under CC BY 4.0.

or other environmental cues are directed toward them. In delusions of thought withdrawal or thought insertion, individuals believe others are reading their mind, their thoughts are being transmitted to others, or outside forces are imposing their thoughts or impulses on them.[32]

Hallucinations may include hearing, seeing, smelling, tasting, or feeling as if they have been touched by things that are not there.[33]

Negative Symptoms

Negative symptoms are those characteristics that should be there but are lacking. Negative symptoms include:

- Apathy (lack of interest in people, things, activities)
- Lack of motivation
- Blunted affect
- Poverty of speech (brief replies)
- Anhedonia (lack of interest in activities once enjoyed)
- Avoidance of relationships

Keep in mind that the inability to show emotion associated with a blunted affect does not reflect an inability to feel emotion. Similarly, it is helpful to understand that withdrawing from others is a coping mechanism for an individual with schizophrenia and not a rejection of those who initiate contact.[34]

Cognitive

Cognitive symptoms are a change in thought pattern and include:

- Poor decision making
- Loss of memory
- Distracted
- Difficulty focusing

Treatment for a patient diagnosed with schizophrenia may include medications to control positive and/or negative signs and symptoms and nonpharmacological interventions such as limit setting, therapeutic communication, ECT, and psychotherapy. Key assessments for a patient with schizophrenia include examination for hallucinations

---

32   This work is a derivative of *Supporting Individuals with Intellectual Disability and Mental Illness* by Sheri Melrose is licensed under CC BY 4.0.

33   This work is a derivative of *Supporting Individuals with Intellectual Disability and Mental Illness* by Sheri Melrose is licensed under CC BY 4.0.

34   This work is a derivative of *Supporting Individuals with Intellectual Disability and Mental Illness* by Sheri Melrose is licensed under CC BY 4.0.

and delusions, use of additional substances (alcohol or drugs), safety, their support system, and a medication review with a focus on compliance with their therapeutic regimen.[35, 36, 37]

Learn more about schizophrenia from the National Institute of Mental Health's website.

Attention-Deficit/Hyperactivity Disorder

Attention-deficit/hyperactivity disorder (ADHD) is characterized by hyperactivity, lack of impulse control, and/or lack of attention that interferes with how a person functions. ADHD is often diagnosed during childhood, but signs and symptoms can last through adulthood.

Signs and Symptoms of ADHD

- Hyperactivity
- Inability to concentrate (see Figure 8.6)[38]
- Difficulty with self-control
- Lack of emotional control

A child with ADHD may have difficulty sitting still and focusing at school or have emotional outbursts. These behaviors often impact their life. Medication, psychotherapy, behavior management, and family support all play a large part in helping an individual with ADHD. Additional resources for parents are also helpful.[39, 40]

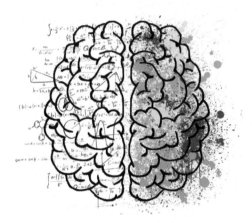

Figure 8.6 Patients with ADHD may have difficulty in focusing on details

35   This work is a derivative of *Principles of Pharmacology* by LibreTexts licensed under CC BY-NC-SA 4.0.

36   Varcarolis, E. M. (2017). *Essentials of psychiatric mental health nursing: a communication approach to evidence-based care.* pp. 255–324. Elsevier.

37   Mayo Clinic Staff. (2020, January 7) *Schizophrenia.* https://www.mayoclinic.org/diseases-conditions/schizophrenia/diagnosis-treatment/drc-20354449.

38   "RightBrainDominant.jpg" by ElisaRiva is licensed under CC0.

39   Mayo Clinic Staff. (2019, June 25). *Attention-deficit/hyperactivity disorder (ADHD) in children.* https://www.mayoclinic.org/diseases-conditions/adhd/symptoms-causes/syc-20350889.

40   McCuistion, L., Vuljoin-DiMaggio, K., Winton, M, and Yeager, J. (2018). *Pharmacology: A patient-centered nursing process approach.* pp. 227–305. Elsevier.

Learn more about ADHD from the National Institute of Mental Health's website.

Seizures

The official definition of a seizure is "a transient occurrence of signs and/or symptoms due to an abnormal excessive or synchronous neuronal activity in the brain." This means that during a seizure, large numbers of brain cells are activated abnormally at the same time. It is like an electrical storm in the brain. They may alter consciousness and produce abnormal motor activity. There are different classifications of seizures based on severity of symptoms.[41]

Signs and Symptoms of Seizures

Motor Symptoms

- Jerking (clonic)
- Muscles becoming limp or weak (atonic)
- Tense or rigid muscles (tonic)
- Brief muscle twitching (myoclonus)
- Epileptic spasms

Non-Motor Symptoms

- Changes in sensation, emotions, thinking, or autonomic functions
- Lack of movement

Classification of Seizures

Seizures are classified in many ways, beginning with whether they are partial or generalized seizures.

Partial Seizures

Partial seizures have focal onset on one side of the brain. They are further classified into simple, complex, or secondarily generalized:

- Simple partial seizures are most common. They may also affect sensory and autonomic systems.
- Complex partial seizures include impairment of consciousness, with or without motor activity or other signs.
- Simple or complex partial seizures may become secondarily generalized, producing a tonic-clonic seizure.

---

41 Epilepsy Foundation. (2016, December 22). *2017 Revised classification of seizures.* https://www.epilepsy.com/article/2016/12/2017-revised-classification-seizures.

Generalized Seizures

Generalized seizures have bilateral onset on both sides of the brain and are typified by petit mal seizures, which can be recognized by clinical characteristics as well as interictal EEG abnormalities. [42, 43, 44, 45]

Status Epilepticus

Status epilepticus is a state of repeated or continuous seizures. It is often defined operationally as a single seizure lasting more than 20 minutes or repeated seizures without recovery of consciousness. Prolonged status epilepticus leads to irreversible brain injury and has a very high rate of mortality. The goal of therapy should be to achieve control of a seizure within 60 minutes or less. Pharmacological treatment of seizures is very successful in the majority of cases, but it requires accurate diagnosis and classification of seizures. Medication management of seizures may include CNS depressants, benzodiazepines or barbiturates, or anticonvulsants such as phenytoin. [46]

Parkinson's Disease

Parkinson's disease is a progressive disease of the nervous system that impairs one's ability to move. The typical onset for Parkinson's disease is middle to later stages of life. This disease worsens over time and has no cure. The cause of this disease is unknown, but it is known that it is characterized by a loss of dopaminergic neurons. [47, 48]

Signs and Symptoms of Parkinson's Disease

- **Tremor** at rest
- **Bradykinesia**
- Muscle **rigidity**
- **Postural instability**
- **Gait disturbance**
- **Dystonia**
- **Ophthalmoplegia**
- Active mood disorders

42   This work is a derivative of *Principles of Pharmacology* by LibreTexts licensed under CC BY-NC-SA 4.0.

43   This work is a derivative of *Pharmacology Notes: Nursing Implications for Clinical Practice* by Gloria Velarde licensed under CC BY-NC-SA 4.0.

44   Mayo Clinic Staff. (2019, June 18). *Seizures*. https://www.mayoclinic.org/diseases-conditions/seizure /symptoms- causes/syc-20365711.

45   Epilepsy Foundation. (2016, December 22). *2017 Revised classification of seizures*. https://www.epilepsy.com/ article/2016/12/2017-revised-classification-seizures.

46   This work is a derivative of *Principles of Pharmacology* by LibreTexts licensed under CC BY-NC-SA 4.0.

47   This work is a derivative of *Neuroscience*: Canadian 1st Edition by Dr. William Ju and is licensed under CC BY 4.0.

48   Mayo Clinic Staff. (2018, June 30). *Parkinson's disease*. https://www.mayoclinic.org/diseases-conditions/ parkinsons-disease/symptoms-causes/syc-20376055.

See Figure 8.7 for a typical posture associated with Parksinon's disease.[49] Treatment for a patient with Parkinson's disease often includes medication to increase dopamine in the brain to slow the progression of the disease.

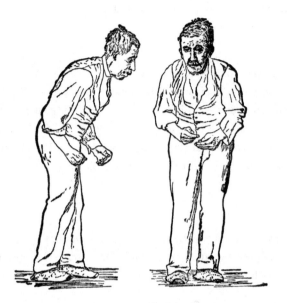

Figure 8.7. The typical stooping posture associated with Parksonson's disease.

Potential new treatment of proteins in Alzheimers and Parkinson's disease

The underlying cause of some neurodegenerative diseases, such as Alzheimer's and Parkinson's, appears to be related to proteins—specifically, to proteins behaving badly. One of the strongest theories of what causes Alzheimer's disease is based on the accumulation of beta-amyloid plaques, dense conglomerations of a protein that is not functioning correctly. Parkinson's disease is linked to an increase in a protein known as alpha-synuclein that is toxic to the cells of the substantia nigra nucleus in the midbrain.

For proteins to function correctly, they are dependent on their three-dimensional shape. The linear sequence of amino acids folds into a three-dimensional shape that is based on the interactions between and among those amino acids. When the folding is disturbed and proteins take on a different shape, they stop functioning correctly. But the disease is not necessarily the result of functional loss of these proteins; rather, these altered proteins start to accumulate and may become toxic. For example, in Alzheimer's the hallmark of the disease is the accumulation of these amyloid plaques in the cerebral cortex. The term coined to describe this sort of disease is "proteopathy" and it includes other diseases. Creutzfeld-Jacob disease, the human variant of the disease known as mad cow disease, also involves the accumulation of amyloid plaques, similar to Alzheimer's. Diseases of other organ systems can fall into this group as well, such as cystic fibrosis or type 2 diabetes. Recognizing the relationship between these diseases has suggested new therapeutic possibilities. Interfering with the accumulation of the proteins, and possibly as early as their original production within the cell, may unlock new ways to alleviate these devastating diseases.[50]

---

49   "Paralysis agitans (1907, after St. Leger).png" by William Richard Gowers is licensed under CC0.

50   This work is a derivative of *Anatomy and Physiology* by OpenStax licensed under CC BY 4.0. Access for free at https://openstax.org/books/anatomy-and-physiology/pages/1-introduction.

8.4   NURSING PROCESS: CNS MEDICATIONS

Now that we have reviewed various CNS disorders and the anatomy and physiology underlying them, let's review the importance of the nursing process in guiding the nurse who administers CNS medication to treat these disorders.

Assessment

When thinking about administering CNS medication, there are many things to consider. Each medication is given for a specific purpose for your patient, and it is your job as a nurse to assess your patients and collect important data before safely administering medication. As a nurse, you will be not only performing the skill of administering medications, but also be expected to think critically about your patient and the safety of any medication at any particular time.

A nursing assessment completed prior to administering CNS medication will likely look different than an assessment for other types of medication because most of the associated assessments are done by collecting subjective data rather than objective data. For example, prior to administering a cardiac medication, a nurse will obtain objective data such as blood pressure and an apical heart rate. However, prior to administering CNS medication, a nurse will use therapeutic communication to ask questions to gather subjective data about how the patient is feeling. After reviewing the possible diseases connecting with the CNS system, you probably noticed that there is usually an associated imbalance of a neurotransmitter. As a nurse, you cannot directly measure a neurotransmitter to determine the effects of the medication, but you can ask questions to determine how your patient is feeling emotionally and perceiving the world, which are influenced by neurotransmitter levels. An example of a nurse using therapeutic communication to perform subjective assessment is asking a question such as, "Tell me more about how you are feeling today?" The nurse may also use general survey techniques such as simply observing the patient to assess for cues of behavior. Examples of data collected by a general survey could be assessing the patient's mood, hygiene, appearance, or movement.

Implementation of Interventions

With the administration of any medications, it is important to always perform the five rights (right patient, medication, dose, route, and time) and to check for allergies prior to administration. It is important to anticipate any common side effects and the expected outcome of the medication. When you administer CNS medication, it is key to perform assessments before administering medication because many patients may have changing behaviors and habits that influence the way they think and feel about taking their medication. Additionally, some medications require assessment of lab values before administration. Many CNS medications may also have cumulative effects when used in conjunction with other medications, so careful assessment of the impact of the medications on one another is needed.

Evaluation

Finally, it is important to always evaluate the patient's response to a medication. Some CNS medications will take weeks to become therapeutic for the patient. It is key to teach the patient about when the medication is expected to produce an effect. Nurses should assess for mood, behavior, and movement improvement. If medications are effective, then patients should report fewer negative thoughts, worry, and symptomatic behaviors, as well as demonstrate fewer abnormal movements. Nurses also need to continually monitor for adverse effects, some of which can be life threatening and require prompt notification to the prescribing provider. Additionally, if symptoms are not improving or the patient's condition is worsening, the nurse should promptly notify the prescribing provider for further orders. For example, a symptom and/or adverse reaction of several CNS medications is increased thoughts of suicide. If a patient is experiencing thoughts of suicide, immediate assistance should be obtained to keep them safe. For more information about suicide, see the link to information about suicide prevention below.

Suicide Prevention

Now that we have reviewed CNS basics and how to use the nursing process related to CNS medications, we will take a closer look at specific classes of CNS medications. We will review classes and specific administration considerations, therapeutic effects, adverse/side effects, and teaching needed for each class of medications.

Medication grids are intended to assist students to learn key points about each medication. Because information about medication is constantly changing, nurses should always consult evidence-based resources to review current recommendations before administering specific medication. Basic information related to each class of medication is outlined below. Detailed information on a specific medication can be found for free at *Daily Med*. On the home page, enter the drug name in the search bar to read more about the medication.

Prototype/generic medications listed in the grids are also hyperlinked directly to a *Daily Med* page.

8.5   CNS DEPRESSANTS

Barbiturates and benzodiazepines are examples of CNS depressants.

Barbiturates

Phenobarbital is an example of a barbiturate primarily used as a sedative and to treat seizure disorders. In high doses it can be used to induce anesthesia, and overdosage can cause death. In the 1960s and 1970s, barbiturates were used to treat anxiety and insomnia, but are no longer used for these purposes due to their serious adverse effects. Barbiturates are a Schedule IV drug under the Federal Controlled Substances Act. However, the abuse of barbiturates continues to occur with street use as a "downer" to counteract the effect of cocaine and methamphetamine.

Mechanism of Action

Barbiturates produce sedation and drowsiness by altering cerebellar function and depressing the actions of the brain and sensory cortex.

Indications for Use

Barbiturates are primarily used for sedation and seizures.

Nursing Considerations Across the Life Span

Do not use for children less than 1 month of age. Barbiturates may harm the fetus during pregnancy. Avoid use in geriatic patients.

Adverse/Side Effects

Patients may experience CNS depression, suicidal thoughts or behaviors, GI disturbances, rashes, or some blood disorders that can be fatal. The concomitant use of alcohol or other CNS depressants may produce additive CNS depressant effects that can cause death. It can be habit forming.

Patient Teaching and Education

The patient should be advised to take the prescribed medication as directed. Patients who undergo prolonged therapy should not discontinue treatment abruptly as this may cause onset of seizure activity. These medications may cause drowsiness and should not be taken with alcohol or other CNS depressants. Female patients using oral contraceptives should also use non-hormonal based contraceptives during therapy.

Overdosage

The onset of symptoms following a toxic oral exposure to phenobarbital may not occur until several hours following ingestion. If overdose occurs, consult with a Certified Poison Control Center (1-800-222-1222) or go to https://www.poisonhelp.org/help for the latest recommendations.[51, 52]

Now let's take a closer look at the medication grid for phenobarbital in Table 8.5a.[53] Medication grids are intended to assist students to learn key points about each medication class. Basic information related to a common generic medication in this class is outlined, including administration considerations, therapeutic effects, and side effects/adverse effects. Prototype/generic medication listed in the med grid is also hyperlinked directly to a free resource from the U.S. National Library of Medicine called *Daily Med*. Because information about medication is constantly changing, nurses should always consult evidence-based resources to review current recommendations before administering specific medication.

Table 8.5a: Phenobarbital Medication Grid

Class/Subclass	Prototype/ Generic	Administration Considerations	Therapeutic Effects	Adverse/Side Effects
Barbiturates	phenobarbital	May be administered orally, IM, or IV High abuse potential Should not be combined with other CNS depressants When therapy is discontinued, the dose should be tapered and not stopped abruptly	Primarily used as an anticonvulsant Also used as a sedative and may also be used as a preanesthetic agent	CNS depression; overdosage can cause death May cause suicidal thoughts or behavior Respiratory depression GI: Nausea and vomiting

Benzodiazepines

Lorazepam, a benzodiazepine with antianxiety, sedative, and anticonvulsant effects, is available for oral, intramuscular, or intravenous routes of administration. Benzodiazepines are a controlled Schedule IV substance because they have a potential for abuse and may lead to dependence.

Mechanism of Action

Benzodiazepines bind to specific GABA receptors to potentiate effects of GABA.

Indications for Use

Benzodiazepines are used for sedation, antianxiety, and anticonvulsant effects. Lorazepam injection is indicated for the treatment of status epilepticus. It may also be used in adult patients for preanesthetic medication to produce sedation (sleepiness or drowsiness), relieve anxiety, and decrease the ability to recall events related to the day of surgery. Oral lorazepam is used to treat anxiety disorders.

---

51 This work is a derivative of *Daily Med* by U.S. National Library of Medicine in the public domain.

52 Drugs.com (2019, February 5). *Barbiturates*. https://www.drugs.com/drug-class/barbiturates.html.

53 This work is a derivative of *Daily Med* by U.S. National Library of Medicine in the public domain.

Nursing Considerations Across the Life Span

Benzodiazepines may cause fetal harm when administered to pregnant women. Children and the elderly are more likely to experience paradoxical reactions to benzodiazepines such as tremors, agitation, or visual hallucinations. Elderly or debilitated patients may be more susceptible to the sedative and respiratory depressive effects of lorazepam. Therefore, these patients should be monitored frequently and have their dosage adjusted carefully according to patient response; the initial dosage should not exceed 2 mg. Dosage for patients with severe hepatic insufficiency should be adjusted carefully according to patient response.

Adverse/Side Effects

A Black Box Warning states that concomitant use of benzodiazepines and opioids may result in profound sedation, respiratory depression, coma, and death.

The most important risk associated with the intravenous use of lorazepam injection is respiratory depression. Accordingly, airway patency must be assured and respiration monitored closely. Ventilatory support should be given as required. The additive central nervous system effects of other drugs, such as phenothiazines, narcotic analgesics, barbiturates, antidepressants, scopolamine, and monoamine-oxidase inhibitors should be considered when these other drugs are used concomitantly with, or during the period of recovery from, lorazepam injection. Sedation, drowsiness, respiratory depression (dose dependant), hypotension, and unsteadiness may occur with oral dosages as well. The use of benzodiazepines may lead to physical and psychological dependence. Abrupt termination of treatment may be accompanied by withdrawal symptoms. Benzodiazepines should be prescribed for short periods only (e.g., 2 to 4 weeks). Extension of the treatment period should not take place without reevaluation of the need for continued therapy.

Overdosage

Overdosage of benzodiazepines is usually manifested by varying degrees of central nervous system depression, ranging from drowsiness to coma.

Treatment of overdosage is mainly supportive until the drug is eliminated from the body. Vital signs and fluid balance should be carefully monitored in conjunction with close observation of the patient. An adequate airway should be maintained and assisted respiration used as needed. The benzodiazepine antagonist flumazenil may be used in hospitalized patients in the management of benzodiazepine overdose. There is a risk of seizure in association with flumazenil treatment, particularly in long-term benzodiazepine users. If overdose occurs, consult with a Certified Poison Control Center (1-800-222-1222) or go to https://www.poisonhelp.org/help for the latest recommendations.

Patient Teaching and Education

Patients who receive lorazepam should be cautioned that driving a motor vehicle, operating machinery, or engaging in hazardous or other activities requiring attention and coordination should be delayed for 24 to 48 hours following administration or until the effects of the drug, such as drowsiness, have subsided. Patients should be advised that getting out of bed unassisted may result in falling and potential injury if undertaken within 8 hours of receiving lorazepam. Alcoholic beverages should not be consumed for at least 24 to 48 hours after receiving lorazepam injectable due to the additive effects on central nervous system depression seen with benzodiazepines in general. Elderly patients should be instructed that lorazepam injection may make them very sleepy for a period longer than 6 to 8 hours following surgery.

Now let's take a closer look at the medication grid for lorazepam in Table 8.5b.[54]

Table 8.5b: Lorazepam Medication Grid

Class/Subclass	Prototype/ Generic	Administration Considerations	Therapeutic Effects	Adverse/Side Effects
Benzodiazepines	lorazepam	Black Box Warning: Concomitant use of benzodiazepines and opioids may result in profound sedation, respiratory depression, coma, and death May cause fetal harm in pregnant women May cause paradoxical effect in children Use cautiously in elderly and with those with liver dysfunction	To relieve anxiety, reduce seizure activity, or as a preanesthetic	Oversedation and drowsiness Respiratory depression Unsteadiness and fall risk Overdosage can cause coma and death Flumazenil used for overdose

Critical Thinking Activity 8.5

A patient who has been experiencing panic attacks is prescribed lorazepam. Upon further discussion with the patient, the nurse discovers that the patient is planning to go on a cruise with her husband next week and plans to use a scopolamine patch to control the nausea. The patient states, "I can't wait to relax on the cruise ship and have a margarita as we leave port!"

What important patient education should the nurse provide to the patient about the new prescription for lorazepam?

Note: Answers to the Critical Thinking activities can be found in the "Answer Key" sections at the end of the book.

---

54   This work is a derivative of *Daily Med* by U.S. National Library of Medicine in the public domain.

8.6   CNS STIMULANTS

Methylphenidate is an example of a CNS stimulant that is often used to treat ADHD. CNS stimulants are Schedule II controlled substances and have a high potential for abuse and dependence.

Mechanism of Action

Methylphenidate stimulates the brain and acts similar to amphetamines. Methylphenidate is thought to block the reuptake of norepinephrine and dopamine into the presynaptic neuron.

Indications for Use

Methylphenidate is used for ADHD.

Nursing Considerations Across the Life Span

Methylphenidate is typically prescribed to patients over the age of 6. It should be avoided in patients with known structural cardiac abnormalities, cardiomyopathy, serious heart rhythm arrhythmias, or coronary artery disease. Blood pressure and heart rate should be monitored in all patients.

CNS stimulants have been associated with weight loss and slowing of growth rate in pediatric patients. It increases the risk of peripheral vasculopathy, such as Raynaud's phenomenon, with signs and symptoms of fingers or toes feeling numb, cool, painful, and/or changing color from pale, to blue, to red.

Methylphenidate is contraindicated in patients using a monoamine oxidase inhibitor (MAOI), or use of an MAOI within the preceding 14 days. If paradoxical worsening of symptoms or other adverse reactions occur, the dosage should be reduced, or if necessary, discontinued.

Administer methylphenidate hydrochloride extended-release capsules orally once daily in the morning. Extended-release capsules should not be crushed, chewed, or divided. Monitor for signs of abuse and dependence while on therapy.

Adverse/Side Effects

Serious cardiovascular events have occurred with sudden death reported in association with CNS-stimulant treatment in pediatric patients with structural cardiac abnormalities or other serious heart problems. Sudden death, stroke, and myocardial infarction have also been reported in adults with CNS-stimulant treatment at recommended doses. Methylphenidate may cause increased blood pressure and increased heart rate. Use of stimulants may cause psychotic or manic symptoms in patients with no prior history and may cause priapism (painful or prolonged penile erections). The most common adverse reactions (greater than 5% incidence) were headache, insomnia, upper abdominal pain, decreased appetite, and anorexia. Alcohol should be avoided because it may cause a rapid release of the drug in extended-release formulations.

Overdose

If overdose occurs, consult with a Certified Poison Control Center (1-800-222-1222) or go to https://www.poisonhelp.org/help for the latest recommendations.

Patient Teaching and Education

There are several important topics to provide patients and/or parents of minor children.

Controlled Substance Status/High Potential for Abuse and Dependence: Advise patients that methylphenidate is a controlled substance, and it can be abused and lead to dependence. Instruct patients that they should not give methylphenidate to anyone else. Advise patients to store methylphenidate in a safe place, preferably locked, to prevent abuse. Advise patients to comply with laws and regulations on drug disposal. Advise patients to dispose of remaining, unused, or expired methylphenidate by a medicine take-back program if available.

Serious Cardiovascular Risks: Advise patients that there is a potential serious cardiovascular risk, including sudden death, myocardial infarction, stroke, and hypertension. Instruct patients to contact a healthcare provider immediately if they develop symptoms such as exertional chest pain or unexplained syncope.

Blood Pressure and Heart Rate Increases: Instruct patients that methylphenidate hydrochloride extended-release capsules can cause elevations of their blood pressure and pulse rate.

Psychiatric Risks: Advise patients that methylphenidate can cause psychotic or manic symptoms, even in patients without prior history of psychotic symptoms or mania.

Priapism: Advise patients of the possibility of painful or prolonged penile erections and to seek immediate medical attention if this occurs.

Circulation Problems in Fingers and Toes: Instruct patients beginning treatment with methylphenidate about the risk of peripheral vasculopathy and associated signs and symptoms: fingers or toes may feel numb, cool, painful, and/or may change color from pale, to blue, to red. Instruct patients to report to their physician any new numbness, pain, skin color change, or sensitivity to temperature in fingers or toes or any signs of unexplained wounds appearing on fingers or toes.

Suppression of Growth: Advise parents that methylphenidate may cause slowing of growth and weight loss.

Alcohol Effect: Advise patients to avoid alcohol while taking extended-release capsules.[55]

Now let's take a closer look at the medication grid for methylphenidate in Table 8.6.[56]

---

55 This work is a derivative of *Daily Med* by U.S. National Library of Medicine in the public domain.

56 This work is a derivative of *Daily Med* by U.S. National Library of Medicine in the public domain.

Table 8.6: Methylphenidate Medication Grid

Class/ Subclass	Prototype/ Generic	Administration Considerations	Therapeutic Effects	Adverse/Side Effects
CNS Stimulant	methylpheni-date	Black Box Warning: High abuse potential Patients should avoid alcohol Monitor BP and HR Monitor growth and weight in children Monitor for signs of abuse Contraindicated with MAOIs or use of an MAOI within the preceding 14 days	Oversedation and drowsiness Respiratory depression Unsteadiness and fall risk Overdosage can cause coma and death Flumazenil used for overdose	Immediately report signs and symptoms of abuse, cardiac or peripheral vascular complications, and priapism Report mania or psychotic episodes Common side effects: headache, insomnia, upper abdominal pain, decreased appetite, and anorexia Gynecomastia

Critical Thinking Activity 8.6

A 12-year-old male child has been diagnosed with ADHD after his parents and teachers became concerned with his inability to concentrate and his poor impulse control in the classroom. The physician has prescribed methylphenidate (Ritalin).

What topics should the nurse reinforce while educating the child and his parents about this medication?

Note: Answers to the Critical Thinking activities can be found in the "Answer Key" sections at the end of the book.

8.7   ANTIDEPRESSANTS

Antidepressants are used to treat depression and other mental health disorders, as well as other medical conditions such as migraine headaches, chronic pain, and premenstrual syndrome. Antidepressants increase levels of neurotransmitters in the CNS, including serotonin (5-HT), dopamine, and norepinephrine. Treatment is based on the belief that alterations in the levels of these neurotransmitters are responsible for causing depression.[57]

This module will discuss four classes of antidepressants: tricyclic antidepressants (TCAs), selective serotonin reuptake inhibitors (SSRIs), serotonin norepinephrine reuptake inhibitors (SNRIs), and monoamine oxidase inhibitors (MAOIs). TCAs and MAOIs are referred to as first-generation antidepressants because they were first marketed in the 1950s. SSRIs, SNRIs, and other miscellaneous medications such as bupropion are called second-generation antidepressants and are popular because of fewer side effects like sedation, hypotension, anticholinergic effects, or cardiotoxicity.[58]

Black Box Warnings are in place for all classes of antidepressants used with children, adolescents, and young adults for a higher risk of suicide. All patients receiving antidepressants should be monitored for signs of worsening depression or changing behavior, especially when the medication is started or dosages are changed.

Tricyclic Antidepressants

Tricyclic antidepressants (TCAs) were one of the original first-generation antidepressants. Due to the popularity of SSRIs and SNRIs, TCAs are now more commonly used to treat neuropathic pain and insomnia.

Mechanism of Action

Amitriptyline is an antidepressant with sedative effects. Its mechanism of action is not known. Amitriptyline inhibits the membrane pump mechanism responsible for uptake of norepinephrine and serotonin in adrenergic and serotonergic neurons. This interference with reuptake of norepinephrine and/or serotonin is believed to underlie the antidepressant activity of amitriptyline.

Indications for Use

TCAs are used to treat depression, neuropathic pain, and insomnia.

Nursing Considerations Across the Life Span

TCAs are often administered at bedtime due to sedating effects and are contraindicated with MAOIs.

Geriatric patients are particularly sensitive to the anticholinergic side effects of tricyclic antidepressants. Peripheral anticholinergic effects include tachycardia, urinary retention, constipation, dry mouth, blurred vision, and exacerbation of narrow-angle glaucoma. Central nervous system anticholinergic effects include cognitive impairment, psychomotor slowing, confusion, sedation, and delirium. Elderly patients taking amitriptyline may be at increased risk for falls. Elderly patients should be started on low doses of amitriptyline and observed closely.

---

57   Lilley, L., Collins, S., and Snyder, J. (2014). *Pharmacology and the Nursing Process.* pp. 246–272. Elsevier.

58   McCuistion, L., Vuljoin-DiMaggio, K., Winton, M, and Yeager, J. (2018). *Pharmacology: A patient-centered nursing process approach.* pp. 227–305. Elsevier.

After prolonged administration, abrupt cessation of treatment may produce nausea, headache, and malaise. The dose should be gradually tapered, but transient symptoms may still occur.

Adverse/Side Effects

Adverse effects of TCAs are a result of their blockade effects on various receptors, often resulting in anticholinergic adverse effects such as constipation, urinary retention, and drowsiness. Blockage of adrenergic and dopaminergic receptors can cause cardiac conduction disturbances and hypotension. Histaminergic blockage can cause sedation, and serotonergic blockage can alter the seizure threshold and cause sexual dysfunction.

Black Box Warnings are in place for all classes of antidepressants used with children, adolescents, and young adults for a higher risk of suicide. Patients receiving antidepressants should be monitored for signs of worsening depression or changing behavior, especially when the medication is started or dosages are changed.

Overdosage

Death may occur from overdosage with this class of drugs. Multiple drug ingestion (including alcohol) is common in deliberate tricyclic antidepressant overdose. If overdose occurs, consult with a Certified Poison Control Center (1-800-222-1222) or go to https://www.poisonhelp.org/help for the latest recommendations.

Patient Teaching and Education

Due to the increased risk of suicidality with antidepressants, patients and their family members or caregivers should be instructed to immediately report any sudden changes in mood, behaviors, thoughts, or feelings. Potential side effects discussed above should be reviewed.[59, 60, 61]

Now let's take a closer look at the medication grid for amitriptyline in Table 8.7a.[62, 63, 64]

59   This work is a derivative of *Daily Med* by U.S. National Library of Medicine in the public domain.

60   McCuistion, L., Vuljoin-DiMaggio, K., Winton, M, and Yeager, J. (2018). *Pharmacology: A patient-centered nursing process approach*. pp. 227–305. Elsevier.

61   Lilley, L., Collins, S., and Snyder, J. (2014). *Pharmacology and the Nursing Process*. pp. 246–272. Elsevier.

62   This work is a derivative of *Daily Med* by U.S. National Library of Medicine in the public domain.

63   McCuistion, L., Vuljoin-DiMaggio, K., Winton, M, and Yeager, J. (2018). *Pharmacology: A patient-centered nursing process approach*. pp. 227–305. Elsevier.

64   Lilley, L., Collins, S., and Snyder, J. (2014). *Pharmacology and the Nursing Process*. pp. 246–272. Elsevier.

My Notes

Table 8.7a: Amitryiptyline Medication Grid

Class/Subclass	Prototype/Generic	Administration Considerations	Therapeutic Effects	Adverse/Side Effects
Tricyclic	amitriptyline	Black Box Warning: Increased risk of suicidality Taper dose when discontinuing; do not stop abruptly Monitor orthostatic blood pressures and consider fall risk precautions	Based on indication: decrease feelings of depression, chronic pain, or insomnia	Immediately report signs or symptoms of suicidality Anticholinergic effects Hypotension May lengthen QT interval; risk for arrhythmias Sedation Sexual dysfunction Altered seizure threshold

Selective Serotonin Reuptake Inhibitor (SSRI)

Selective Serotonin Reuptake Inhibitors (SSRIs) are a second-generation antidepressant and have fewer side effects than TCAs and MAOIs. Fluoxetine and citalopram are commonly used SSRIs.

Mechanism of Action

SSRIs inhibit the reuptake of serotonin.

Indications for Use

SSRIs are primarily used to treat depression, but are also used to treat obsessive compulsive disorder, bulimia, panic disorder, posttraumatic stress disorder, other forms of anxiety, premenstrual syndrome, and migraines.

Nursing Considerations Across the Life Span

The onset of fluoxetine's antidepressant effect develops slowly for up to 12 weeks.

Use with caution in patients who are taking other CNS medications or who have liver dysfunction. This drug is contraindicated with MAOIs. Monitor for increased suicide ideation in all populations, as well as for the development of serotonin syndrome. Patients should avoid grapefruit juice due to its effect on the CYP3A4 enzyme that affects the bioavailability of the medication.

Adverse/Side Effects

Black Box Warnings are in place for all classes of antidepressants used with children, adolescents, and young adults for a higher risk of suicide. Patients receiving antidepressants should be monitored for signs of worsening depression or changing behavior, especially when the medication is started or dosages are changed.

The development of a potentially life-threatening serotonin syndrome or neuroleptic malignant syndrome (NMS)-like reactions have been reported with SNRIs and SSRIs, particularly with concomitant use of serotonergic drugs, drugs that impair metabolism of serotonin (including MAOIs), or with antipsychotics or other dopamine antagonists. Symptoms of **serotonin syndrome** may include mental status changes (e.g., agitation, hallucinations, coma), autonomic instability (e.g., tachycardia, labile blood pressure, hyperthermia), neuromuscular aberrations (e.g., hyperreflexia, incoordination), and/or gastrointestinal symptoms (e.g., nausea, vomiting, diarrhea). Serotonin syndrome, in its most severe form, can resemble **neuroleptic malignant syndrome** (NMS), which includes hyperthermia, muscle rigidity, autonomic instability with possible rapid fluctuation of vital signs, and mental status changes. Patients should be monitored for the emergence of serotonin syndrome or NMS-like signs and symptoms.[65]

Other side effects include rash; mania; seizures; decreased appetite and weight; increased bleeding associated with the concomitant use of fluoxetine and NSAIDs, aspirin, warfarin, or other drugs that affect coagulation; hyponatremia; anxiety; and insomnia.

Abrupt discontinuation may cause several adverse effects, so a gradual reduction in the dose rather than abrupt cessation is recommended whenever possible.[66, 67, 68]

Patient Teaching and Education

Patients should be careful to take medications as directed. Abrupt discontinuation may cause anxiety, insomnia, and increased nervousness. Additionally, orthostatic blood pressure changes are common during medication therapy. Patients may also be increasingly drowsy or exhibit some confusion. Use of SSRI medications with alcohol or other CNS depressant drugs should be avoided.

Patients, family, and caregivers should monitor patients carefully for suicidality. Other side effects include possible decreased libido, urinary retention, constipation, and increased photosensitivity.

Now let's take a closer look at the medication grid for fluoxetine and citalopram in Table 8.7b.[69, 70, 71]

65   This work is a derivative of *Daily Med* by U.S. National Library of Medicine in the public domain.

66   This work is a derivative of *Daily Med* by U.S. National Library of Medicine in the public domain.

67   McCuistion, L., Vuljoin-DiMaggio, K., Winton, M, and Yeager, J. (2018). *Pharmacology: A patient-centered nursing process approach*. pp. 227–305. Elsevier.

68   Lilley, L., Collins, S., and Snyder, J. (2014). *Pharmacology and the Nursing Process*. pp. 246–272. Elsevier.

69   This work is a derivative of *Daily Med* by U.S. National Library of Medicine in the public domain.

70   McCuistion, L., Vuljoin-DiMaggio, K., Winton, M, and Yeager, J. (2018). *Pharmacology: A patient-centered nursing process approach*. pp. 227–305. Elsevier.

71   Lilley, L., Collins, S., and Snyder, J. (2020). *Pharmacology and the Nursing Process*.

My Notes

Table 8.7b: Fluoxetine and Citalopram Medication Grid

Class/ Subclass	Prototype/ Generic	Administration Considerations	Therapeutic Effects	Adverse/Side Effects
SSRI	fluoxetine citalopram	Black Box Warning: Monitor for increased risk of suicidality Do not stop abruptly; taper dose when discontinuing Contraindicated with MAOIs Use caution with liver dysfunction May take up to 12 weeks before achieve therapeutic effect	Based on indication: primarily decreases feelings of depression	Immediately report signs/symptoms of increased suicidality or serotonin syndrome Rash, mania, seizures, decreased appetite and weight, increased bleeding, hyponatremia, anxiety, and insomnia

Critical Thinking Activity 8.7

A 32-year-old female visits the nurse practitioner with concerns about "feeling tired all the time," "having difficulty concentrating," "problems sleeping," and "just generally feeling down." The nurse practitioner prescribed fluoxetine.

The patient tells the nurse, "One of my friends told me I have to be careful or I might get serotonin syndrome if I take medication."

1. What places a patient at risk for serotonin syndrome, and what symptoms should the nurse teach the patient about this condition?

2. The nurse knows that anyone starting an antidepressant is at risk for suicidal thoughts. How should the nurse therapeutically discuss this potential adverse effect with the patient?

3. What potential common side effects should the nurse discuss with the patient?

4. The patient states, "I can't wait to feel better again. How soon will this medication work?" What is the nurse's best response?

Note: Answers to the Critical Thinking activities can be found in the "Answer Key" sections at the end of the book.

Serotonin Norepinephrine Reuptake Inhibitor (SNRI)

Venlafaxine is an example of a Serotonin Norepinephrine Reuptake Inhibitor (SNRI).

Mechanism of Action

Venlafaxine inhibits the reuptake of serotonin and norepinephrine, with weak inhibition of dopamine reuptake.

Indications for Use

SNRIs are indicated for treatment of a major depressive disorder.

Nursing Considerations Across the Life Span

SNRIs are contraindicated with MAOIs or within 14 days of use of an MAOI. Dosage adjustment is required for use in patients with renal and/or liver disease. Elderly patients are at greater risk for developing hyponatremia. Use with caution with other serotonin medications.

Adverse/Side Effects

Black Box Warnings are in place for all classes of antidepressants used with children, adolescents, and young adults for a higher risk of suicide. Patients receiving antidepressants should be monitored for signs of worsening depression or changing behavior, especially when the medication is started or dosages are changed.

SNRI medication may cause sustained increase in blood pressure. Other side effects include serotonin syndrome, insomnia, anxiety, decreased appetite, weight loss, mania, hyponatremia, increased bleeding (especially with the concomitant use of fluoxetine and NSAIDs, aspirin, warfarin, or other drugs that affect coagulation), elevated serum cholesterol, somnolence, and nausea.[72]

Patient Teaching and Education

Patients should be careful to take medications as directed. The dose should be tapered prior to discontinuation. Patients may also be increasingly drowsy or dizzy. Use of SNRI medications with alcohol or other CNS depressant drugs should be avoided. Patients, family, and caregivers should monitor patients carefully for suicidality.

---

72   This work is a derivative of *Daily Med* by U.S. National Library of Medicine in the public domain.

Now let's take a closer look at the medication grid for venlafaxine in Table 8.7c.[73]

Table 8.7c: Medication Grid for Venlafaxine				
Class/ Subclass	Prototype/ Generic	Administration Considerations	Therapeutic Effects	Adverse/Side Effects
SNRI	venlafaxine	Black Box Warning: Monitor for increased risk of suicidality Monitor BP Gradually reduce dose when discontinuing when possible Use with caution with patients with liver or renal disease	May take up to 8 weeks before therapeutic effect is recognized Decrease feelings of depression	Increased suicidality Serotonin syndrome Elevated BP Anxiety Insomnia Decreased appetite Weight loss Mania Hyponatremia Increased bleeding Elevated cholesterol Somnolence GI: Nausea and constipation

Monoamine Oxidase inhibitors (MAOI)

Monoamine oxidase inhibitors (MAOIs) are a first-generation antidepressant. Tranylcypromine is an example of a MAOI. A significant disadvantage to MAOIs is their potential to cause a hypertensive crisis when taken with stimulant medications or foods containing tyramine.

Mechanism of Action

The mechanism of action of tranylcypromine tablets as an antidepressant is not fully understood, but is presumed to be linked to potentiation of monoamine neurotransmitter activity in the central nervous system resulting from its irreversible inhibition of the enzyme monoamine oxidase (MAO).[74] MAO inactivates norepinephrine, dopamine, epinephrine, and serotonin. By inhibiting MAO, the levels of these transmitters rise.[75]

Indications for Use

Tranylcypromine is indicated for the treatment of major depressive disorder in adult patients who have not responded adequately to other antidepressants. The drug may also be used to treat Parkinson's disease.

Nursing Considerations Across the Life Span

Serious interactions with several medications, as well as foods and beverages containing tyramine, have been reported; check drug labelling before administering. Safety has not been established with the pediatric population.

---

73 This work is a derivative of *Daily Med* by U.S. National Library of Medicine in the public domain.

74 This work is a derivative of *Daily Med* by U.S. National Library of Medicine in the public domain.

75 McCuistion, L., Vuljoin-DiMaggio, K., Winton, M, and Yeager, J. (2018). *Pharmacology: A patient-centered nursing process approach.* pp. 227–305. Elsevier.

The elderly population is at increased risk for postural hypotension and serious adverse effects. Abuse and dependence have been reported. Withdrawal effects can continue for several weeks after discontinuation.

Adverse/Side Effects

Black Box Warnings are in place for all classes of antidepressants used with children, adolescents, and young adults for a higher risk of suicide. Patients receiving antidepressants should be monitored for signs of worsening depression or changing behavior, especially when the medication is started or dosages are changed.

Use with caution due to the risks of hypertensive crisis, serotonin syndrome, and increased suicidality. **Hypertensive crisis** is defined by severe hypertension (blood pressure greater than 180/120 mm Hg) with evidence of organ dysfunction. Symptoms may include occipital headache (which may radiate frontally), palpitations, neck stiffness or soreness, nausea or vomiting, sweating, dilated pupils, photophobia, shortness of breath, or confusion. Either tachycardia or bradycardia may be present and may be associated with constricting chest pain. Seizures may also occur. Intracranial bleeding, sometimes fatal, has been reported in association with the increase in blood pressure. See more information about serotonin syndrome in the "SSRI" section.

Other potential side effects include mania, **orthostatic hypotension**, hepatotoxicity, seizures, hypoglycemia in diabetic patients, decreased appetite and weight loss, dizziness, headache, drowsiness, and restlessness. Patients should be advised it may impair ability to operate machinery or drive. MAOIs should be discontinued if hepatotoxicity occurs.[76]

Patient Teaching and Education

Patients should be careful to take medications as directed. They should avoid abrupt cessation of therapy to avoid withdrawal symptoms. Patients should avoid alcohol, other CNS depressants, and tyramine-containing products for two weeks after therapy is discontinued. Patients should be advised regarding the signs of hypertensive crisis and to immediately report headache, chest or throat tightness, and palpitations to the provider.

---

76   This work is a derivative of *Daily Med* by U.S. National Library of Medicine in the public domain.

Now let's take a closer look at the medication grid for tranylcypromine in Table 8.7d.[77]

Table 8.7d: Medication Grid for Tranylcypromine

Class/ Subclass	Prototype/ Generic	Administration Considerations	Therapeutic Effects	Adverse/Side Effects
MAOI	tranylcypromine	Black Box Warning: Monitor for hypertensive crisis and increased suicide ideation Avoid foods containing tyramine Many drug interactions Monitor BP Do not stop abruptly; taper dose when discontinuing Discontinue if hepatotoxicity	Based on indication: decreased feeling symptoms of Parkinson's disease	Increased suicidality Hypertensive crisis Serotonin syndrome Mania Orthostatic hypotension Hepatotoxicity Seizures Hypoglycemia in diabetic patients Decreased appetite and weight loss CNS: dizziness, headache, drowsiness, and restlessness May impair ability to operate machinery or drive

---

77 This work is a derivative of *Daily Med* by U.S. National Library of Medicine in the public domain.

8.8   ANTIMANIA

Mood stabilizers are used to treat bipolar affective disorder. Lithium was the first medication used to treat this disorder and is sometimes referred to as an anti-mania drug because it can help control the mania that occurs in bipolar disorder. Lithium must be closely monitored with a narrow therapeutic range.[78]

Lithium

Mechanism of Action

Lithium alters sodium transport in **nerve** and muscle cells and effects a shift toward intraneuronal metabolism of catecholamines, but the specific biochemical mechanism of lithium action in mania is unknown.[79]

Indications for Use

Lithium is indicated in the treatment of manic episodes of bipolar disorder and as a maintenance treatment for individuals with a diagnosis of bipolar disorder.

Nursing Considerations Across the Life Span

Lithium must be closely monitored with a narrow therapeutic serum range of 0.8 to 1.2 mEq/L. Serum sodium levels should also be monitored for potential hyponatremia.[80]

The drug is contraindicated in renal or cardiovascular disease, severe dehydration or sodium depletion, and to patients receiving diuretics because the risk of lithium toxicity is very high in such patients.

Lithium can cause fetal harm in pregnant women. Safety has not been established for children under 12 and is not recommended.

When given to a patient experiencing a manic episode, lithium may produce a normalization of symptomatology within 1 to 3 weeks.[81]

Adverse/Side Effects

Black Box Warning: Lithium toxicity is closely related to serum lithium levels and can occur at doses close to therapeutic levels at 1.5 mEq/L. Facilities for prompt and accurate serum lithium determinations should be available before initiating therapy. Lithium can cause abnormal electrocardiographic (ECG) findings and risk of sudden death. Patients should be advised to seek immediate emergency assistance if they experience fainting, lightheadedness, abnormal heartbeats, or shortness of breath.

---

78   McCuistion, L., Vuljoin-DiMaggio, K., Winton, M, and Yeager, J. (2018). *Pharmacology: A patient-centered nursing process approach*. pp. 227–305. Elsevier.

79   This work is a derivative of *Daily Med* by U.S. National Library of Medicine in the public domain.

80   McCuistion, L., Vuljoin-DiMaggio, K., Winton, M, and Yeager, J. (2018). *Pharmacology: A patient-centered nursing process approach*. pp. 227–305. Elsevier.

81   This work is a derivative of *Daily Med* by U.S. National Library of Medicine in the public domain.

My Notes

Signs of early lithium toxicity include diarrhea, vomiting, drowsiness, muscular weakness, and lack of coordination. At higher levels, giddiness, ataxia, blurred vision, tinnitus, and a large output of dilute urine may be seen. No specific antidote for lithium poisoning is known; treatment focuses on the elimination of the medication.

Fine hand tremor, polyuria, and mild thirst may also persist throughout treatment.[82, 83]

Patient Teaching and Education

Patients should take medication as directed. It is important to note the antimanic drugs may increase dizziness and drowsiness. Additionally, if individuals have low sodium levels, it may predispose the patient toxicity. Patients should also be advised that weight gain may occur.

Now let's take a closer look at the medication grid for lithium in Table 8.8.[84, 85]

Table 8.8: Lithium Medication Grid

Class/ Subclass	Prototype/ Generic	Administration Considerations	Therapeutic Effects	Adverse/Side Effects
Antimanic	lithium	Black Box Warning: Monitor for signs of lithium toxicity Monitor serum lithium and sodium levels Contraindicated in renal and cardiovascular disease and in dehydration	When given during a manic episode, symptoms may resolve in 1-3 weeks When given for maintenance therapy, it should reduce the frequency and intensity of manic episodes	Lithium toxicity Hyponatremia Tremor Cardiac arrhythmia Polyuria Thirst

82 This work is a derivative of *Daily Med* by U.S. National Library of Medicine in the public domain.

83 McCuistion, L., Vuljoin-DiMaggio, K., Winton, M, and Yeager, J. (2018). *Pharmacology: A patient-centered nursing process approach.* pp. 227–305. Elsevier.

84 This work is a derivative of *Daily Med* by U.S. National Library of Medicine in the public domain.

85 McCuistion, L., Vuljoin-DiMaggio, K., Winton, M, and Yeager, J. (2018). *Pharmacology: A patient-centered nursing process approach.* pp. 227–305. Elsevier.

Critical Thinking Activity 8.8

A 42-year-old male was recently diagnosed with bipolar disorder after his partner became concerned about his extreme highs and lows in moods. His high mood swings were often associated with grandiose ideas, gambling, risky sexual behavior, and shopping sprees that were causing the couple to go bankrupt. The physician prescribed lithium.

1. The patient states, "The doctor told me I am having manic episodes. What does that mean?" What is the nurse's best response?

2. The nurse knows that there is a risk of lithium toxicity. What are the symptoms of lithium toxicity, and how will it be prevented?

3. The patient's partner asks, "How quickly will the lithium work?" What is the nurse's best response?

Note: Answers to the Critical Thinking activities can be found in the "Answer Key" sections at the end of the book.

8.9 ANTIPSYCHOTICS

Antipsychotic drugs are used to treat drug-induced psychosis, schizophrenia, extreme mania, depression that is resistant to other therapy, and other CNS conditions. Antipsychotics are sometimes referred to as tranquilizers because they produce a state of tranquility. First-generation antipsychotics, also called conventional antipsychotics, have similar mechanisms of action. An example of a conventional antipsychotic is haloperidol. Conventional antipsychotics have several potential adverse effects, and selection of a medication is based on the patient's ability to tolerate the adverse effects. Second-generation antipsychotics, also referred to as atypical antipsychotics, have fewer adverse effects. An example of an atypical antipsychotic is risperidone.[86] Both conventional and atypical antipsychotics have a Black Box Warning indicating that elderly patients with dementia-related psychosis treated with antipsychotic drugs are at an increased risk of death.

Mechanism of Action

All antipsychotics block dopamine receptors in the brain. However, the precise mechanism of action has not been clearly established. Conventional antipsychotics, such as haloperidol, block dopamine receptors in certain areas of the CNS, such as the limbic system and the basal ganglia. These areas are associated with emotions, cognitive function, and motor function, and blockage thus produces a tranquilizing effect in psychotic patients. However, several adverse effects are also caused by this dopamine blockade.

Second-generation, or atypical, antipsychotics block specific dopamine 2 receptors and specific serotonin 2 receptors, thus causing fewer adverse effects.

Indications for Use

Haloperidol is primarily indicated for schizophrenia and Tourette's disorder. Risperidone is primarily indicated for schizophrenia but is also used for acute manic episodes and for irritability caused by autism. Some atypical antipsychotics are also used as adjunct therapy for depression.

Nursing Considerations Across the Life Span

Elderly patients with dementia-related psychosis treated with antipsychotic drugs should be closely monitored for signs and symptoms of cardiovascular events or infections such as pneumonia.

Haloperidol is contraindicated in patients with Parkinson's disease or dementia with lewy bodies.

Patients who are concurrently taking lithium and antipsychotics should be monitored closely for neurotoxicity (weakness, lethargy, fever, tremulousness, confusion, and extrapyramidal symptoms) and symptoms should be immediately reported.

Adverse/Side Effects

Elderly patients with dementia-related psychosis treated with antipsychotic drugs are at an increased risk of death due to cardiovascular or infection-related causes.

Conventional antipsychotic medications have several potential serious adverse effects such as **tardive dyskinesia**, neuroleptic malignant syndrome (NMS), and **extrapyramidal symptoms.** These adverse effects are due to the

---

86   McCuistion, L., Vuljoin-DiMaggio, K., Winton, M, and Yeager, J. (2018). *Pharmacology: A patient-centered nursing process approach.* pp. 227–305. Elsevier.

blockage of alpha-adrenergic, dopamine, endocrine, histamine, and muscarinic receptors. For additional details about these types of receptors, see the "Autonomic Nervous System" chapter. Figure 8.8 describes adverse effects associated with conventional antipsychotics. Patients should be warned to not consume alcohol and that their ability to operate machinery or drive may be impaired.

Figure 8.8 Potential Adverse Effects of Antipsychotic Medication

Adverse Effect	Definition
Tardive Dyskinesia	Involuntary contraction of the oral and facial muscles (such as tongue thrusting) and wavelike movements of the extremities.
Neuroleptic Malignant Syndrome (NMS)	Potentially life-threatening adverse effect that includes high fever, unstable blood pressure, and myoglobinemia.
Extrapyramidal Symptoms	Involuntary motor symptoms similar to those associated with Parkinson's disease. Includes symptoms such as **akathisia** (distressing motor restlessness) and **acute dystonia** (painful muscle spasms.) Often treated with anticholinergic medications such as benztropine and trihexyphenidyl.

Figure 8.8 Potential Adverse Effects of Antipsychotic Medication[87]

Second-generation, or atypical, antipsychotics are less likely to cause adverse effects, but have a potential to do so. Atypical antipsychotics may also cause metabolic changes such as hyperglycemia, hyperlipidemia, and weight gain.

Patient Teaching and Education

Advise patient to take medication at directed. Medication doses should be evenly spaced throughout the day. This drug may require several weeks to obtain desired effects. Patients should be advised regarding the possibility of extrapyramidal symptoms and that abrupt withdrawal may cause dizziness, nausea and vomiting, uncontrolled movements of mouth, tongue, or jaw. Additionally, the patient should be careful to avoid alcohol or other CNS depressants while using the medication.

---

87 McCuistion, L., Vuljoin-DiMaggio, K., Winton, M, and Yeager, J. (2018). *Pharmacology: A patient-centered nursing process approach.* pp. 227–305. Elsevier.

Now let's take a closer look at the medication grid for haloperidol and risperidone in Table 8.9.[88, 89]

Table 8.9: Haloperidol and Risperidone Medication Grid

Class/Subclass	Prototype/ Generic	Administration Considerations	Therapeutic Effects	Adverse/Side Effects
1st generation (conventional) antipsychotic 2nd generation (atypical) antipsychotic	haloperidol risperidone	Black Box Warning: Monitor elderly patients with dementia closely for symptoms of cardiovascular events or infection Advise patients to avoid alcohol, operate machinery, or drive	Decrease symptoms of psychosis, hallucinations, delusions, and delirium	Life-threatening cardiovascular events or infections Tardive dyskinesia Neuroleptic Malignant Syndrome Extrapyramidal symptoms Hypersensitivity reactions Falls related to sedation, motor instability, and postural hypotension

88 This work is a derivative of *Daily Med* by U.S. National Library of Medicine in the public domain.

89 McCuistion, L., Vuljoin-DiMaggio, K., Winton, M, and Yeager, J. (2018). *Pharmacology: A patient-centered nursing process approach.* pp. 227–305. Elsevier.

8.10 ANTICONVULSANTS

Medications used for seizures are called anticonvulsants or antiseizure drugs. Antiseizure drugs stabilize cell membranes and suppress the abnormal electric impulses in the cerebral cortex. These drugs prevent seizures but do not provide a cure. Antiseizure drugs are classified as CNS depressants. There are many types of medications used to treat seizures such as phenytoin, phenobarbital, benzodiazepines, carbamazepine, valproate, and levetiracetam.[90]

There are three main pharmacological effects of antiseizure medications. First, they increase the threshold of activity in the motor cortex, thus making it more difficult for a nerve to become excited. Second, they limit the spread of a seizure discharge from its origin by suppressing the transmission of impulses from one nerve to the next. Third, they decrease the speed of the nerve impulse conduction within a given neuron.

Some drugs work by enhancing the effects of the inhibitory neurotransmitter gamma-aminobutyric acid (GABA), which plays a role in regulating neuron excitability in the brain.[91] Gabapentin, although structurally similar to GABA and classified as an anticonvulsant, is commonly used to control chronic neuropathic pain. Neuropathic pain is defined by the International Association for the Study of Pain as "pain caused by a lesion or disease of the somatosensory nervous system."[92] An example of neuropathic pain is tingling or burning in the lower extremities that often occurs in patients with diabetes.

Phenytoin

Phenytoin, which was discovered in 1938, was the first anti-seizure medication and is still being used to control seizures.[93]

Mechanism of Action

Phenytoin improves evidence of seizures by interfering with sodium channels in the brain, resulting in a reduction of sustained high-frequency neuronal discharges.

Indications for Use

Phenytoin is indicated for the treatment of tonic-clonic (grand mal) and psychomotor (temporal lobe) seizures and for the prevention and treatment of seizures occurring during or following neurosurgery.

Nursing Considerations Across the Life Span

Phenytoin should not be administered to pregnant women because it will cause harm to the fetus. When given intravenously, there is a Black Box Warning that the rate of administration should not exceed 50 mg per minute in adults and 1 to 3 mg/kg/min (or 50 mg per minute, whichever is slower) in pediatric patients because of the risk of

---

90   McCuistion, L., Vuljoin-DiMaggio, K., Winton, M, and Yeager, J. (2018). *Pharmacology: A patient-centered nursing process approach.* pp. 227–305. Elsevier.

91   Lilley, L., Collins, S., and Snyder, J. (2020). *Pharmacology and the Nursing Process.* pp. 246–272. Elsevier.

92   Murnion B. P. (2018, June 1). Neuropathic pain: current definition and review of drug treatment. *Australian prescriber, 41*(3), 60–63. https://www.ncbi.nlm.nih.gov/pmc/articles/PMC6003018/.

93   McCuistion, L., Vuljoin-DiMaggio, K., Winton, M, and Yeager, J. (2018). *Pharmacology: A patient-centered nursing process approach.* pp. 227–305. Elsevier.

severe hypotension and cardiac arrhythmias. Careful cardiac monitoring is needed during and after administering intravenous phenytoin.

Phenytoin has a narrow therapeutic drug level, usually between 10-20 mcg/ml, so serum drug monitoring is required. Serum levels of phenytoin sustained above the therapeutic range may produce confusional states referred to as delirium, psychosis, or encephalopathy. Accordingly, at the first sign of acute toxicity, serum levels should be immediately checked.

Abrupt discontinuation can cause status epilepticus, so in the event of an allergic or hypersensitivity reaction, rapid substitution of alternative therapy may be necessary.

Use with caution in patients with renal or hepatic impairment. Elderly patients may require dosage adjustment.

There are many potential drug interactions with phenytoin. Read drug label information before administering. Phenytoin is extensively bound to plasma proteins and is prone to competitive displacement. Phenytoin is metabolized by hepatic cytochrome P450 enzymes, so it is susceptible to inhibitory drug interactions, which may produce significant increases in circulating phenytoin concentrations and enhance the risk of drug toxicity.

Adverse/Side Effects

Serious and sometimes fatal dermatologic reactions, including toxic epidermal necrolysis (TEN) and Stevens-Johnson syndrome (SJS), have been reported with phenytoin treatment. The onset of symptoms is usually within 28 days, but can occur later. Phenytoin should be discontinued at the first sign of a rash.

Drug Reaction with Eosinophilia and Systemic Symptoms (DRESS) has been reported in patients taking anti-epileptic drugs, including phenytoin. Some of these events have been fatal or life threatening. DRESS typically presents with fever, rash, lymphadenopathy, and/or facial swelling, in association with other organ system involvement. These findings should be immediately reported to the provider. Acute hepatotoxicity has been reported with phenytoin. These events may be part of the spectrum of DRESS or may occur in isolation.

Hematopoietic complications, some fatal, have occasionally been reported in association with administration of phenytoin. These have included thrombocytopenia, leukopenia, granulocytopenia, agranulocytosis, and pancytopenia with or without bone marrow suppression.

The most common adverse reactions encountered with phenytoin therapy are nervous system reactions and are usually dose-related. Reactions include nystagmus, ataxia, slurred speech, decreased coordination, somnolence, and mental confusion.[94]

Patient Teaching and Education

Patients should be advised to take medications as directed and that doses should be evenly spaced throughout the day. It may take several weeks to obtain the desired medication effect. Abrupt withdrawal of medication may cause status epilepticus. Patients should avoid alcohol and other CNS depressants while taking anticonvulsant drug therapy. Additionally, diabetic patients should monitor their blood glucose levels carefully.

Now let's take a closer look at the medication grid for phenytoin in Table 8.10a.[95]

---

94 This work is a derivative of *Daily Med* by U.S. National Library of Medicine in the public domain.

95 This work is a derivative of *Daily Med* by U.S. National Library of Medicine in the public domain.

Table 8.10a: Phenytoin Medication Grid

Class/Subclass	Prototype/ Generic	Administration Considerations	Therapeutic Effects	Adverse/Side Effects
Anticonvulsant	phenytoin	Careful cardiac monitoring is needed during and after administering intravenous phenytoin For IV infusions, an in-line filter (0.22 to 0.55 microns) should be used. Cannot be given with D5W due to preciptiation and no faster than 50 mg/minute in adults Monitor serum drug levels Contraindicated with patient with heart block Use cautiously in patients with hepatic or renal impairment Taper dose; do not stop abruptly	Decrease or prevent seizure activity	Cardiovascular risk associated with rapid IV infusion Discontinue and notify the provider if a rash occurs Notify the provider immediately if fever, rash, lymphadenopathy, and/or facial swelling occur Cardiovascular: arrhythmia and hypotension CNS: Nystagmus, ataxia, slurred speech, decreased coordination, somnolence, and mental confusion GI: Constipation, gingival hyperplasia, and hepatotoxicity Hematology: Thrombocytopenia, pancytopenia, and agranulocytosis

Levetiracetam

Levetiracetam is indicated as adjunctive therapy in the treatment of partial onset seizures in patients 12 years of age and older with epilepsy. It is generally well tolerated.

Mechanism of Action

The exact mechanism of action is unknown. This medication may interfere with sodium, calcium, potassium, or GABA transmission.[96]

Indications for Use

Levetiracetam is used for partial onset seizures in patients with epilepsy.

Nursing Considerations Across the Life Span

Plasma levels can gradually decrease during pregnancy and should be monitored closely. Safety and effectiveness in pediatric patients 12 years of age and older have been established.

Levetiracetam immediate release and solution can be used in patients as young as 1 month.

Levetiracetam should not be stopped abruptly or withdrawal seizures may occur. Use with caution in patients with renal impairment.

---

96   This work is a derivative of *Daily Med* by U.S. National Library of Medicine in the public domain.

Adverse/Side Effects

Behavioral abnormalities including psychotic symptoms, suicidal ideation, irritability, and aggressive behavior have been observed; monitor patients for psychiatric signs and symptoms.

The most common adverse reactions are somnolence and irritability. Advise patients not to drive or operate machinery until they have gained sufficient experience on levetiracetam.

This drug can cause anaphylaxis or angioedema after the first dose or at any time during treatment. Serious dermatological reactions, including Stevens-Johnson syndrome (SJS) and toxic epidermal necrolysis (TEN), have been reported, as well as coordination difficulties and hematologic abnormalities.

Patient Teaching and Education

Medications should be taken as directed and may cause increased dizziness and somnolence. Patients, family, and caregivers should also monitor carefully for suicidality during medication therapy.

Now let's take a closer look at the medication grid for levetiracetam in Table 8.10b.[97]

Table 8.10b: Levetiracetam Medication Grid				
Class/Subclass	**Prototype/ Generic**	**Administration Considerations**	**Therapeutic Effects**	**Adverse/Side Effects**
Anticonvulsant	levetiracetam	Taper dose; do not stop abruptly or seizures may occur Monitor plasma levels for pregnant women Use cautiously if renal impairment	Decrease seizure activity	Behavioral/mood changes (psychotic symptoms, suicidal ideation, irritability, and aggressive behavior) Anaphylaxis or angioedema Somnolence, fatigue, and irritability Serious skin conditions Coordination difficulties Hematopoietic abnormalities

Gabapentin

Gabapentin is indicated as an adjunct treatment for partial seizures, but is most commonly used to treat neuropathic pain.

Mechanism of Action

The exact mechanism of action is unknown. It is structurally similar to GABA, but does not act on GABA receptors or influence GABA.

Indications for Use

---

97 This work is a derivative of *Daily Med* by U.S. National Library of Medicine in the public domain.

Gabapentin is used for partial seizures and neuropathic pain.[98]

Nursing Considerations Across the Life Span

This drug can cause harm to the fetus of pregnant women.

Gabapentin use in pediatric patients with epilepsy 3 to 12 years of age is associated with the occurrence of central nervous system related adverse events. The most significant of these can be classified into the following categories: 1) emotional lability (primarily behavioral problems); 2) hostility, including aggressive behaviors; 3) thought disorder, including concentration problems and change in school performance; and 4) hyperkinesia (primarily restlessness and hyperactivity).

In elderly patients, peripheral edema and ataxia tended to increase in incidence with age. Fall precautions should be considered.

Antiepileptic drugs should not be abruptly discontinued because of the possibility of increasing seizure frequency.

Adverse/Side Effects

Antiepileptic drugs, including gabapentin, increase the risk of suicidal thoughts or behavior in patients taking these drugs for any indication. Patients should be monitored for the emergence or worsening of depression, suicidal thoughts or behavior, and/or any unusual changes in mood or behavior.

Drug Reaction with Eosinophilia and Systemic Symptoms (DRESS), also known as multiorgan hypersensitivity, has been reported in patients taking antiepileptic drugs, including gabapentin. Some of these events have been fatal or life threatening. DRESS typically, although not exclusively, presents with fever, rash, and/or lymphadenopathy, in association with other organ system involvement. If these symptoms occur, they should be immediately reported to the provider.

Gabapentin may cause dizziness, somnolence, and other symptoms and signs of CNS depression. Patients should be advised neither to drive a car nor to operate other complex machinery until they have gained sufficient experience on gabapentin to gauge whether or not it affects their mental and/or motor performance adversely.[99]

---

98   Lilley, L., Collins, S., and Snyder, J. (2020). *Pharmacology and the Nursing Process.* pp. 246–272. Elsevier.

99   This work is a derivative of *Daily Med* by U.S. National Library of Medicine in the public domain.

Patient Teaching and Education

Patients receiving gabapentin therapy should take medication as directed and be careful to not exceed dosage recommendations. Patients should not take gabapentin within 2 hours of antacid medications. Additionally, gabapentin may cause increased drowsiness and dizziness. Patients, family, and caregivers should also monitor for suicidality.

Now let's take a closer look at the medication grid for gabapentin in Table 8.10c.[100]

Table 8.10c: Gabapentin Medication Grid

Class/Subclass	Prototype/ Generic	Administration Considerations	Therapeutic Effects	Adverse/Side Effects
Anticonvulsant	gabapentin	Administer first dose at bedtime to decrease dizziness and drowsiness Monitor for worsening depression, suicidal thoughts or behavior, and/or any unusual changes in mood or behavior Taper dose; do not stop abruptly	Decreased neuropathic pain or seizures	Increased suicidal ideation Immediately report fever, rash, and/or lymphadenopathy CNS depression: dizziness, somnolence, and ataxia

Critical Thinking Activity 8.10

A 70-year-patient in a long-term care center has diabetes and has been prescribed gabapentin for neuropathic pain.

1. The patient states, "I have never had a seizure. Why has the doctor prescribed an antiseizure medication for me?" What is the nurse's best response?

2. The nurse plans to implement additional fall precautions for this patient. Why are additional fall precautions needed?

3. What potential adverse effects should the nurse plan to monitor? What adverse effects would require immediate notification of the provider?

Note: Answers to the Critical Thinking activities can be found in the "Answer Key" sections at the end of the book.

---

100   This work is a derivative of *Daily Med* by U.S. National Library of Medicine in the public domain.

8.11   ANTIPARKINSON MEDICATIONS

Parkinson's disease is believed to be related to an imbalance of dopamine and acetylcholine and a deficiency of dopamine in certain areas of the brain, so drug therapies are aimed at increasing levels of dopamine and/or antagonizing the effects of acetylcholine. Drug therapy does not cure the disease, but is used to slow the progression of symptoms. Common medications used to treat Parkinson's disease are carbidopa/levodopa, selegiline, and amantadine.[101]

Carbidopa/Levodopa

Carbidopa/levodopa is the most common drug used to treat Parkinson's disease and is usually started as soon as the patient becomes functionally impaired.

Mechanism of Action

Administration of dopamine is ineffective in the treatment of Parkinson's disease because it does not cross the **blood-brain barrier**, but levodopa, the metabolic precursor of dopamine, does cross the blood-brain barrier and presumably is converted to dopamine in the brain. Carbidopa is combined with levodopa to help stop the breakdown of levodopa before it is able to cross the blood-brain barrier. Additionally, the incidence of levodopa-induced nausea and vomiting is less when it is combined with carbidopa.

Indications for Use

Carbidopa/levodopa is indicated for Parkinson's disease. It is also used to treat restless leg syndrome.

Nursing Considerations Across the Life Span

Carbidopa/Levodopa is recommended for use in patients older than age 18. It can take several weeks to see positive effects and this should be explained to patients and their caregivers.

The drug is contraindicated for use with MAOIs. All patients should be observed carefully for the development of depression with concomitant suicidal tendencies.

Patients taking carbidopa and levodopa have reported suddenly falling asleep without prior warning of sleepiness while engaged in activities of daily living (including operation of motor vehicles). Patients should be advised to exercise caution while driving or operating machines during treatment with carbidopa and levodopa.

Sporadic cases of symptoms resembling neuroleptic malignant syndrome (NMS) have been reported in association with dose reductions or withdrawal of certain antiparkinsonian agents. Therefore, patients should be observed carefully when the dosage of levodopa is reduced abruptly or discontinued.

Periodic evaluations of hepatic, hematopoietic, cardiovascular, and renal functions are recommended during extended therapy. The most common adverse effect of carbidopa/levodopa is dyskinesia, which may require dosage reduction.

Patients should be instructed to plan their meal times around medication times to improve the ability to use their utensils and to avoid diets high in protein due to decreased absorption of the medication.

---

101   Lilley, L., Collins, S., and Snyder, J. (2020). *Pharmacology and the Nursing Process*. pp. 246–272. Elsevier.

Adverse/Side Effects

Hallucinations and psychotic-like behavior have been reported with dopaminergic medications. Patients taking dopaminergic medications may experience intense gambling urges, increased sexual urges, intense urges to spend money, binge eating, and/or other intense urges, and the inability to control these urges. These urges stopped when the dosage was decreased or the medication discontinued.

A higher risk for melanoma has been reported. Occasionally, dark red, brown, or black color may appear in saliva, urine, or sweat after ingestion of carbidopa and levodopa. Although the color appears to be clinically insignificant, garments may become discolored.[102, 103, 104]

Patient Teaching and Education

Patients should take their medications at regular intervals as directed. If gastric irritation is experienced, patients may eat food shortly after taking medications but high-protein foods may impair drug action. Medications may cause increased drowsiness, dizziness, and orthostatic changes. Patients should carefully assess their skin to monitor for new lesions and any abnormality should be reported to the healthcare provider.

Now let's take a closer look at the medication grid for carbidopa-levodopa in Table 8.11.[105]

Table 8.11a: Carbidopa-Levodopa Medication Grid

Class/subclass	Prototype/ Generic	Administration Considerations	Therapeutic Effects	Adverse/Side Effects
Antiparkinson agent	carbidopa/ levodopa	Avoid high-protein diets due to decreased absorption Monitor for sudden somnolence and increased depression Contraindicated with MAOIs Periodically monitor hepatic, renal, and hematopoietic functions	Slow progression of symptoms of Parkinson's disease (tremors, rigidity, and mobility issues)	Depression, suicidal ideation, hallucinations, and intense urges with inability to control them Somnolence and fatigue NMS symptoms with dose reductions or when discontinued Dyskinesia Discolored body fluids Hypomobility with long-term use

102 This work is a derivative of *Daily Med* by U.S. National Library of Medicine in the public domain.

103 McCuistion, L., Vuljoin-DiMaggio, K., Winton, M, and Yeager, J. (2018). *Pharmacology: A patient-centered nursing process approach.* pp. 227–305. Elsevier.

104 Lilley, L., Collins, S., and Snyder, J. (2020). *Pharmacology and the Nursing Process.* pp. 246–272. Elsevier.

105 This work is a derivative of *Daily Med* by U.S. National Library of Medicine in the public domain.

Selegiline

Selegiline is often used conjunction with carbidopa-levodopa when patients demonstrate a deteriorating response to this treatment. It is helpful to control symptom fluctuations.[106]

Mechanism of Action

Selegiline inhibits MAO-B, blocking the breakdown of dopamine.[107]

Indications for Use

Selegiline capsules are indicated as an adjunct in the management of Parkinsonian patients being treated with levodopa/carbidopa who exhibit deterioration in the quality of their response to this therapy. There is no evidence from controlled studies that selegiline has any beneficial effect in the absence of concurrent levodopa therapy.

Nursing Considerations Across the Life Span

Large doses of selegiline may inhibit MAO-A that promotes metabolism of tyramine in the GI tract, which can cause a hypertensive crisis.

Adverse/Side Effects

Side effects are dose dependent, with larger doses posing a hypertensive crisis risk if there is consumption of food or beverages with tyramine.

Patient Teaching and Education

Patients should be advised to avoid foods high in tyramine. Additionally, medications may cause increased drowsiness, dizziness, and orthostatic changes. If patients experience abnormal behaviors such as hallucination, sexual urges, gambling, etc., this should be reported promptly to the healthcare provider.

Now let's take a closer look at the medication grid for selegiline in Table 8.11b.[108]

Table 8.11b: Selegiline Medication Grid

Class/Subclass	Prototype/ Generic	Administration Considerations	Therapeutic Effects	Adverse/Side Effects
Antiparkinson agent, MAO Type B Inhibitor	selegiline	Avoid food with tyramine if on a large dose (above 10mg/ day)	Minimize progression of Parkinson's disease symptoms	Higher doses increase risk for hypertensive crisis

---

106   Lilley, L., Collins, S., and Snyder, J. (2020). *Pharmacology and the Nursing Process*. pp. 246–272. Elsevier.

107   This work is a derivative of *Daily Med* by U.S. National Library of Medicine in the public domain.

108   This work is a derivative of *Daily Med* by U.S. National Library of Medicine in the public domain.

Amantadine

Amantadine is used in early stages of Parkinson's disease but can be effective in moderate or advanced stages in reducing tremor and muscle rigidity.[109]

Mechanism of Action

The exact mechanism of action is unknown. Amantadine is an antiviral drug that acts on dopamine receptors.[110]

Indications for Use

Amantadine is used for Parkinson's disease, medication-induced extrapyramidal symptoms, and influenza A.

Nursing Considerations Across the Life Span

Use cautiously with renal impairment. This drug may cause suicidal ideation and should not be stopped abruptly or can cause Parkinsonian crisis. Neuroleptic Malignant Syndrome (NMS) has been reported in association with dose reduction or withdrawal of amantadine therapy.

Adverse/Side Effects

Suicide ideation, congestive heart failure, and peripheral edema can occur. This drug can cause intense gambling urges, increased sexual urges, intense urges to spend money uncontrollably, and other intense urges with an inability to control them. There is an increased risk of melanoma.

Adverse reactions reported most frequently are nausea, dizziness (lightheadedness), and insomnia. This drug can also cause anticholinergic side effects, impaired thinking, and orthostatic hypotension.[111]

Patient Teaching and Education

Patients should take medications as directed and ensure they do not skip or double doses. Medications may cause drowsiness, dizziness, and orthostatic blood pressure changes. Patients should avoid using this medication with OTC cold medications or alcoholic beverages. If patients, family, or caregivers note worsening depression or suicidality, this should be reported immediately to the healthcare provider.

---

109   Lilley, L., Collins, S., and Snyder, J. (2020). *Pharmacology and the Nursing Process.* pp. 246–272. Elsevier.

110   McCuistion, L., Vuljoin-DiMaggio, K., Winton, M, and Yeager, J. (2018). *Pharmacology: A patient-centered nursing process approach.* pp. 227–305. Elsevier.

111   This work is a derivative of *Daily Med* by U.S. National Library of Medicine in the public domain.

Now let's take a closer look at the medication grid for amantadine in Table 8.11c.[112]

Table 8.11c: Amantadine Medication Grid

Class	Prototype/ Generic	Administration Considerations	Therapeutic Effects	Adverse/Side Effects
Anti-Parkinson Agent, Antiviral	amantadine	Monitor renal function Monitor mental state Assess blood pressure	Improve Parkinson's disease symptoms	Increased suicidal ideation and urges Congestive heart failure and peripheral edema Neuromalignant syndrome (NMS) when dosage decreased Orthostatic hypotension Nausea, dizziness, and insomnia Anticholinergic side effects

Critical Thinking Activity 8.11

A 76-year-old patient in a long-term care center has developed a shuffling gait with a stooped posture, along with a hand tremor at rest. The nurse practitioner prescribed carbidopa/levodopa.

1. The nurse knows that Parkinson's disease is related to dopamine, but dopamine can't cross the blood-brain barrier. How will carbidopa/levodopa assist with dopamine levels?

2. The patient states, "I am looking forward to spending next weekend with my grandson. He even said he would let me drive his new Mustang!" What teaching should the nurse provide the patient and his grandson (with the patient's permission) regarding the new medication and his weekend plans?

3. The nurse reads that the most common side effect of carbidopa-levodopa is dyskinesia. What is dyskinesia? If it occurs, what is the likely treatment?

Note: Answers to the Critical Thinking activities can be found in the "Answer Key" sections at the end of the book.

---

112   This work is a derivative of *Daily Med* by U.S. National Library of Medicine in the public domain.

8.12 MODULE LEARNING ACTIVITIES

Interactive Activities

 An interactive or media element has been excluded from this version of the text. You can view it online here: https://wtcs.pressbooks.pub/pharmacology/?p=1824

GLOSSARY

Action potential: A change in voltage of a cell membrane in response to a stimulus that results in transmission of an electrical signal; unique to neurons and muscle fibers.

Acute dystonia: Painful muscle spasms.

Affective mood disorders: Mental illness such such as major depression.

Akathisia: Distressing motor restlessness.

Blood-brain barrier (BBB): A physiological barrier between the circulatory system and the central nervous system that establishes a privileged blood supply, restricting the flow of substances into the CNS.

Bradykinesia: Slowness in initiation and execution of voluntary movements.

Central nervous system (CNS): Anatomical division of the nervous system located within the cranial and vertebral cavities, namely the brain and spinal cord.

Chemical synapse: Connection between two neurons, or between a neuron and its target, where a neurotransmitter diffuses across a very short distance.

Drug Reaction with Eosinophilia and Systemic Symptoms (DRESS): A condition reported in patients taking antiepileptic drugs. Some of these events have been fatal or life threatening. DRESS typically presents with fever, rash, lymphadenopathy, and/or facial swelling.

Dystonia: Inappropriate and continuous muscle contraction.

Electrical synapse: Connection between two neurons, or any two electrically active cells, where ions flow directly through channels spanning their adjacent cell membranes.

Extrapyramidal symptoms: Involuntary motor symptoms similar to those associated with Parkinson's disease. Includes symptoms such as akathisia (distressing motor restlessness) and acute dystonia (painful muscle spasms). Often treated with anticholinergic medications such as benztropine and trihexyphenidyl.

Gait disturbance: An abnormal way of walking, such as shuffling feet.

Hypertensive crisis: Severe hypertension (blood pressure greater than 180/120 mm Hg) with evidence of organ dysfunction. Symptoms may include occipital headache (which may radiate frontally), palpitations, neck stiffness or soreness, nausea or vomiting, sweating, dilated pupils, photophobia, shortness of breath, or confusion. Either tachycardia or bradycardia may be present and may be associated with constricting chest pain. Seizures may also occur. Intracranial bleeding, sometimes fatal, has been reported in association with the increase in blood pressure.

Mania: Periods of extreme highs in bipolar disorder. Manic episodes may include these symptoms: rapid speech, hyperactivity, reduced need for sleep, flight of ideas, grandiosity, poor judgement, aggression/hostility, risky sexual behavior, neglected basic self-care, or decreased impulse control.

Nerve: Cord-like bundle of axons located in the peripheral nervous system that transmits sensory input and response output to and from the central nervous system.

Neuroleptic malignant syndrome (NMS): Potentially life-threatening adverse effect that includes high fever, unstable blood pressure, and myoglobinemia.

Neuron(s): Neural tissue cell that is primarily responsible for generating and propagating electrical signals into, within, and out of the nervous system.

Neurotransmitter: Chemical signal that is released from the synaptic end bulb of a neuron to cause a change in the target cell.

Ophthalmoplegia: Weakness in eye muscles.

Orthostatic hypotension: A significant change in blood pressure from lying to sitting to standing.

Peripheral nervous system (PNS): An anatomical division of the nervous system that is largely outside the cranial and vertebral cavities, namely all parts except the brain and spinal cord.

Postural instability: Abnormal fixation of posture (stoop when standing), problems with equilibrium, and righting reflex.

Rigidity: Increased muscle tone and increase resistance to movement. As severity increases, there may be cogwheel rigidity.

Serotonin syndrome: May occur when taking serotonin medications.

Includes mental status changes (e.g., agitation, hallucinations, coma), autonomic instability (e.g., tachycardia, labile blood pressure, hyperthermia), neuromuscular aberrations (e.g., hyperreflexia, incoordination) and/or gastrointestinal symptoms (e.g., nausea, vomiting, diarrhea). Serotonin syndrome, in its most severe form, can resemble neuroleptic malignant syndrome, which includes hyperthermia, muscle rigidity, autonomic instability with possible rapid fluctuation of vital signs, and mental status changes.

Status epilepticus: A state of repeated or continuous seizures.

Tardive dyskinesia: Involuntary contraction of the oral and facial muscles (such as tongue thrusting) and wavelike movements of the extremities.

Thalamus: The region of the central nervous system that acts as a relay for sensory pathways.

Threshold: The membrane voltage at which an action potential is initiated.

Tremor: Usually tremor at rest; when person sits, the arms shake, but tremor stops when person attempts to grab something.

Chapter IX

Endocrine

9.1   ENDOCRINE INTRODUCTION

Learning Objectives

- Cite the classifications and actions of endocrine system drugs

- Give examples of when, how, and to whom endocrine system drugs may be administered

- Identify the side effects and special considerations associated with endocrine system drug therapy

- Identify the considerations and implications of using endocrine system medications across the life span

- Apply evidence-based concepts when using the nursing process

- Identify indications, side effects, and potential drug interactions associated with the use of herbal supplements

- Identify and interpret related laboratory tests

Have you ever wondered how your body controls functions such as digestion, metabolism, and the stress response? The endocrine system is always working behind the scenes, regulating various organs by releasing hormones and using feedback loops. This chapter will discuss medications that affect three of the major endocrine glands: the adrenal glands, the pancreas, and the thyroid. But before we get started with discussing medications, let's review some key endocrine system concepts to understand the mechanism of action of endocrine medications.

9.2   ENDOCRINE SYSTEM BASICS

You may never have thought of it this way, but when you send a text message to two friends to meet you at a restaurant at six, you're sending digital signals that you hope will affect their behavior—even though they are some distance away. Similarly, certain cells send chemical signals to other cells in the body that influence their behavior. This long-distance intercellular communication, coordination, and control are critical for homeostasis, and it is the fundamental function of the endocrine system.

Whereas the nervous system uses neurotransmitters to communicate, the endocrine system uses **hormones** for chemical signaling. These hormone signals are sent by the endocrine organs. Hormones are transported primarily via the bloodstream throughout the body, where they bind to receptors on target cells, inducing a characteristic response. Some of the glands in the endocrine system include the pituitary, thyroid, parathyroid, adrenal, and pineal glands. See Figure 9.1 for an illustration of the endocrine system.[1] Some of these glands have both endocrine and nonendocrine functions. For example, the pancreas contains cells that function in digestion, as well as cells that secrete the hormones insulin and glucagon, which regulate blood glucose levels.[2]

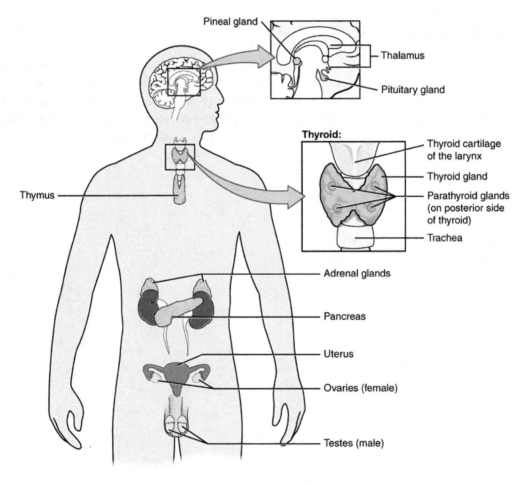

Figure 9.1 Overview of the Endocrine System

---

1   "1801 The Endocrine System.jpg" by OpenStax is licensed under CC BY 4.0 Access for free at https://openstax.org /books/anatomy-and-physiology/pages/17-1-an-overview-of-the-endocrine-system.

2   This work is a derivative of *Anatomy and Physiology* by OpenStax licensed under CC BY 4.0. Access for free at https:// openstax.org/books/anatomy-and-physiology/pages/1-introduction.

This module will focus on medications that affect three major endocrine glands and their hormones: the adrenal glands, the pancreas, and the thyroid. See Table 9.1 for a list of hormones associated with each of these glands and their effects.[3]

Table 9.1: Hormones Associated with Adrenal Gland, Pancreas, and Thyroid and Their Effects

Endocrine gland	Hormone	Effect
Adrenal (cortex)	Aldosterone	Increases blood Na+ levels
Adrenal (cortex)	Cortisol	Increases blood sugar levels
Adrenal (medulla)	Epinephrine and Norepinephrine	Stimulates fight-or-flight response
Pancreas	Insulin	Reduces blood glucose levels
Pancreas	Glucagon	Increases blood glucose levels
Thyroid	Thyroxine (T4), triiodothyronine (T3)	Stimulates basal metabolic rate
Thyroid	Calcitonin	Reduces blood Ca+ levels

Regulation of Hormone Secretion

To prevent abnormal hormone levels and a potential disease state, hormone levels must be tightly controlled. Feedback loops govern the initiation and maintenance of hormone secretion in response to various stimuli.

The most common method of hormone regulation is the **negative feedback loop.** Negative feedback is characterized by the inhibition of further secretion of a hormone in response to adequate levels of that hormone. This allows blood levels of the hormone to be regulated within a narrow range. An example of a negative feedback loop is the release of glucocorticoid hormones from the adrenal glands, as directed by the hypothalamus and pituitary gland. As glucocorticoid concentrations in the blood rise, the hypothalamus and pituitary gland reduce their signaling to the adrenal glands to prevent additional glucocorticoid secretion.[4] See Figure 9.2 for an illustration of a negative feedback loop.[5]

---

3   This work is a derivative of *Anatomy and Physiology* by OpenStax licensed under CC BY 4.0. Access for free at https://openstax.org/books/anatomy-and-physiology/pages/1-introduction.

4   This work is a derivative of *Anatomy and Physiology* by OpenStax licensed under CC BY 4.0. Access for free at https://openstax.org/books/anatomy-and-physiology/pages/1-introduction.

5   "1805 Negative Feedback Loop.jpg" by OpenStax is licensed under CC BY 4.0 Access for free at https://openstax.org/books/anatomy-and-physiology/pages/17-2-hormones.

My Notes

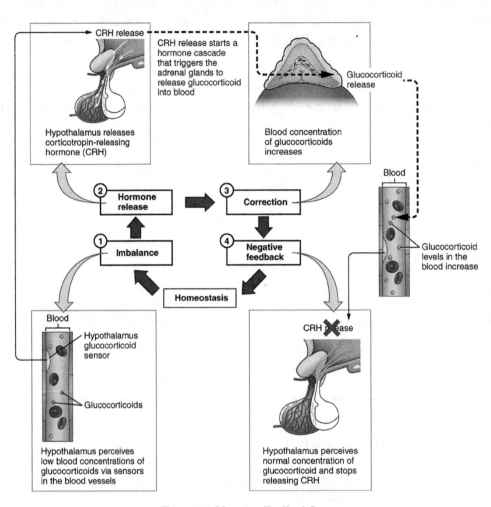

Figure 9.2 Negative Feedback Loop

Endocrine Gland Stimuli

Endocrine glands can be stimulated by humoral stimuli, by stimulation of another hormone, or by neural stimuli. **Humoral stimuli** are changes in blood levels of non-hormone chemicals that cause the release or inhibition of a hormone to maintain homeostasis. For example, osmoreceptors in the hypothalamus detect changes in **blood osmolarity** (the concentration of solutes in the blood plasma). If blood osmolarity is too high, meaning that the blood is not dilute enough, osmoreceptors signal the hypothalamus to release ADH (antidiuretic hormone). ADH causes the kidneys to reabsorb more water and reduce the volume of urine produced. This reabsorption causes a reduction of the osmolarity of the blood by diluting the blood to the appropriate level. Another example of humoral stimuli is the regulation of blood glucose. High blood glucose levels cause the release of insulin from the pancreas, which increases glucose uptake by cells and liver storage of glucose as glycogen.

An endocrine gland may also secrete a hormone in response to the presence of another hormone produced by a different endocrine gland. For example, the thyroid gland secretes T4 into the bloodstream when triggered by thyroid-stimulating hormone (TSH) that is released from the anterior pituitary gland.

In addition to these chemical signals, hormones can also be released in response to **neural stimuli**. An example of neural stimuli is the activation of the fight-or-flight response by the sympathetic nervous system. When an individual perceives danger, sympathetic neurons signal the adrenal glands to secrete norepinephrine and epinephrine.

The two hormones dilate blood vessels, increase the heart and respiratory rate, and suppress the digestive and immune systems. These responses boost the body's transport of oxygen to the brain and muscles, thereby improving the body's ability to fight or flee.[6]

The Hypothalamus–Pituitary Complex

The **hypothalamus–pituitary complex** can be thought of as the "command center" of the endocrine system. This complex secretes several hormones that directly produce responses in target tissues, as well as hormones that regulate the synthesis and secretion of hormones of other glands. In addition, the hypothalamus–pituitary complex coordinates the messages of the endocrine and nervous systems. In many cases, a stimulus received by the nervous system must pass through the hypothalamus–pituitary complex to be translated into hormones that can initiate a response. See Figure 9.3 for an illustration of the hypothalamus–pituitary complex.[7] The hypothalamus connects to the pituitary gland by the stalk-like infundibulum. The pituitary gland consists of an anterior and posterior lobe, with each lobe secreting different hormones in response to signals from the hypothalamus.

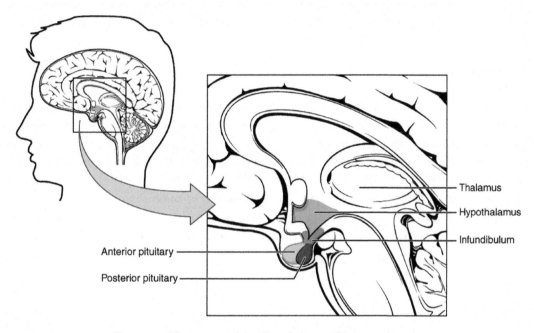

Figure 9.3 Illustration of the Hypothalamus–Pituitary Complex

Posterior Pituitary

The posterior pituitary gland does not produce hormones, but stores and secretes two hormones produced by the hypothalamus: oxytocin and antidiuretic hormone (ADH).

---

6   This work is a derivative of *Anatomy and Physiology* by OpenStax licensed under CC BY 4.0. Access for free at https://openstax.org/books/anatomy-and-physiology/pages/1-introduction.

7   "1806 The Hypothalamus-Pituitary Complex.jpg" by OpenStax is licensed under CC BY 4.0 Access for free at https://openstax.org/books/anatomy-and-physiology/pages/17-3-the-pituitary-gland-and-hypothalamus.

My Notes

Antidiuretic Hormone (ADH)

Blood osmolarity, the concentration of sodium ions and other solutes, is constantly monitored by **osmoreceptors** in the hypothalamus. Blood osmolarity may change in response to the consumption of certain foods and fluids, as well as in response to disease, injury, medications, or other factors. In response to high blood osmolarity, which can occur during dehydration or following a very salty meal, the osmoreceptors signal the posterior pituitary to release antidiuretic hormone (ADH). Its effect is to cause increased water reabsorption by the kidneys. As more water is reabsorbed by the kidneys, a greater amount of water is returned to the blood, thus causing a decrease in blood osmolarity. The release of ADH is controlled by a negative feedback loop. As blood osmolarity decreases, the hypothalamic osmoreceptors sense the change and prompt a corresponding decrease in the secretion of ADH. As a result, less water is reabsorbed by the kidneys.

Drugs can also affect the secretion of ADH or imitate its effects. For example, alcohol consumption inhibits the release of ADH, resulting in increased urine production that can eventually lead to dehydration and a hangover. Vasopressin is a synthetic ADH medication used to treat very low blood pressure. It is called vasopressin because in very high concentrations it also causes constriction of blood vessels in addition to the retention of water. Vasopressin is also used to treat a disease called **diabetes insipidus (DI)** that causes dehydration due to an under-production of ADH.[8]

Anterior Pituitary

In contrast to the posterior pituitary, the anterior pituitary does manufacture hormones. However, the secretion of hormones from the anterior pituitary is regulated by two classes of hormones secreted by the hypothalamus called releasing hormones. Releasing hormones then stimulate the secretion of hormones from the anterior pituitary (see Figure 9.4[9]). The anterior pituitary produces seven hormones. These are the growth hormone (GH), thyroid-stimulating hormone (TSH), adrenocorticotropic hormone (ACTH), follicle-stimulating hormone (FSH), luteinizing hormone (LH), beta endorphin, and prolactin. Of the hormones of the anterior pituitary, TSH, ACTH, FSH, and LH are collectively referred to as **tropic hormones** (trope- = "turning") because they turn on or off the function of other endocrine glands. This module will focus on the effects of TSH and ACTH.

---

8   This work is a derivative of *Anatomy and Physiology* by OpenStax licensed under CC BY 4.0. Access for free at https://openstax.org/books/anatomy-and-physiology/pages/1-introduction.

9   "1808 The Anterior Pituitary Complex.jpg" by OpenStax is licensed under CC BY 4.0 Access for free at https://openstax.org/books/anatomy-and-physiology/pages/17-3-the-pituitary-gland-and-hypothalamus.

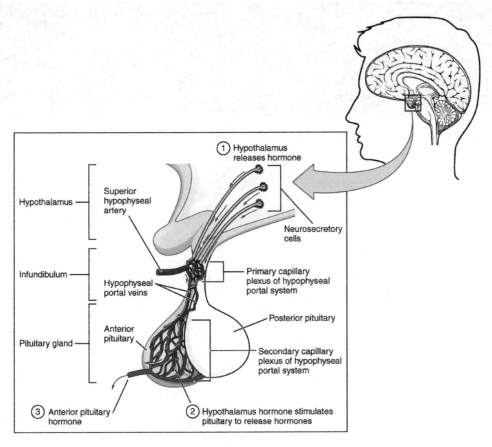

Figure 9.4 The hypothalamus releases hormones to regulate the release of hormones from the anterior pituitary

Thyroid-Stimulating Hormone (TSH)

The activity of the thyroid gland is regulated by the thyroid-stimulating hormone (TSH). TSH is released from the anterior pituitary in response to the thyrotropin-releasing hormone (TRH) from the hypothalamus and triggers the secretion of thyroid hormones by the thyroid gland. In a classic negative feedback loop, elevated levels of thyroid hormones in the bloodstream then trigger a drop in production of TRH and subsequently, the production of TSH. TSH is further discussed in the "Thyroid" submodule.

Adrenocorticotropic Hormone (ACTH)

The adrenocorticotropic hormone (ACTH) is released from the anterior pituitary in response to the corticotropin-releasing hormone (CRH) from the hypothalamus. ACTH then stimulates the adrenal cortex to secrete corticosteroid hormones such as cortisol. A variety of stressors can also influence the release of ACTH, and the role of ACTH in the stress response is discussed under the "Adrenal" submodule.[10]

---

10   This work is a derivative of *Anatomy and Physiology* by OpenStax licensed under CC BY 4.0. Access for free at https://openstax.org/books/anatomy-and-physiology/pages/1-introduction.

Interactive Activity

 An interactive or media element has been excluded from this version of the text. You can view it online here: https://wtcs.pressbooks.pub/pharmacology/?p=1678

9.3   CORTICOSTERIODS

Adrenal: A&P Basics Review

The adrenal gland consists of the adrenal cortex that is composed of glandular tissue and the adrenal medulla that is composed of nervous tissue. Each region secretes its own set of hormones.

The adrenal cortex is a component of the **hypothalamic-pituitary-adrenal (HPA) axis**. The hypothalamus stimulates the release of ACTH from the pituitary, which then stimulates the adrenal cortex to produce steroid hormones that are important for the regulation of the stress response, blood pressure and blood volume, nutrient uptake and storage, fluid and electrolyte balance, and inflammation.

The **adrenal medulla** is neuroendocrine tissue composed of postganglionic sympathetic nervous system (SNS) neurons that secretes the hormones epinephrine and norepinephrine. It is an extension of the autonomic nervous system, which regulates homeostasis in the body. See Figure 9.5 for an illustration of the adrenal gland and associated hormones.[11]

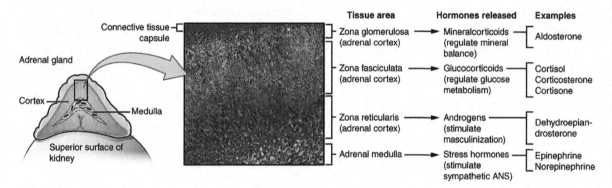

Figure 9.5 The Adrenal Gland and Associated Hormones

One of the major functions of the adrenal gland is to respond to stress. The body responds in different ways to short-term stress and long-term stress following a pattern known as the **general adaptation syndrome (GAS)**. Stage one of GAS is called the alarm reaction. This is short-term stress, also called the fight-or-flight response, and is mediated by the hormones epinephrine and norepinephrine from the adrenal medulla. Their function is to prepare the body for extreme physical exertion. If the stress is not soon relieved, the body adapts to the stress in the second stage called the stage of resistance. If a person is starving for example, the body may send signals to the gastrointestinal tract to maximize the absorption of nutrients from food. If the stress continues for a longer term however, the body responds with symptoms such as depression, suppressed immune response, or severe fatigue. These symptoms are mediated by the hormones of the adrenal cortex, especially cortisol.

Adrenal hormones also have several non–stress-related functions, including the increase of blood sodium and glucose levels, which will be described in further detail below.

---

11   "1818 The Adrenal Glands.jpg" by OpenStax is licensed under CC BY 4.0 Access for free at https://openstax.org/books/anatomy-and-physiology/pages/17-6-the-adrenal-glands.

Mineralocorticoids: Aldosterone

The most superficial region of the adrenal cortex is the zona glomerulosa, which produces a group of hormones collectively referred to as **mineralocorticoids** because of their effect on body minerals, especially sodium and potassium. These hormones are essential for fluid and electrolyte balance.

Aldosterone is the major mineralocorticoid that is important in the regulation of the concentration of sodium and potassium ions in the body. The secretion of aldosterone by the adrenal cortex is prompted by the HPA axis when the hypothalamus triggers ACTH release from the anterior pituitary. It is released in response to elevated blood levels of potassium (K+), low blood levels of sodium (Na+), low blood pressure, or low blood volume.

Aldosterone targets the kidneys and increases the excretion of K+ and the retention of Na+, which, in turn, causes the retention of water, thus increasing blood volume and blood pressure.

Aldosterone is also a key component of the renin-angiotensin-aldosterone system (RAAS) in which specialized cells of the kidneys secrete renin in response to low blood volume or low blood pressure. Renin then catalyzes the conversion of the blood protein angiotensinogen, which is produced by the liver, to the hormone Angiotensin I. Angiotensin I is converted in the lungs to Angiotensin II by the angiotensin-converting enzyme (ACE). Angiotensin II has three major functions: initiating vasoconstriction of the arterioles, thus decreasing blood flow; stimulating kidney tubules to reabsorb sodium and water, thus increasing blood volume; and signaling the adrenal cortex to secrete aldosterone, which further increases blood volume and blood pressure. It is important to understand these effects because many cardiac medications target the effects of aldosterone and the RAAS system. For example, drugs that block the production of Angiotensin II are known as ACE inhibitors. ACE inhibitors are used to help lower blood pressure in patients with hypertension by blocking the ACE enzyme from converting Angiotensin I to Angiotensin II, which, in turn, causes vasodilation of the arterioles. Another medication called spironolactone is used as a diuretic because it blocks the effects of aldosterone and, thus, causes the kidneys to eliminate water and sodium to decrease blood volume and blood pressure.

Glucocorticoids: Cortisol

The intermediate region of the adrenal cortex produces hormones called glucocorticoids because of their role in glucose metabolism. In response to long-term stressors, the HPA axis triggers the release of glucocorticoids. Their overall effect is to inhibit tissue building while stimulating the breakdown of stored nutrients to maintain adequate fuel supplies. In conditions of long-term stress, cortisol promotes the catabolism of glycogen to glucose, stored triglycerides into fatty acids and glycerol, and muscle proteins into amino acids. These raw materials can then be used to synthesize additional glucose and ketones for use as body fuels. However, the negative effects of catabolism for energy can result in muscle breakdown and weakness, poor wound healing, and the suppression of the immune system.

Many medications contain glucocorticoids to treat various conditions, such as cortisone injections for inflamed joints; prednisone tablets, IV medication, and steroid-based inhalers to manage inflammation that occurs in asthma; and hydrocortisone creams that are applied to relieve itchy skin rashes.

Androgens

The deepest region of the adrenal cortex produces small amounts of a class of steroid sex hormones called androgens. During puberty and most of adulthood, androgens are produced in the gonads. The androgens produced in the adrenal cortex supplement the gonadal androgens.

Adrenal Medulla: Epinephrine and Norepinephrine

As noted earlier, the adrenal cortex releases glucocorticoids in response to long-term stress such as severe illness. In contrast, the adrenal medulla releases its hormones in response to acute, short-term stress mediated by the sympathetic nervous system (SNS). The medullary tissue is composed of unique postganglionic SNS neurons called chromaffin cells that produce the neurotransmitters epinephrine (also called adrenaline) and norepinephrine (also called noradrenaline), which are chemically classified as catecholamines. Epinephrine is produced in greater quantities and is the more powerful hormone.

The secretion of medullary epinephrine and norepinephrine is controlled by a neural pathway that originates from the hypothalamus in response to danger or stress. Both epinephrine and norepinephrine increase the heart rate, pulse, and blood pressure to prepare the body to fight the perceived threat or flee from it. In addition, the pathway dilates the airways, raising blood oxygen levels. It also prompts vasodilation, further increasing the oxygenation of important organs such as the lungs, brain, heart, and skeletal muscle while also prompting vasoconstriction to blood vessels serving less essential organs such as the gastrointestinal tract, kidneys, and skin. It also downregulates some components of the immune system. Other effects include a dry mouth, loss of appetite, pupil dilation, and a loss of peripheral vision.

Disorders Involving the Adrenal Glands

Several disorders are caused by the dysregulation of the hormones produced by the adrenal glands. For example, Cushing's disease is a disorder characterized by high blood glucose levels, the development of a moon-shaped face, a buffalo hump on the back of the neck, rapid weight gain, and hair loss. It is caused by hypersecretion of cortisol. Cushing's syndrome can also be caused by long-term use of corticosteroid medications.

In contrast, the hyposecretion of corticosteroids can result in Addison's disease, a disorder that causes low blood glucose levels and low blood sodium levels. Addisonian crisis is a life-threatening condition due to severely low blood pressure resulting from a lack of corticosteroid levels. [12, 13, 14, 15]

A supplementary video about ACTH and the adrenal gland is provided below.

---

12   This work is a derivative of *Anatomy and Physiology* by OpenStax licensed under CC BY 4.0. Access for free at https://openstax.org/books/anatomy-and-physiology/pages/1-introduction.

13   This work is a derivative of *Daily Med* by U.S. National Library of Medicine in the public domain.

14   Nieman, L., Biller, B., Findling, J., Murad, M., Newell-Price, J., Savage, M, and Tabarin, A. (2015, August 1). Treatment of Cushing's Sydnrome: an endocrine clinical practice guideline. *The Journal of Clinical Endocrinology and Metabolism, 100*(8). pp. 2807–2831. https://academic.oup.com/jcem/article/100/8/2807/2836065.

15   Liu, D., Ahmet, A., Ward, L., et al (2013). A practical guide to the monitoring and management of the complications of systemic corticosteroid therapy. *Allergy, Asthma and Clinical Immunology, 9*, 30. https://aacijournal.biomedcentral.com/articles/10.1186/1710-1492-9-30.

ACTH and the Adrenal Gland[16]

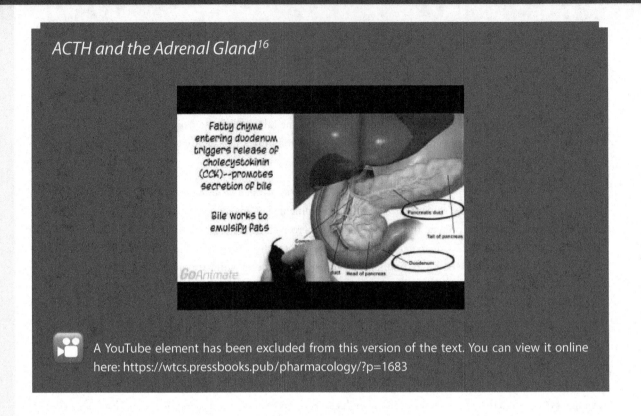

Nursing Considerations for Adrenal Medications

Assessment

Before initiating long-term systemic corticosteroid therapy, a thorough history and physical examination should be performed to assess for risk factors or pre-existing conditions that may potentially be exacerbated by glucocorticoid therapy, such as diabetes, dyslipidemia, cerebrovascular disease (CVD), GI disorders, affective disorders, or osteoporosis. At a minimum, baseline measures of body weight, height, bone mineral density, and blood pressure should be obtained, along with laboratory assessments that include a complete blood count (CBC), blood glucose values, and lipid profile. In children, nutritional and pubertal status should also be examined. Symptoms of and/or exposure to serious infections should also be assessed as corticosteroids are contraindicated in patients with untreated systemic infections. Concomitant use of other medications should also be assessed before initiating therapy as significant drug interactions have been noted between glucocorticoids and several drug classes. Females of childbearing age should also be questioned about the possibility of pregnancy because use in pregnancy may increase the risk of cleft palate in offspring.[17]

16 Forciea, B. (2015, May 12). *Anatomy and Physiology: Endocrine System: ACTH* (Adrenocorticotropin Hormone) V2.0. [Video]. YouTube. All rights reserved. Video used with permission. https://youtu.be/4m7XflJzm2w.

17 Liu, D., Ahmet, A., Ward, L., Krishnamoorthy, P., Mandelcorn, E., Leigh, R., Brown, J., Cohen, A., and Kim, H. (2013, August 15). A practical guide to the monitoring and management of the complications of systemic corticosteroid therapy. *Allergy, Asthma and Clinical Immunology, 9*(30). https://doi.org/10.1186/1710-1492-9-30.

Implementation

My Notes

Long-term corticosteroid therapy should never be stopped abruptly due to its effect on the hypothalamic-pituitary-adrenal (HPA) axis and potential adrenal suppression. Instead, the dose should be tapered to allow the body to resume natural production of adrenal hormone levels.

Patients on long-term corticosteroid therapy who are also at high risk for fractures are recommended to receive concurrent pharmacological treatment for osteoporosis. Alendronate, a bisphosphonates class of medication, is often used in addition to other osteoporosis preventative measures such as weight-bearing exercise and calcium/Vitamin D supplementation.[18]

Evaluation

The lowest effective dose should be used for treatment of the underlying condition, and the dose should be re-evaluated regularly to determine if further reductions can be instituted.

The parameters described under "Assessment" should be monitored regularly. Health care professionals should monitor for adrenal suppression in patients who have been treated with corticosteroids for greater than two weeks or in multiple short courses of high-dose therapy. Symptoms of adrenal insufficiency include weakness/fatigue, malaise, nausea, vomiting, diarrhea, abdominal pain, headache (usually in the morning), poor weight gain and/or growth in children, myalgia, arthralgia, psychiatric symptoms, hypotension, and hypoglycemia. If these symptoms occur, further lab work, such as an early morning cortisol test, should be performed.[19]

Adrenal Medication: Corticosteroids

Indications

Corticosteroids are used as replacement therapy in adrenal insufficiency, as well as for the management of various dermatologic, ophthalmologic, rheumatologic, pulmonary, hematologic, and gastrointestinal (GI) disorders. In respiratory conditions, systemic corticosteroids are used for the treatment of acute exacerbations of chronic obstructive pulmonary disease (COPD) and severe asthma. Mineralocorticoids are primarily involved in the regulation of electrolyte and water balance. Glucocorticoids are predominantly involved in carbohydrate, fat, and protein metabolism and also have anti-inflammatory, immunosuppressive, anti-proliferative, and vasoconstrictive effects. Prednisone is perhaps the most widely used of the systemic corticosteroids. It is generally used as an anti-inflammatory and immunosuppressive agent. Hydrocortisone is a commonly used topical cream for itching, and its oral formulation is used to treat Addison's disease.[20] Methylprednisolone is a commonly used injectable

---

18 Liu, D., Ahmet, A., Ward, L., Krishnamoorthy, P., Mandelcorn, E., Leigh, R., Brown, J., Cohen, A., Kim, H. (2013, August 15). A practical guide to the monitoring and management of the complications of systemic corticosteroid therapy. *Allergy, Asthma and Clinical Immunology, 9*(30). https://doi.org/10.1186/1710-1492-9-30.

19 Liu, D., Ahmet, A., Ward, L., Krishnamoorthy, P., Mandelcorn, E., Leigh, R., Brown, J., Cohen, A., Kim, H. (2013, August 15). A practical guide to the monitoring and management of the complications of systemic corticosteroid therapy. *Allergy, Asthma and Clinical Immunology, 9*(30). https://doi.org/10.1186/1710-1492-9-30.

20 This work is a derivative of *Daily Med* by U.S. National Library of Medicine in the public domain.

My Notes

corticosteroid. Fludrocortisone has much greater mineralocorticoid potency and, therefore, is commonly used to replace aldosterone in Addison's disease.[21] See Figure 9.6 for images of various formulations of corticosteroids.[22, 23, 24]

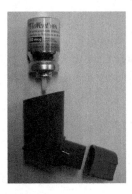 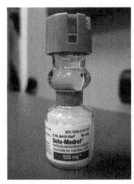 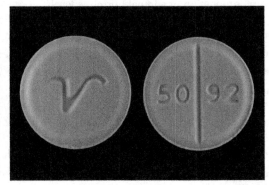

Figure 9.6 Examples of Corticosteroid Medications (fluticasone inhaler, intravenous methylprednisolone, and prednisone tablets)

Corticosteroids are used for a variety of disorders such as:

- Endocrine disorders such as adrenocortical insufficiency
- Rheumatic disorders such as rheumatoid arthritis
- Collagen diseases such as systemic lupus erythematosus
- Dermatologic diseases such as severe psoriasis
- Allergic states such as contact dermatitis or drug hypersensitivity reactions
- Ophthalmic diseases such as optic neuritis
- Respiratory diseases such as asthma or COPD
- Neoplastic diseases such as leukemia
- Gastrointestinal diseases such as ulcerative colitis
- Nervous system diseases such as multiple sclerosis[25]

21   Liu, D., Ahmet, A., Ward, L., Krishnamoorthy, P., Mandelcorn, E., Leigh, R., Brown, J., Cohen, A., and Kim, H. (2013, August 15). A practical guide to the monitoring and management of the complications of systemic corticosteroid therapy. *Allergy, Asthma and Clinical Immunology, 9*(30). https://doi.org/10.1186/1710-1492-9-30.

22   "Fluticasone.JPG" by James Heilman, MD is licensed under CC BY-SA 3.0.

23   "Methylprednisolone vial.jpg" by Intropin is licensed under CC BY 3.0.

24   "006035339lg Prednisone 20 MG Oral Tablet.jpg" by NLM is licensed under CC0.

25   This work is a derivative of *Daily Med* by U.S. National Library of Medicine in the public domain.

Mechanism of Action

Glucocorticoids cause profound and varied metabolic effects as described in the "Adrenal A&P Basics Review" section earlier. In addition, they modify the body's immune responses.[26]

Specific Administration Considerations

Despite their beneficial effects, long-term systemic use of corticosteroids is associated with well-known adverse events, including osteoporosis and fractures, adrenal suppression, hyperglycemia and diabetes, cardiovascular disease and dyslipidemia, dermatological and GI events, psychiatric disturbances, and immunosuppression. One side effect that is unique to children is growth suppression.[27] Therefore, the lowest possible dose of corticosteroid should be used to control the condition under treatment to avoid the development of these adverse effects. When reduction in dosage is possible, the reduction should be gradual and should not be stopped abruptly because of the associated HPA suppression that occurs with long-term administration. This hypothalamus-pituitary-adrenal (HPA) suppression can cause an impaired stress response, which may persist for months after discontinuation of therapy; therefore, in any situation of stress occurring during that period, hormone therapy should be reinstituted. Alternate day therapy is a corticosteroid dosing regimen in which twice the usual daily dose of corticoid is administered every other morning. The purpose of this mode of therapy is to minimize undesirable effects that can occur during long-term administration.

Dosages are variable and tailored to the disease process and the individual.

Adverse/Side Effects

Adverse/side effects of corticosteroids include fluid and electrolyte imbalances; muscle weakness; peptic ulcers; thin, fragile skin that bruises easily; poor wound healing; and the development of Cushing's syndrome. Corticosteroids may mask some signs of infection, and new infections may appear during their use. Psychic derangements may appear when corticosteroids are used, ranging from euphoria, insomnia, mood swings, personality changes to severe depression.

Patient Teaching and Education

Teach patients taking long-term prednisone therapy to never abruptly stop taking the medication and to report any adverse/side effects or new signs of infection.[28]

Glucocorticoid medication can cause immunosuppression, which makes it more difficult to detect signs of infection. Patients should seek advice from healthcare providers regarding vaccination administration while on glucocorticoids. Patients should report unusual swelling, weight gain, fatigue, bone pain, bruising, non-healing sores, visual and behavioral disturbances to the provider.

Use of glucocorticoid therapy may cause an increase in blood glucose levels. Patients should be advised to consume diets that are high in protein, calcium, and potassium.

---

26   This work is a derivative of *Daily Med* by U.S. National Library of Medicine in the public domain.

27   Liu, D., Ahmet, A., Ward, L., Krishnamoorthy, P., Mandelcorn, E., Leigh, R., Brown, J., Cohen, A., and Kim, H. (2013, August 15). A practical guide to the monitoring and management of the complications of systemic corticosteroid therapy. *Allergy, Asthma and Clinical Immunology, 9*(30). https://doi.org/10.1186/1710-1492-9-30.

28   This work is a derivative of *Daily Med* by U.S. National Library of Medicine in the public domain.

Now let's take a closer look at the medication grid comparing different formulations of corticosteroids in Table 9.3.[29, 30, 31, 32, 33]

Medication grids are intended to assist students to learn key points about each medication. Because information about medication is constantly changing, nurses should always consult evidence-based resources to review current recommendations before administering specific medication. Basic information related to each class of medication is outlined below. Detailed information on a specific medication can be found for free at *Daily Med* at https://dailymed.nlm.nih.gov/dailymed/index.cfm. On the home page, enter the drug name in the search bar to read more about the medication.

Prototype/generic medications listed in the grids below are also hyperlinked directly to a *Daily Med* page.

29   This work is a derivative of *Daily Med* by U.S. National Library of Medicine in the public domain.

30   AHFS Patient Medication Information [Internet]. Bethesda (MD): American Society of Health-System Pharmacists, Inc.; c2019. *Neomycin, Polymyxin, Bacitracin, and Hydrocortisone Topical;* [reviewed 2018 Jun 15]. https://medlineplus.gov /druginfo/meds/a601061.html.

31   Bornstein, S., Allolio, B., Arlt., W., Barthel., A., Don-Wauchope, A., Hammer, G., Husebye, E., Merke, D., Murad, M., Stratakis, C., and Tropy, D. (2016, February 1). Diagnosis and treatment of primary adrenal insufficiency: an endocrine society clinical practice guideline. *The Journal of Clinical Endocrinology and Metabolism, 101*(2). pp. 364–389. https://doi.org /10.1210/jc.2015-1710.

32   Nieman, L., Biller, B., Findling, J., Murad, M., Newell-Price, J., Savage, M, and Tabarin, A. (2015, August 1). Treatment of Cushing's Sydnrome: an endocrine clinical practice guideline. *The Journal of Clinical Endocrinology and Metabolism, 100*(8). pp. 2807–2831. https://academic.oup.com/jcem/article/100/8/2807/2836065.

33   Liu, D., Ahmet, A., Ward, L., Krishnamoorthy, P., Mandelcorn, E., Leigh, R., Brown, J., Cohen, A., and Kim, H. (2013, August 15). A practical guide to the monitoring and management of the complications of systemic corticosteroid therapy. *Allergy, Asthma and Clinical Immunology, 9*(30). https://doi.org/10.1186/1710-1492-9-30.

Table 9.3: Medication Grid Comparing Prednisone, Methylprednisolone, Hydrocortisone, and Fludrocortisone

Class	Prototypes/ generics	Administration Considerations	Therapeutic Effects	Adverse/Side Effects
Gluco-corticoid	prednisone (PO) methylpred-nisolone (IV)	Never abruptly stop corticosteroid therapy Use the lowest dose possible to control disorder and taper when feasible May require concurrent treatment for osteoporosis or elevated blood glucose levels Regularly monitor for development of symptoms of adrenal suppression Contraindicated in patients with untreated systemic infections	Often used to reduce inflammation or for immunosu	Fluid and electrolyte imbalances Increase in blood glucose Muscle weakness Peptic ulcers Thin, fragile skin that bruises easily Poor wound healing Development of Cushing's syndrome May mask some signs of infection, and new infections may appear Psychic derangements may appear when corticosteroids are used, ranging from euphoria, insomnia, mood swings, personality changes to severe depression
Topical Gluco-corticoid	hydrocortisone cream	Cream is only for use on the skin. Do not use in eyes Apply a small amount of medication to cover the affected area of skin with a thin, even film and rub in gently Do not wrap or bandage the treated area unless included in the prescription Symptoms should begin to improve during the first few days of treatment; do not use this medication longer than 7 days unless directed	Cream: topical relief of itching, redness, and swelling	Contact the provider if no improvement within 7 days
Mineralo-corticoid	fludrocortisone	Often administered in conjunction with cortisone or hydrocortisone Contraindicated if systemic fungal infection present Continually monitor for signs that indicate dosage adjustment is necessary, such as exacerbations of the disease or stress (surgery, infection, trauma)	Aldosterone replacement in Addison's disease	Potential adverse effects from retention of sodium and water: hypertension, edema, cardiac enlargement, congestive heart failure, potassium loss, and hypokalemic alkalosis

Critical Thinking Activity 9.3

A patient in a long-term care facility who has COPD receives prednisone 10 mg daily to help manage her respiratory status. Upon reviewing the patient's chart, the nurse notices that the patient was diagnosed with osteoporosis in the past, but is not currently receiving medications indicated for osteoporosis. The nurse is concerned because the patient requires assistance and is a fall risk so the nurse plans to call the provider.

1. What cues in the patient's medical history cause the nurse to be concerned about the risk for a fracture?

2. What medication(s) may be prescribed concurrently with prednisone to reduce the risk for a fracture?

3. What other patient teaching can the nurse provide to help reduce the patient's risk for a fracture?

4. Bedside glucose testing with sliding scale insulin is ordered for this patient, although she has no history of diabetes mellitus. What is the rationale for these orders?

5. What cues would cause the nurse to contact the provider with the hypothesis that adrenal suppression is occurring?

Note: Answers to the Critical Thinking activities can be found in the "Answer Key" sections at the end of the book.

9.4   ANTIDIABETICS

Pancreatic Basics: A&P Review

Pancreas

The pancreas is a long, slender organ located near the stomach (see Figure 9.7).[34] Although it is primarily an **exocrine gland**, secreting a variety of digestive enzymes, the pancreas also has an endocrine function. Pancreatic islets, clusters of cells formerly known as the islets of Langerhans, secrete glucagon and insulin. Glucagon plays an important role in blood glucose regulation because low blood glucose levels stimulate its release. On the other hand, elevated blood glucose levels stimulate the release of insulin.

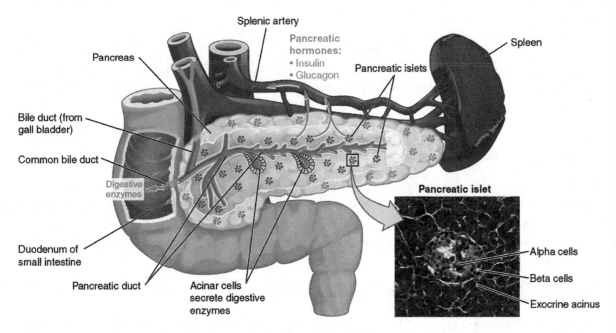

Figure 9.7 Pancreas

Regulation of Blood Glucose Levels by Glucagon and Insulin

Glucose is the preferred fuel for all body cells. The body derives glucose from the breakdown of the carbohydrate-containing foods and drinks we consume. Glucose not immediately taken up by cells for fuel can be stored by the liver and muscles as glycogen or converted to triglycerides and stored in the adipose tissue. Hormones regulate both the storage and the utilization of glucose as required. Receptors located in the pancreas sense blood glucose levels, and subsequently, the pancreatic cells secrete glucagon or insulin to maintain normal levels.

Glucagon

Receptors in the pancreas can sense the decline in blood glucose levels, such as during periods of fasting or during prolonged labor or exercise. In response, the alpha cells of the pancreas secrete the hormone glucagon, which has several effects:

---

34 "1820 The Pancreas.jpg"" by OpenStax is licensed under CC BY 4.0. Access for free at https://openstax.org/books/anatomy-and-physiology/pages/17-9-the-endocrine-pancreas.

- It stimulates the liver to convert stores of glycogen back into glucose. This response is known as glycogenolysis. The glucose is then released into the circulation for use by body cells.

- It stimulates the liver to take up amino acids from the blood and convert them into glucose. This response is known as gluconeogenesis.

- It stimulates lipolysis, the breakdown of stored triglycerides into free fatty acids and glycerol. Some of the free glycerol released into the bloodstream travels to the liver, which converts it into glucose. This is also a form of gluconeogenesis.

Taken together, these actions increase blood glucose levels. The activity of glucagon is regulated through a negative feedback mechanism; rising blood glucose levels inhibit further glucagon production and secretion. (See Figure 9.8 for an illustration of homeostatic regulation of blood glucose levels.)[35]

Insulin

Insulin facilitates the uptake of glucose into skeletal and adipose body cells. The presence of food in the intestine triggers the release of gastrointestinal tract hormones. This, in turn, triggers insulin production and secretion by the beta cells of the pancreas. Once nutrient absorption occurs, the resulting surge in blood glucose levels further stimulates insulin secretion.

Insulin triggers the rapid movement of glucose transporter vesicles to the cell membrane, where they are exposed to the extracellular fluid. The transporters then move glucose by facilitated diffusion into the cell interior.

Insulin also reduces blood glucose levels by stimulating **glycolysis**, the metabolism of glucose for generation of ATP. It further stimulates the liver to convert excess glucose into glycogen for storage, and it inhibits enzymes involved in glycogenolysis and gluconeogenesis. Finally, insulin promotes triglyceride and protein synthesis. The secretion of insulin is regulated through a negative feedback mechanism. As blood glucose levels decrease, further insulin release is inhibited.

Disorders of the Endocrine System: Diabetes Mellitus

Dysfunction of insulin production and secretion, as well as the target cells' responsiveness to insulin, can lead to a condition called diabetes mellitus, a common disease that affects the ability of the body to produce and/or utilize insulin. There are two main forms of diabetes mellitus. **Type 1 diabetes** is an autoimmune disease affecting the beta cells of the pancreas. The beta cells of people with type 1 diabetes do not produce insulin; thus, synthetic insulin must be administered by injection or infusion. **Type 2 diabetes** accounts for approximately 95 percent of all cases. It is acquired, and lifestyle factors such as poor diet and inactivity greatly increase a person's risk. In type 2 diabetes, the body's cells become resistant to the effects of insulin. In response, the pancreas increases its insulin secretion, but over time, the beta cells become exhausted. In many cases, type 2 diabetes can be reversed by moderate weight loss, regular physical activity, and consumption of a healthy diet. However, if blood glucose levels cannot be controlled, oral diabetic medication is implemented and eventually the type 2 diabetic may require insulin.

Diabetes is diagnosed when lab tests reveal that blood glucose levels are higher than normal, a condition called **hyperglycemia**.[36] According to the American Diabetes Association (ADA), normal fasting blood glucose levels

---

35 "1822 The Homostatic Regulation of Blood Glucose Levels.jpg" by OpenStax is licensed under CC BY 4.0. Access for free at https://openstax.org/books/anatomy-and-physiology/pages/17-9-the-endocrine-pancreas.

36 This work is a derivative of *Anatomy and Physiology* by OpenStax licensed under CC BY 4.0. Access for free at https://openstax.org/books/anatomy-and-physiology/pages/1-introduction.

are 80-130 mg/dL. Glycosylated hemoglobin, also called A1C, is used to assess long-term blood glucose levels over 3 months. The ADA states that A1C target levels vary according to age and health, but the generalized A1C target is less than 7%.[37]

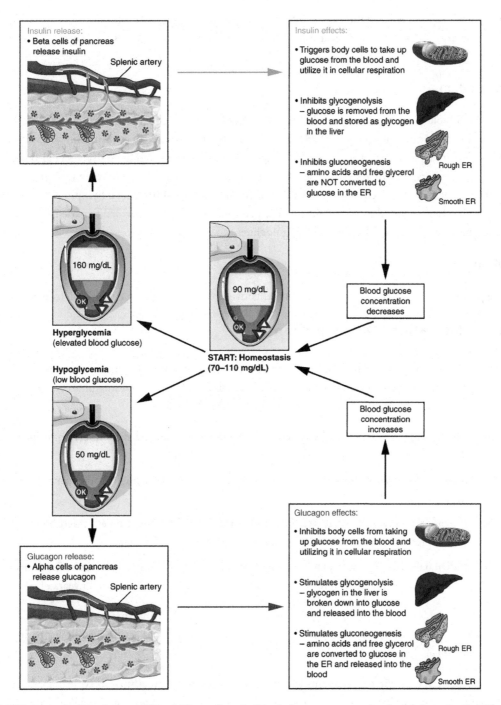

Figure 9.8 Homeostatic Regulation of Blood Glucose Levels. Blood glucose concentration is tightly maintained between 70 mg/dL and 110 mg/dL. If blood glucose concentration rises above this range, insulin is released, which stimulates body cells to remove glucose from the blood. If blood glucose concentration drops below this range, glucagon is released, which stimulates body cells to release glucose into the blood.

37   American Diabetes Association. (2019). The Big Picture: Checking your Blood Glucose. https://www.diabetes.org /diabetes/medication-management/blood-glucose-testing-and-control/checking- your-blood-glucose.

My Notes

Nursing Considerations

Assessment

Diabetic patients should be continuously monitored for signs of hypoglycemia and hyperglycemia. When a diabetic patient is experiencing stress or an infection, the nurse should plan to assess the blood glucose levels more frequently.

Implementation

The nurse should follow agency policy and ISMP guidelines for safe insulin administration. See the "Legal Ethical" chapter for more information about ISMP guidelines. Onset and peak times of insulin and sulfonylureas, in association with anticipated meal times, should always be considered to avoid hypoglycemia episodes. If a hypoglycemia episode occurs, the nurse should intervene quickly using the agency's established hypoglycemia protocol, and the event should be reported to the provider and in the shift-to-shift report. Symptomatic hyperglycemia should be immediately reported to the provider. Patient education should be provided to patients, family members, and/or caregivers according to ADA and ISMP guidelines.

Evaluation

The nurse should evaluate A1C levels to determine effectiveness (and compliance with) the treatment regimen.

Diabetic Medication Classes: Insulins

Because the hallmark of type 1 diabetes is absent or near-absent β-cell function, insulin treatment is essential for individuals with type 1 diabetes. Current evidence-based recommendations regarding pharmacological treatment of type 1 diabetes from the American Diabetes Association (ADA) include:

- Most people with type 1 diabetes should be treated with multiple daily injections of prandial and basal insulin or continuous subcutaneous insulin infusion.

- Most individuals with type 1 diabetes should use rapid-acting insulin analogs to reduce hypoglycemia risk.

- Individuals with type 1 diabetes on prandial insulin doses should be educated on carbohydrate intake, premeal blood glucose levels, and anticipated physical activity.

- Individuals with type 1 diabetes who have been successfully using continuous subcutaneous insulin infusion should have continued access to this therapy after they turn 65 years of age.

Basal insulin can be long-acting (insulin glargine or insulin detemir) or intermediate-acting (insulin isophane suspension [NPH]). **Prandial insulins** are used with meals and may be rapid acting (insulin lispro, insulin aspart, or insulin glulisine) or short acting (regular insulin).

According to the ADA, insulin requirements can be estimated based on weight, with typical doses ranging from 0.4 to 1.0 units/kg/day. Higher amounts are required during puberty, pregnancy, and medical illness. Physiologic insulin secretion varies with glycemia, meal size, and tissue demands for glucose. To approach this variability in people using insulin treatment, strategies have evolved to adjust meal-time doses based on predicted needs. Thus, education of patients on how to adjust insulin to account for carbohydrate intake, premeal glucose levels, and anticipated activity is important. Ensuring that patients and/or caregivers understand correct insulin injection technique is also important to optimize glucose control and insulin use safety.[38]

Patients on insulin therapy are at risk for **hypoglycemia**. It is essential for the nurse to monitor for signs of hypoglycemia and to intervene appropriately. See Figure 9.9 for symptoms of hypoglycemia. Hypoglycemia is defined as a blood glucose level below 70 mg/dL; severe hypoglycemia refers to a blood glucose level below 40 mg/dL.

Hypoglycemia Symptoms

Mild-to-Moderate	Severe
• Shaky or jittery	Unable to eat or drink
• Sweaty	Seizures or convulsions (jerky movements)
• Hungry	Unconsciousness
• Headache	
• Blurred vision	
• Sleepy or tired	
• Dizzy or lightheaded	
• Confused or disoriented	
• Pale	
• Uncoordinated	
• Irritable or nervous	
• Argumentative or combative	
• Changed behavior or personality	
• Trouble concentrating	
• Weak	
• Fast or irregular heart beat	

If a patient with diabetes shows a sudden change in mood or mental status or other symptoms of hypoglycemia, the nurse should immediately check the blood glucose level. Healthcare agencies use hypoglycemia protocols so that the nurse can react quickly to episodes of hypoglycemia before they become severe. Hypoglycemia protocols contain orders for immediate treatment by the nurse. For instance, in patients who can tolerate oral intake, 15 grams of rapidly digested carbohydrates (such as 4 ounces of fruit juice) are recommended. In patients who are NPO or can't take oral treatment, dextrose 50% IV or glucagon IM or subcutaneously are administered. Patients who have had a hypoglycemic episode should be monitored closely for the following 24 hours because they are at increased risk for another episode. The provider and the oncoming nurse should be notified of hypoglycemia episodes to discuss the possible cause of the hypoglycemic event and make insulin adjustments, if needed, to avoid additional hypoglycemia. Tracking hypoglycemia episodes and analyzing causes are important performance improvement activities.[39]

---

38   American Diabetes Association. (2019). 9. Pharmacologic Approaches to Glycemic Treatment: Standards of Medical Care in Diabetes—2019. *Diabetes Care 42*(S1). https://doi.org/10.2337/dc19-S009.

39   Seggelke, S., Everhart, B. (2012, September 11) Managing glucose levels in hospital patients. *American Nurse Today.* https://www.americannursetoday.com/managing-glucose-levels-in-hospital-patients/.

The arrival of continuous glucose monitors to clinical practice has been proven to reduce nocturnal hypoglycemia in people using insulin pumps with glucose sensors due to automatic suspension of insulin delivery at a preset glucose level. The U.S. Food and Drug Administration has also approved the first hybrid closed-loop pump system.[40] A hybrid closed-loop pump system automatically adjusts basal insulin delivery every 5 minutes based on sensor glucose to maintain blood glucose levels as close to a specific target as possible.[41]

According to the ADA, lifestyle modifications that improve health should be emphasized, along with any pharmacologic therapy. Lifestyle modifications include healthy food choices to stabilize blood glucose levels, as well as daily exercise.

Hypokalemia

All insulin products cause a shift in potassium from the extracellular to intracellular space, which can possibly lead to hypokalemia. Untreated hypokalemia may cause respiratory paralysis, ventricular arrhythmia, and death. Monitor potassium levels in patients at risk for hypokalemia due to other medications such as diuretics.

Insulin Pens

Insulin pens are often used in inpatient settings, as well as for self-administration, to facilitate safe and accurate self-administration of insulin. See Figure 9.10 for an image of an insulin pen.[42] According to the ISMP, insulin pens offer several advantages over vials beyond dosing accuracy, convenience, and ease of use:

- Each pen is already labeled by the manufacturer with the product name and product barcode (whereas syringes of insulin prepared on the patient care unit from vials run the risk of being unlabeled).

- Each pen can be individually labeled with the patient's name (and ideally with a patient-specific barcode).

- The pen provides the patient's insulin in a form ready for administration.

- The pen lessens nursing time needed to prepare and administer insulin.

- Insulin pens reduce medication waste that can occur when dispensing 10 mL-sized insulin vials for each patient.

However, improper sharing of insulin pens among multiple patients has exposed patients to bloodborne pathogens. Insulin pens should never be reused for multiple patients; even if the needle is changed between patients, there can still be body fluid exposure.[43]

---

40   American Diabetes Association. (2019). 9. Pharmacologic Approaches to Glycemic Treatment: Standards of Medical Care in Diabetes—2019. *Diabetes Care* 42(S1). https://doi.org/10.2337/dc19-S009.

41   Weaver, H., Hirsch, I (2018, June 6). The Hybrid Closed Loop System: Evolution and Practical Applications. *Diabetes Technology and Therapeutics* 20(S2). https://www.liebertpub.com/doi/10.1089/dia.2018.0091.

42   "Human insulin 100 IU-1ml pen yellow background (02).jpg" by Wesalius is licensed under CC BY 4.0.

43   Institute for Safe Medication Practices. (2017). *ISMP Guidelines for Optimizing Safe Subcutaneous Insulin Use in Adults.* https://www.ismp.org/sites/default/files/attachments/2017-11/ISMP138-Insulin%20Guideline-051517-2-WEB.pdf.

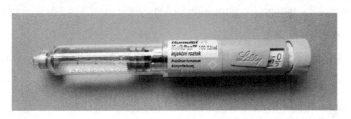

Figure 9.10 Insulin Pens

High-Alert Medication and Prevention of Errors

Insulin is a high-alert medication that can be associated with significant patient harm when used in error. A variety of error types have been associated with insulin therapy, including administration of the wrong insulin product, improper dosing (underdosing and overdosing), dose omissions, incorrect use of insulin delivery devices, wrong route (intramuscular versus subcutaneous), and improper patient monitoring. Many errors result in serious hypoglycemia or hyperglycemia. Hypoglycemia is often caused by a failure to adjust insulin therapy in response to a reduction in nutritional intake or an excessive insulin dose stemming from a prescribing or dose measurement error. Other factors that contribute to serious hypoglycemia include inappropriate timing of insulin doses with food intake, creatinine clearance, body weight, changes in medications that affect blood glucose levels, poor communication during patient transfer to different care teams, and poor coordination of blood glucose testing with insulin administration at meal time.

In an inpatient setting, manifestations of poor glycemic control, including severe hypoglycemia and hyperglycemia, are deemed hospital-acquired conditions by the Centers for Medicare and Medicaid Services (CMS). CMS notes that poor glycemic control can be reasonably prevented with implementation of evidence-based guidelines; thus, the CMS denies payment for diabetic ketoacidosis, hypoglycemic coma, and other serious conditions related to poor glycemic control. Agency policies and procedures should be closely followed to avoid these errors and manifestations of poor glycemic control.

One strategy for look-alike medications such as Humalog and Humalin is tall man lettering on the label. Tall man lettering describes a method for differentiating the unique letter characters of similar drug names known to be confused with one another, such as HumaLOG and HumaLIN.

ISMP recommends the following safe practice guidelines for the administration of insulin by the nurse:

- Patient-specific insulin pens are stored on clinical units in a manner that prevents their inadvertent use on more than one patient.

- A coordinated process is developed to ensure timely blood glucose checks and administration of prandial insulin in conjunction with meal delivery.

- Verbal communication of point-of-care blood glucose value results are avoided as much as possible and are NEVER routinely used as the only source of information when determining insulin doses.

- Appropriately label all clinician-prepared syringes of subcutaneous insulin, unless the medication is prepared at the patient's bedside and is immediately administered to the patient without any break in the process.

- Prior to subcutaneous insulin administration, the practitioner:
  - Confirms that there is an appropriate indication
  - Assesses the patient's most current blood glucose value

My Notes

- Assesses the patient for symptoms of hypoglycemia

- Informs the patient of their most current blood glucose level

- Informs the patient of their dose, the full name of the product, and the insulin's intended action

- An individual insulin pen is never used for more than one patient.

- Barcode scanning is used to verify that a patient-specific pen is used to administer the correct insulin to the correct patient.

- Prior to transitions of care, a process is in place to ensure that patients will have the necessary prescriptions, supplies, a follow-up care plan, and printed instructions for all prescribed insulin and blood glucose monitoring.

- Patients discharged on insulin are assessed for understanding of their self-management, including:

  - Demonstration of proper dose measurement and self-administration using the same administration device that will be used at home (e.g., vial and syringe, pen, pump)

- Correct monitoring of blood glucose values

- The signs and symptoms of hyper- and hypoglycemia and how to respond if these symptoms occur

- Common types of errors possible with their insulin therapy and how to prevent or detect these errors

- The importance of regular follow-up with their primary care provider/specialist, including the date of their next appointment

- Patients who self-administer concentrated U-500 insulin using a vial and syringe are taught to use only a U-500 syringe and communicate their doses in terms of the name and concentration of the insulin and the actual dose in units using only the U-500 syringe[44]

Life Span Considerations

Elderly

The elderly are at higher risk for hypoglycemia episodes. The ADA has the following recommendations for elderly patients with diabetes:

- In older adults at increased risk of hypoglycemia, medication classes with low risk of hypoglycemia are preferred.

- Overtreatment of diabetes is common in older adults and should be avoided.

- Deintensification (or simplification) of complex regimens is recommended to reduce the risk of hypoglycemia, if it can be achieved within the individualized A1C target.[45]

---

44   Institute for Safe Medication Practices. (2017). ISMP Guidelines for Optimizing Safe Subcutaneous Insulin Use in Adults. https://www.ismp.org/sites/default/files/attachments/2017-11/ISMP138-Insulin%20Guideline-051517-2-WEB .pdf.

45   American Diabetes Association (2019) 12. Older adults: Standards of Medical Care in Diabetes—2019. *Diabetes Care* 42(S1). https://doi.org/10.2337/dc19-S012.

Children and Adolescents

Type 1 diabetes is the most common form of diabetes in youth. Unique aspects of care and management of children and adolescents with type 1 diabetes must be considered, such as changes in insulin sensitivity related to physical growth and sexual maturation, ability to provide self-care, supervision in the child care and school environment, neurological vulnerability to hypoglycemia and hyperglycemia in young children, as well as possible adverse neurocognitive effects of diabetic ketoacidosis (DKA). Evidence-based ADA recommendations for glycemic control for children and adolescents include:

- The majority of children and adolescents with type 1 diabetes should be treated with intensive insulin regimens, either via multiple daily injections or continuous subcutaneous insulin infusion.

- All children and adolescents with type 1 diabetes should self-monitor glucose levels multiple times daily (up to 6–10 times/day), including pre-meal, pre-bedtime, and as needed for safety in specific situations such as exercise, driving, or the presence of symptoms of hypoglycemia.

- Continuous glucose monitoring should be considered in all children and adolescents with type 1 diabetes, whether using injections or continuous subcutaneous insulin infusion, as an additional tool to help improve glucose control. Benefits of continuous glucose monitoring correlate with adherence to ongoing use of the device.

- Automated insulin delivery systems appear to improve glycemic control and reduce hypoglycemia in children and should be considered in children with type 1 diabetes.

- An A1C target of <7.5% should be considered in children and adolescents with type 1 diabetes but should be individualized based on the needs and situation of the patient and family.[46]

There are several different types of insulins that vary in terms of onset, peak, and duration. It is critical for the nurse to be knowledgeable of these differences to help prevent episodes of hypoglycemia due to mismatched administration of insulin with food intake.

Rapid-Acting Insulin

Rapid-acting insulins include insulin lispro (Humalog) and insulin aspart (Novolog) and are also available via inhalation (Afrezza). See Figure 9.11 for an image of Novolog insulin.[47]

---

46   American Diabetes Association. (2019). 13. Children and adolescents: Standards of Medical Care in Diabetes—2019. *Diabetes Care* 42(S1). https://doi.org/10.2337/dc19-S013.

47   "Untitled" from Pxhere website is licensed under CC0.

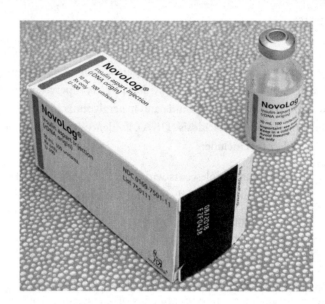

Figure 9.11 Novolog insulin

Indications

Rapid-acting insulins are also called prandial insulins because they are administered with meals to mimic the effects of endogenous insulin release when food is eaten. Dosages of rapid-acting insulin are individualized based on carbohydrate intake, premeal glucose levels, and anticipated activity.

Mechanism of Action

Insulins lower blood glucose by stimulating peripheral glucose uptake by skeletal muscle and fat and by inhibiting hepatic glucose production.

Specific Administration Considerations

Humalog-100 (100 units per ml) and Humalog-200 (200 units per ml) are administered subcutaneously; however, only Humalog-100 is administered via continuous subcutaneous injection or intravenously. Humalog-100 can only be mixed with NPH insulin, but Humalog-200 should not be mixed with other insulin. Inspect insulin visually before use. It should appear clear and colorless; do not use if particulate matter or coloration is seen. Humalog-100 is available in vials, KwikPens, and cartridges; Humalog-200 is only available in KwikPens. Administer subcutaneously into the outer lateral aspect of the upper arm, the abdomen (from below the costal margin to the iliac crest and more than two inches from the umbilicus), the anterior upper thighs, or the buttocks. Rotate injection sites within the same region from one injection to the next to reduce the risk of lipodystrophy. Lipodystrophy can be a lump or small dent in the skin that forms when a person performs injections repeatedly in the same spot.

Because of the rapid onset of insulin lispro and insulin aspart and the potential for hypoglycemia, these insulins should be administered within 15 minutes before or right after eating a meal. Peak serum levels are seen 30 to 90 minutes after dosing. Inhaled insulin enters the bloodstream within 1 minute and peaks in 30-60 minutes. Inhaled insulin is contraindicated in patients with chronic lung disease such as asthma or COPD.

Adverse effects of all insulins include hypoglycemia and hypokalemia. Inhaled insulin has a Black Box Warning for potentially causing acute bronchoconstriction.

Patient Teaching and Education

See ISMP guidelines for patient teaching in the previous section titled "High Risk Medications and Prevention of Errors."

Short-Acting Insulin

Short-acting insulins include regular insulin with a brand name of Humulin R or Novolin R. A concentrated formulation of Humulin R u-500 is also available. See Figure 9.12 for an image of Humulin R insulin.[48]

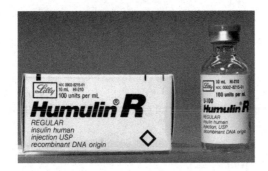

Figure 9.12 Humulin R insulin

Indications

Short-acting insulins are given with meals to mimic the effects of endogenous insulin release when food is eaten. Dosages of short-acting insulin are individualized based on carbohydrate intake, premeal glucose levels, and anticipated activity levels.

Mechanism of Action

The primary activity of insulin is the regulation of glucose metabolism. Insulin lowers blood glucose by stimulating peripheral glucose uptake, especially by skeletal muscle and fat, and by inhibiting hepatic glucose production.

Specific Administration Considerations

Regular insulin is generally administered subcutaneously. It is the only insulin that can be administered intravenously under close supervision of blood glucose and potassium levels. It is available in vials and insulin pens. Inspect insulin visually before use. It should appear clear and colorless; do not use if particulate matter or coloration is seen. Administer subcutaneously into the outer lateral aspect of the upper arm, the abdomen (from below the costal margin to the iliac crest and more than two inches from the umbilicus), the anterior upper thighs, or the buttocks. Rotate injection sites within the same region from one injection to the next to reduce the risk of lipodystrophy. Subcutaneous doses should be administered approximately 30 minutes before meals because this is the typical onset of action. Peak effects occur in 3 hours with a duration of 8 hours. Do not mix with insulin preparations other than NPH.

Humulin R u-500 should only be administered in u-500 insulin syringes to avoid dosage calculation errors.

Adverse effects of insulin include hypoglycemia and hypokalemia.

---

48   "Humulin R, Insulin, 1987" by National Museum of American History Smithsonian Institution is licensed under CC BY-NC-ND 2.0.

Patient Teaching and Education

See IMSP guidelines for patient teaching in the previous section entitled "High Risk Medications and Prevention of Errors."

Intermediate-Acting Insulin

NPH insulin, also known as isophane insulin, is an intermediate–acting insulin. Brand names include Humulin-N or Novolin-N. Mixtures of short- and intermediate-acting insulin include Humulin 70/30 or Novolin 70/30.

Indications

Intermediate insulins are administered once or twice daily to mimic endogenous basal insulin levels.

Mechanism of Action

Insulins lower blood glucose by stimulating peripheral glucose uptake by skeletal muscle and fat and by inhibiting hepatic glucose production.

Specific Administration Considerations

NPH insulin is a white and cloudy suspension. Gently roll or invert vial/pen several times to re-suspend the insulin before administration. It should only be administered subcutaneously. It may be mixed with rapid-acting or short-acting insulins, but those insulins should be drawn into the syringe before the NPH is added. Administer subcutaneously into the outer lateral aspect of the upper arm, the abdomen (from below the costal margin to the iliac crest and more than two inches from the umbilicus), the anterior upper thighs, or the buttocks. Rotate injection sites within the same region from one injection to the next to reduce the risk of lipodystrophy. The onset of action and peak are affected by the site of injection, physical activity level, and other variables but the median peak level occurs in 4 hours. See Figure 9.13 for an image of Novolin-N (a cloudy insulin) that can be mixed with Novolin R (a clear insulin).[49]

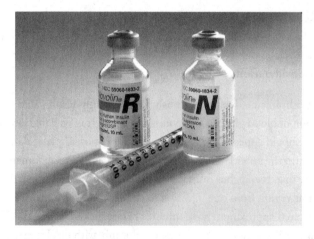

Figure 9.13 Comparison of Novolin-N (a cloudy insulin) that can be mixed with Novolin-R (a clear insulin)

Mixed medications such as Humulin 70/30 should be administered subcutaneously approximately 30 minutes before a meal. They are typically dosed twice daily (with each dose intended to cover 2 meals or a meal and a snack).

---

49 "The Gift of Life" by Melissa Johnson is licensed under CC BY 2.0.

Unopened vials should be stored in the refrigerator until the expiration date. Opened vials should be labelled with the open date and stored in the refrigerator for up to 28-42 days (depending on the formulation/insulin type) and then discarded. Unopened pens should be stored in the refrigerator until the expiration date. Used pens should be stored at room temperature, but kept away from heat and light, for up to 10-28 days (depending on the formulation/insulin type) and then discarded.

Patient Teaching and Education

See IMSP guidelines for patient teaching in the previous section titled "High Risk Medications and Prevention of Errors."

Long-Acting Insulin

Insulin glargine (Lantus) and insulin devemir (Levemir) are long-acting insulins given once or twice daily. See Figure 9.14 for an image of a levemir insulin pen.[50]

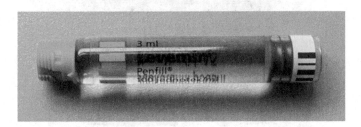

Figure 9.14 Vial used for Levemir insulin pen

Indications

Long-acting insulins are given once or twice daily. In type 1 diabetics, long-acting insulin should be used concomitantly with rapid- or short-acting insulin at mealtimes.

Mechanism of Action

Insulins lower blood glucose by stimulating peripheral glucose uptake by skeletal muscle and fat and by inhibiting hepatic glucose production.

Specific Administration Considerations

Long-acting insulin has a relatively constant concentration/time profile over 24 hours with no pronounced peak in comparison to NPH insulin. It should only be administered subcutaneously and is available in vials and insulin pens. Inspect insulin visually before use. It should appear clear and colorless; do not use if particulate matter or coloration is seen. Administer subcutaneously into the outer lateral aspect of the upper arm, the abdomen (from below the costal margin to the iliac crest and more than two inches from the umbilicus), the anterior upper thighs, or the buttocks. Rotate injection sites within the same region from one injection to the next to reduce the risk of lipodystrophy.

Patient Teaching and Education

See ISMP guidelines for patient teaching in the previous section titled "High Risk Medications and Prevention of Errors."

---

50   "Insulin analog 100 IU-1ml penfill levemir yellow background.jpg" by Wesalius is licensed under CC BY 4.0.

Glucagon

Indications

Glucagon is indicated as a treatment for severe hypoglycemia (low blood sugar), which may occur in patients with diabetes mellitus. Glucagon injection is used for patients who are unable to safely swallow carbohydrates to treat hypoglycemia due to the effects of hypoglycemia or other medical conditions.

Mechanism of Action

Glucagon increases blood glucose concentration during an episode of hypoglycemia. See Figure 9.15 for an image of an emergency glucagon kit.[51]

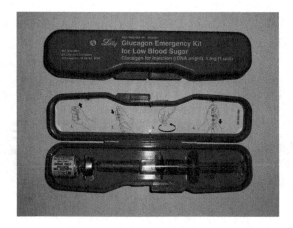

Figure 9.15 Emergency glucagon kit

Specific Administration Considerations

Glucagon may be administered subcutaneously, intramuscularly, or intravenously. Peak glucose levels occur within 13-20 minutes of subcutaneous or IM injection.

Patient Teaching and Education

Patients with type 1 diabetes may have less of an increase in blood glucose levels compared with a stable type 2 patient, so a supplementary carbohydrate should be given as soon as possible, especially to a pediatric patient.[52]

---

51 "Glucagon emergency rescue kit.JPG" by mbbradford is licensed under CC0.

52 This work is a derivative of *Daily Med* by U.S. National Library of Medicine in the public domain.

Now let's take a closer look at the medication grid comparing insulins in Table 9.4a.[53]

Table 9.4a: Insulins Medication Grid

Class/Subclass	Prototypes/ Generics	Onset/Peak/ Duration	Administration Considerations	Therapeutic Effects	Adverse/Side Effects
Rapid-Acting Insulin	insulin lispro (Humalog) insulin aspart (Novolog) inhaled insulin (Afreeza)	Onset: 15-30 minutes Peak effect: 1-3 hours Duration: 3 – 5 hours	Administer within 15 minutes before a meal or immediately after a meal Afrezza is contraindicated in patients with asthma or COPD	Maintain serum blood glucose in normal range and achieve individualized target level of A1C (often 7%)	Hypoglycemia Hypokalemia Afrezza can cause acute bronchospasm
Short-Acting Insulin	Humulin R Novolin R	Onset: 30 minutes Peak effect: 3 hours Duration: 8 hours	Administer 30 minutes before a meal	Maintain serum blood glucose in normal range and achieve individualized target level of A1C (often 7%)	Hypoglycemia Hypokalemia
Intermediate-Acting Insulin	Humulin N Novolin N	Onset: 1-2 hours Peak effect: 6 hours (range 2.8-13 hours) Duration: up to 24 hours	Administer once or twice daily Only administer subcutaneously Gently roll or invert vial/pen several times to re-suspend the insulin before administration Do not mix with other insulin	Maintain serum blood glucose in normal range and achieve individualized target level of A1C (often 7%)	Hypoglycemia Hypokalemia
Combination: Intermediate-Acting/ Rapid-Acting	Humalog Mix 50/50 Humalog Mix 75/25 Novolog Mix 70/30 *First number is % intermediate-acting insulin, second number is % rapid-acting	Onset: 15-30 minutes Peak effect: 50/50: 1-5 hours Duration: 11-22 hours	Administer twice daily, 15 minutes before a meal or immediately after a meal Only administer subcutaneously Gently roll or invert vial/pen several times to re-suspend the insulin before administration	Maintain serum blood glucose in normal range and achieve individualized target level of A1C (often 7%)	Hypoglycemia Hypokalemia

---

53   This work is a derivative of *Daily Med* by U.S. National Library of Medicine in the public domain.

My Notes

Combination: Intermediate-Acting/ Short-Acting	Humulin 70/30 Novolin 70/30	Onset: 30-90 minutes Peak effect: 1.5-6.5 hours Duration: 18-24 hours	Administer twice daily, 30-45 minutes before a meal Only administer subcutaneously Gently roll or invert vial/pen several times to re-suspend the insulin before administration Do not mix with other insulin	Maintain serum blood glucose in normal range and achieve individualized target level of A1C (often 7%)	Hypoglycemia Hypokalemia
Long-Acting Insulin	insulin glargine (Lantus) insulin detemir (Levemir)	Onset: 3-4 hours Peak effect: none Duration: >24 hours	Administer once daily (sometimes dose is split and administered twice daily) Only administer subcutaneously Do not mix with other insulin	Maintain serum blood glucose in normal range and achieve individualized target level of A1C (often 7%)	Hypoglycemia Hypokalemia
Hyperglycemic	glucagon		May be administered subcutaneously, IM, or IV Supplementary carbohydrate should be given as soon as possible, especially to a pediatric patient Used to reverse hypoglycemic episode if NPO administration is not appropriate	Used to reverse hypoglycemic episode if NPO administration is not appropriate	Hyperglyce-mia

General adminstration considerations:

- Review orders closely because they may include a standard meal dose, a "sliding scale" dose, and a carb-related dose.

- Always read drug labelling closely as there are several types of dosages and formulations.

- See agency policies and ISMP guidelines for safe administration of insulin.

- When administering with an insulin pen, after inserting the pen count to 5 before removing the needle.

General therapeutic effects:

- Maintain serum blood glucose in normal range and achieve individualized target level of A1C (often 7%)

General side effects:

- Hypoglycemia and hypokalemia

Diabetic Medication: Oral Antihyperglycemics

There are several different classes of oral antihyperglycemic drugs used in conjunction with a healthy diet and exercise for the management of type 2 diabetes. According to the American Diabetes Association, metformin is the preferred initial pharmacologic agent for the treatment of type 2 diabetes.[54] Three of the most commonly used antihyperglycemic classes and prototypes are sulfonylureas (glipizide), biguanide (metformin), and DPP-IV (sitagliptin). The mechanism of action and administration considerations for each of these prototypes are described below.

Glipizide

Mechanism of Action

Glipizide is in the sulfonylurea class of antihyperglycemic medication. The mechanism of action is the stimulation of insulin secretion from the beta cells of pancreatic islet tissue and is thus dependent on functioning beta cells in the pancreatic islets. Peak plasma concentrations occur 1 to 3 hours after a single oral dose.

Specific Administration Considerations

All sulfonylurea drugs are capable of producing severe hypoglycemia. Hypoglycemia may be difficult to recognize in the elderly and in people who are taking beta-adrenergic blocking drugs. Sulfonylurea medications should be given 30 minutes before a meal due to hypoglycemic effects.

Glipizide is contraindicated in type 1 diabetics or for use of diabetic ketoacidosis; insulin should be used to treat this condition. Treatment of patients with glucose 6-phosphate dehydrogenase (G6PD) deficiency with sulfonylurea agents can lead to hemolytic anemia.

The hypoglycemic action of sulfonylureas may be potentiated by certain drugs such as nonsteroidal anti-inflammatory agents and other drugs that are highly protein bound.

Patient Teaching and Education

Patients should take the medication at the same time each day. It is important that patients understand that the medication helps control episodes of hyperglycemia but does not cure diabetes. Patients should be instructed regarding the signs of hyperglycemia and hypoglycemia. The use of sulfonylureas and alcohol may cause a disulfiram-like reaction.

---

54   American Diabetes Association. (2019). 9. Pharmacologic Approaches to Glycemic Treatment: Standards of Medical Care in Diabetes—2019. *Diabetes Care 42*(S1). https://doi.org/10.2337/dc19-S009.

Metformin

Mechanism of Action

Metformin is in the biguanide class of antihyperglycemics. It decreases hepatic glucose production, decreases intestinal absorption of glucose, and improves insulin sensitivity by increasing peripheral glucose uptake and utilization. Unlike sulfonylureas, metformin does not produce hypoglycemia. See Figure 9.16 for an image of a metformin tablet.[55]

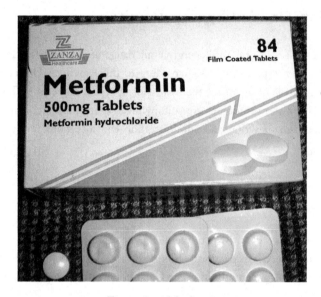

Figure 9.16 Metformin

Specific Administration Considerations

Metformin hydrochloride should be given in divided doses with meals. The therapeutic goal should be to decrease both fasting plasma glucose and glycosylated hemoglobin levels to near normal by using the lowest effective dose of metformin, either when used as monotherapy or in combination with sulfonylurea or insulin.

Common adverse reactions include diarrhea, nausea/vomiting, weakness, flatulence, indigestion, abdominal discomfort, and headache.

Metformin is contraindicated in patients with kidney disease (e.g., serum creatinine levels ≥1.5 mg/dL [males] or ≥1.4 mg/dL [females]) and should be temporarily discontinued in patients undergoing radiologic studies involving intravascular administration of iodinated contrast materials because use of such products may result in acute alteration of renal function. It is also contraindicated in patients with metabolic acidosis.

Lactic acidosis is a rare, but serious, metabolic complication that can occur due to metformin accumulation during treatment with metformin; when it occurs, it is fatal in approximately 50% of cases. The risk of lactic acidosis increases with the degree of renal dysfunction and the patient's age. Metformin should be promptly withheld in the presence of any condition associated with hypoxemia, dehydration, or sepsis. Because impaired hepatic function may significantly limit the ability to clear lactate, metformin should be avoided in patients with hepatic

---

55 "Metformin 500mg Tablets.jpg" by User:Ash is licensed under CC0.

disease. The onset of lactic acidosis often is subtle and accompanied only by nonspecific symptoms such as malaise, myalgias, respiratory distress, increasing somnolence, and nonspecific abdominal distress.

Patient Teaching and Education

Patients should take the medication at the same time each day. It is important that patients understand that the medication helps control episodes of hyperglycemia but does not cure diabetes. Patients should be instructed regarding the signs of hyperglycemia and hypoglycemia. The patient may be at risk for lactic acidosis and should report chills, low blood pressure, muscle pain, or dyspnea immediately to the healthcare provider. The use of medications like metformin can cause a metallic taste in the mouth.

Sitagliptin

Mechanism of Action

Sitagliptin is an orally-active inhibitor of dipeptidyl peptidase-4 (DPP-4) enzyme that slows the inactivation of incretin hormones involved in the regulation of glucose homeostasis and thus, increases insulin release and decreases glucagon levels in the circulation. See Figure 9.17 for an image of sitagliptin.[56]

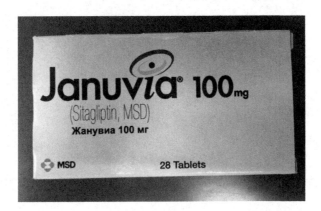

Figure 9.17 Sitagliptin

Specific Administration Considerations

Sitagliptin is taken once daily and can be taken with or without food. It can cause hypoglycemia. Dose adjustment should occur for patients with kidney disease depending on their glomerular filtration rate. Report hypersensitivity reactions, blisters/erosions, headache, or symptoms of pancreatitis, heart failure, severe arthralgia, and upper respiratory infection.

Patient Teaching and Education

Patients should take the medication at the same time each day. It is important that patients understand that the medication helps control episodes of hyperglycemia but does not cure diabetes. Patients should be instructed regarding the signs of hyperglycemia and hypoglycemia. Patients should stop taking the medication if symptoms of hypersensitivity occur and follow up immediately with their provider to determine the next course of treatment.

---

56   "Januvia sitagliptin.jpg" by Kimivanil is licensed under CC BY-SA 4.0.

Now let's take a closer look at the medication grid comparing oral antihyperglycemics in Table 9.4b.[57]

Table 9.4b: Medication Grid Comparing Oral Antihyperglycemics

Class	Prototype	Administration Considerations	Therapeutic Effects	Adverse/Side Effects
Sulfonylureas	glipizide	Time with meals; peak plasma concentrations occur 1 to 3 hours after administration	Reduce fasting blood sugar and glycosylated hemoglobin to near normal	Hypoglycemia; may be potentiated by nonsteroidal anti-inflammatory agents and other drugs that are highly protein bound
Biguanide	metformin	Contraindicated in renal and hepatic disease Should be temporarily discontinued in patients undergoing radiologic studies involving intravascular administration of iodinated contrast materials	Reduce fasting blood sugar and glycosylated hemoglobin to near normal	Stop immediately if signs of lactic acidosis or any condition associated with hypoxemia, dehydration, or sepsis occurs Common adverse effects: diarrhea, nausea/vomiting, weakness, flatulence, indigestion, abdominal discomfort, and headache
DPP-IV inhibitor	sitagliptin	Can be given with or without food	Reduce fasting blood sugar and glycosylated hemoglobin to near norm	Hypoglycemia Report hypersensitivity reactions, blisters/erosions, headache, or symptoms of pancreatitis, heart failure, severe arthralgia, or upper respiratory infection

---

57 This work is a derivative of *Daily Med* by U.S. National Library of Medicine in the public domain.

Critical Thinking Activity 9.4

A patient with diabetes mellitus type 2 is admitted to the hospital for hip replacement surgery. The nurse reviews the following orders:

Diabetic diet with carb counting

Bedside blood glucose testing before meals and at bedtime with sliding scale Humalog insulin

Sliding scale Humalog insulin based on preprandial glucose level:

- 0–150: No coverage
- 151–175: 2 units
- 176–200: 4 units
- 201–225: 6 units
- 226–250: 8 units
- Over 250: call the provider

Insulin coverage per carbohydrate intake at meals: Humalog 2 units/carb

Metformin 1000 mg twice daily

Humulin-N 20 units at breakfast and at bedtime Hypoglycemia protocol

1. Explain the difference between type 1 and type 2 diabetes.

2. The patient states that he usually does not take insulin at home. What is the likely rationale for insulin therapy while hospitalized?

3. The patient's blood sugar before breakfast is 223 and he eats 3 carbs at breakfast. What types and amounts of insulin will the nurse administer?

4. The nurse reviews the patient's morning lab results and finds a creatinine of 1.8. She plans to call the provider to discuss the impact of the results on the medications ordered. Which medication may require a dosage adjustment based on these results?

5. When the nurse enters the room around 4 p.m., she discovers that the patient has become irritable and is shaky. The nurse performs a bedside blood glucose and obtains a value of 60. What is the nurse's best response?

6. What is the likely cause of the patient's condition? Explain using the onset and peak actions of the insulin orders.

7. On admission, the patient's A1C level was 10%. What does this lab value indicate?

8. The provider states the discharge plan is to initiate Lantus insulin therapy at home, based on the admitting A1C level. What patient teaching should the nurse plan to provide before discharge?

Note: Answers to the Critical Thinking activities can be found in the "Answer Key" sections at the end of the book.

9.5 THYROID MEDICATIONS

Thyroid Basics: A&P Review

The thyroid is a butterfly-shaped organ located anterior to the trachea, just inferior to the larynx (see Figure 9.18).[58] Each of the thyroid lobes are embedded with parathyroid glands.

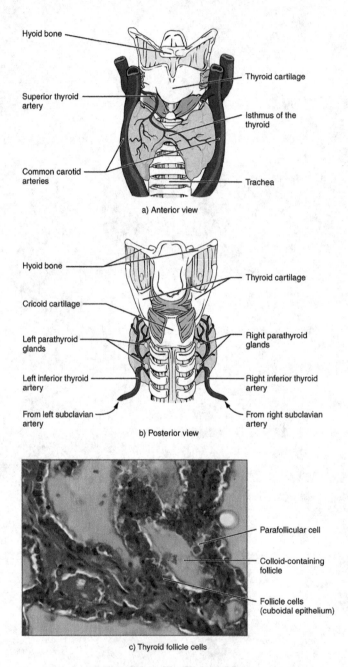

Figure 9.18 The Thyroid Gland

---

58 "1811 The Thyroid Gland.jpg" by OpenStax College is licensed under CC BY 3.0. Access for free at https://openstax .org/books/anatomy-and-physiology/pages/17-4-the-thyroid-gland.

Synthesis and Release of Thyroid Hormones

Thyroid hormone production is dependent on the hormone's essential component: iodine. T3 and T4 hormones are produced when iodine attaches to a glycoprotein called thyroglobulin. The following steps outline the hormone's assembly: Binding of TSH to thyroid receptors causes the cells to actively transport iodide ions across their cell membrane from the bloodstream. As a result, the concentration of iodide ions "trapped" in the thyroid cells is many times higher than the concentration in the bloodstream. The iodide ions undergo oxidation (i.e., their negatively charged electrons are removed) and enzymes link the iodine to tyrosine to produce triiodothyronine (T3), a thyroid hormone with three iodines, or thyroxine (T4), a thyroid hormone with four iodines. These hormones remain in the thyroid follicles until TSH stimulates the release of free T3 and T4 into the bloodstream. In the bloodstream, less than one percent of the circulating T3 and T4 remains unbound. This free T3 and T4 can cross the lipid bilayer of cell membranes and be taken up by cells. The remaining 99 percent of circulating T3 and T4 is bound to specialized transport proteins called thyroxine-binding globulins (TBGs), to albumin, or to other plasma proteins. This "packaging" prevents their free diffusion into body cells. When blood levels of T3 and T4 begin to decline, bound T3 and T4 are released from these plasma proteins and readily cross the membrane of target cells. T3 is more potent than T4, and many cells convert T4 to T3 through the removal of an iodine atom.

Regulation of Thyroid Hormone Synthesis

A negative feedback loop controls the regulation of thyroid hormone levels. As shown in Figure 9.19,[59] low blood levels of T3 and T4 stimulate the release of thyrotropin-releasing hormone (TRH) from the hypothalamus, which triggers secretion of TSH from the anterior pituitary. In turn, TSH stimulates the thyroid gland to secrete T3 and T4. The levels of TRH, TSH, T3, and T4 are regulated by a negative feedback system in which increasing levels of T3 and T4 decrease the production and secretion of TSH.

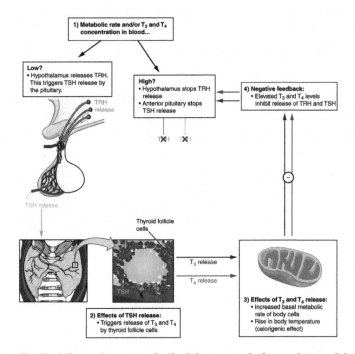

Figure 9.19 Negative Feedback Loop. A negative feedback loop controls the regulation of thyroid hormone levels

---

Functions of Thyroid Hormones

The thyroid hormones T3 and T4 are often referred to as metabolic hormones because their levels influence the body's basal metabolic rate, which is the amount of energy used by the body at rest. When T3 and T4 bind to intracellular receptors located on the mitochondria, they cause an increase in nutrient breakdown and the use of oxygen to produce ATP. In addition, T3 and T4 initiate the transcription of genes involved in glucose oxidation. Although these mechanisms prompt cells to produce more ATP, the process is inefficient, and an abnormally increased level of heat is released as a byproduct of these reactions. This calorigenic effect (calor- = "heat") raises body temperature.

Adequate levels of thyroid hormones are also required for protein synthesis and for fetal and childhood tissue development and growth. They are especially critical for normal development of the nervous system both in utero and in early childhood, and they continue to support neurological function in adults. Thyroid hormones also have a complex interrelationship with reproductive hormones, and deficiencies can influence libido, fertility, and other aspects of reproductive function. Finally, thyroid hormones increase the body's sensitivity to catecholamines (epinephrine and norepinephrine) from the adrenal medulla by upregulation of receptors in the blood vessels. When levels of T3 and T4 hormones are excessive, this effect accelerates the heart rate, strengthens the heartbeat, and increases blood pressure. Because thyroid hormones regulate metabolism, heat production, protein synthesis, and many other body functions, thyroid disorders can have severe and widespread consequences.

Disorders of the Thyroid Gland: Iodine Deficiency, Hypothyroidism, and Hyperthyroidism

As discussed above, dietary iodine is required for the synthesis of T3 and T4. For much of the world's population, foods do not provide adequate levels of iodine because the amount varies according to the level in the soil in which the food was grown, as well as the irrigation and fertilizers used. Marine fish and shrimp tend to have high levels because they concentrate iodine from seawater, but many people in landlocked regions lack access to seafood. Thus, the primary source of dietary iodine in many countries is iodized salt. Fortification of salt with iodine began in the United States in 1924, and international efforts to iodize salt in the world's poorest nations continue today.

Dietary iodine deficiency can result in the impaired ability to synthesize T3 and T4, leading to a variety of severe disorders. When T3 and T4 cannot be produced, TSH is secreted in increasing amounts. As a result of this hyperstimulation, thyroglobulin and colloid accumulate in the thyroid gland and increase the overall size of the thyroid gland, a condition called a **goiter** (see Figure 9.20[60]). A goiter is only a visible indication of the deficiency. Other disorders related to iodine deficiency include impaired growth and development, decreased fertility, and prenatal and infant death. Moreover, iodine deficiency is the primary cause of preventable mental retardation worldwide. Neonatal hypothyroidism (cretinism) is characterized by cognitive deficits, short stature, and sometimes deafness and muteness in children and adults born to mothers who were iodine-deficient during pregnancy.

---

60   "Goitre.jpg" by Almazi is licensed under CC0.

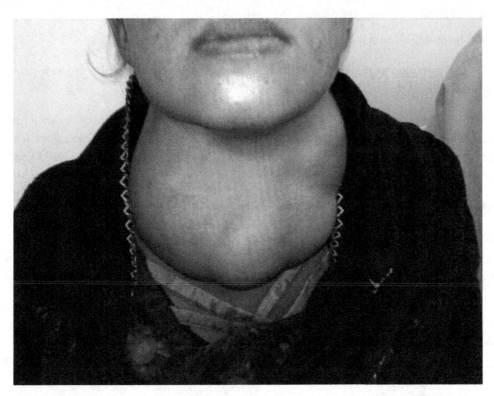

Figure 9.20 Goiter

In areas of the world with access to iodized salt, dietary deficiency is rare. Instead, inflammation of the thyroid gland is a common cause of **hypothyroidism**, or low blood levels of thyroid hormones. Hypothyroidism is a disorder characterized by a low metabolic rate, weight gain, cold extremities, constipation, reduced libido, menstrual irregularities, and reduced mental activity, and requires long-term thyroid hormone replacement therapy. In contrast, **hyperthyroidism**—an abnormally elevated blood level of thyroid hormones—is often caused by a pituitary or thyroid tumor. In Graves' disease, the hyperthyroid state results from an autoimmune reaction in which antibodies overstimulate the follicle cells of the thyroid gland. Hyperthyroidism can lead to an increased metabolic rate, excessive body heat and sweating, diarrhea, weight loss, tremors, and increased heart rate. The person's eyes may bulge (called exophthalmos) as antibodies produce inflammation in the soft tissues of the orbits. The person may also develop a goiter. Hyperthyroidism is often treated by thyroid surgery or with radioactive iodine (RAI) therapy. Patients are asked to follow radiation precautions after RAI treatment to limit radiation exposure to others, especially pregnant women and young children, such as sleeping in a separate bed and flushing the toilet 2-3 times after use. The RAI treatment may take up to several months to have its effect. The end result of thyroid surgery or RAI treatment is often hypothyroidism, which is treated by thyroid hormone replacement therapy.[61]

Calcitonin

The thyroid gland also secretes another hormone called calcitonin. Calcitonin is released in response to elevated blood calcium levels. It decreases blood calcium concentrations by:

- Inhibiting the activity of osteoclasts (bone cells that breakdown bone matrix and release calcium into the circulation)

---

61   American Thyroid Association. (2019). *Radioactive iodine*. https://www.thyroid.org/radioactive-iodine/.

My Notes

- Decreasing calcium absorption in the intestines

- Increasing calcium loss in the urine

Pharmaceutical preparations of calcitonin are prescribed to reduce osteoclast activity in people with osteoporosis. Osteoporosis is a disease that can be caused by glucocorticoids.

Calcium is critical for many other biological processes. It is a second messenger in many signaling pathways and is essential for muscle contraction, nerve impulse transmission, and blood clotting. Given these roles, it is not surprising that blood calcium levels are tightly regulated by the endocrine system. The parathyroid glands are primarily involved in calcium regulation.

Calcium Regulation: Parathyroid Glands

The parathyroid glands are four tiny, round structures usually embedded in the posterior surface of the thyroid gland (see Figure 9.21).[62] The primary function of the parathyroid glands is to regulate blood calcium levels by producing and secreting **parathyroid hormone (PTH)** in response to low blood calcium levels.

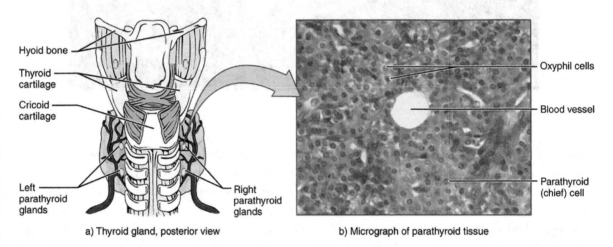

Figure 9.21 The Parathyroid Glands

PTH secretion causes the release of calcium from the bones by stimulating osteoclasts that degrade bone and then release calcium into the bloodstream. PTH also inhibits osteoblasts, the cells involved in bone deposition, thereby keeping calcium in the blood. PTH also causes increased reabsorption of calcium (and magnesium) in the kidney and initiates the production of the steroid hormone calcitriol, which is the active form of vitamin D3. Calcitriol then stimulates increased absorption of dietary calcium by the intestines. A negative feedback loop regulates the levels of PTH, with rising blood calcium levels inhibiting further release of PTH. (See Figure 9.22 for an illustration of the role of parathyroid hormone in maintaining blood calcium homeostasis.)[63]

---

62   "1814 The Parathyroid Glands.jpg" by OpenStax College is licensed under CC BY 3.0. Access for free at https://openstax.org/books/anatomy-and-physiology/pages/17-5-the-parathyroid-glands.

63   "1817 The Role of Parathyroid Hormone in Maintaining Blood Calcium Homeostasis.jpg" by OpenStax is licensed under CC BY 4.0. Access for free at https://openstax.org/books/anatomy-and-physiology/pages/ 17-5-the-parathyroid-glands.

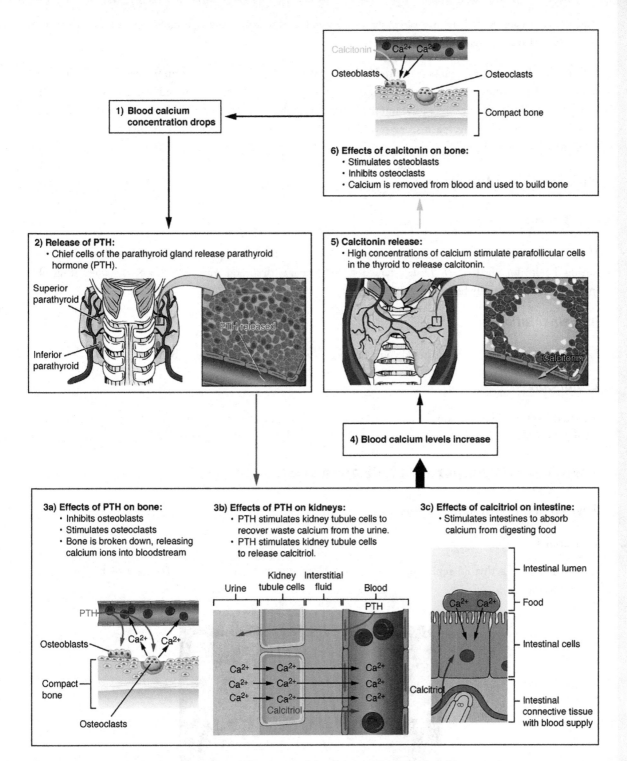

Figure 9.22 Parathyroid Hormone in Maintaining Blood Calcium Homeostasis

Disorders of the Parathyroid Glands

Abnormally high activity of the parathyroid gland can cause **hyperparathyroidism,** a disorder caused by an over-production of PTH that results in excessive degradation of bone and elevated blood levels of calcium, also called hypercalcemia. Hyperparathyroidism can thus significantly decrease bone density, which can lead to spontaneous fractures or deformities. As blood calcium levels rise, cell membrane permeability to sodium is also decreased, and thus the responsiveness of the nervous system is reduced. At the same time, calcium deposits may collect in the body's tissues and organs, impairing their functioning.

In contrast, abnormally low blood calcium levels may be caused by parathyroid hormone deficiency, called **hypo-parathyroidism**, which may develop following injury or surgery involving the thyroid gland. Low blood calcium increases membrane permeability to sodium, thus increasing the responsiveness of the nervous system, resulting in muscle twitching, cramping, spasms, or convulsions. Severe deficits can paralyze muscles, including those involved in breathing, and can be fatal.

Nursing Considerations

Assessment

When administering thyroid replacement medications, the nurse should plan to monitor TSH levels before and during therapy for effectiveness. Drug interactions may occur with several other medications, so review drug labeling information carefully before administering.

Implementation

Levothyroxine should be administered consistently every morning 30-60 minutes before a meal.

Evaluation

Elevated levels of thyroid hormone can cause cardiac dysrhythmias; immediately report any symptoms of tachycardia, chest pain, or palpitations to the provider.

Thyroid and Osteoporosis Medication Classes

Thyroid Replacement Medication

Indications

Levothyroxine is a thyroid replacement drug used to treat hypothyroidism. See Figure 9.23 for an image of levothyroxine.[64]

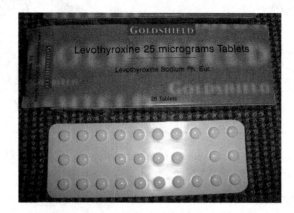

Figure 9.23 Levothyroxine

---

64 "Levothyroxine 25mcg Tablets.jpg" by User:Ash is licensed under CC0.

Mechanism of Action

Oral levothyroxine sodium is a synthetic T4 hormone that exerts the same physiologic effect as endogenous T4, thereby maintaining normal T4 levels when a deficiency is present.

Specific Administration Considerations

Levothyroxine tablets should be taken with a full glass of water as the tablet may rapidly disintegrate. It should be administered as a single daily dose, on an empty stomach, one-half to one hour before breakfast, and at least 4 hours before or after drugs known to interfere with levothyroxine absorption.

Levothyroxine is contraindicated for patients with hyperthyroidism and adrenal insufficiency until the condition is corrected. Many patients who undergo treatment for hyperthyroidism may develop hypothyroidism. Overtreatment with levothyroxine may cause symptoms of hyperthyroidism with increased heart rate, cardiac wall thickness, and cardiac contractility that may precipitate angina or arrhythmias, particularly in patients with cardiovascular disease and in elderly patients. Levothyroxine therapy in this population should be initiated at lower doses. If cardiac symptoms develop or worsen, the nurse should withhold the medication, contact the health care provider, and anticipate a lower dose prescribed or the medication to be withheld for one week then restarted at a lower dose.

Addition of levothyroxine therapy in patients with diabetes mellitus may worsen glycemic control and result in the need for higher dosages of antidiabetic medication. Carefully monitor glycemic control, especially when thyroid therapy is started, changed, or discontinued.

Levothyroxine increases the response to oral anticoagulant therapy. Therefore, a decrease in the dose of anticoagulant may be warranted with correction of the hypothyroid state or when the levothyroxine dose is increased. Closely monitor INR results and anticipate dosage adjustments.

Levothyroxine can affect, or be affected by, several other medications, so carefully read drug label information when therapy is initiated.

Pregnancy: There are risks to the mother and fetus associated with untreated hypothyroidism in pregnancy. Because TSH levels may increase during pregnancy, TSH should be monitored and levothyroxine dosage may require adjustment during pregnancy.[65]

Patient Teaching and Education

Patients should take thyroid replacement medications at the same time each day. Patients should be aware that thyroid replacement medications do not cure hypothyroidism and therapy is lifelong. Patients should notify their healthcare provider if they experience signs of headache, diarrhea, sweating, or heat intolerance. Medications should be spaced four hours apart from medications like antacid, iron, or calcium supplements. Patients will be followed closely by their healthcare provider regarding their response to medication therapy and serum thyroid levels will be taken.[66]

---

65   This work is a derivative of *Daily Med* by U.S. National Library of Medicine in the public domain.

66   uCentral from Unbound Medicine. https://www.unboundmedicine.com/ucentral.

Antithyroid Medication

Indications

Propylthiouracil (PTU) is an antithyroid medication used to treat hyperthyroidism or to ameliorate symptoms of hyperthyroidism in preparation for thyroidectomy or radioactive iodine therapy.

Mechanism of Action

Propylthiouracil inhibits the synthesis of thyroid hormones.

Specific Administration Considerations

Propylthiouracil is administered orally. The total daily dosage is usually given in 3 equal doses at approximately 8-hour intervals. Propylthiouracil can cause hypothyroidism necessitating routine monitoring of TSH and free T4 levels, with adjustments in dosing to maintain a euthyroid state.

Liver injury resulting in liver failure, liver transplantation, or death has been reported. Patients should be instructed to report any symptoms of hepatic dysfunction (anorexia, pruritus, and right upper quadrant pain), particularly in the first six months of therapy.

Agranulocytosis is a potentially life-threatening side effect of propylthiouracil therapy. Agranulocytosis typically occurs within the first 3 months of therapy. Patients should be instructed to immediately report any symptoms suggestive of agranulocytosis, such as fever or sore throat.

Cases of vasculitis resulting in severe complications and death have been reported in patients receiving propylthiouracil therapy. If vasculitis is suspected, discontinue therapy and initiate appropriate intervention.

Pregnancy: Propylthiouracil crosses the placenta and can cause fetal liver failure, goiter, and cretinism if administered to a pregnant woman.

Patient Teaching and Education

Patients should take the medication as directed at regular dosing intervals. They should monitor their weight 2-3 times per week. Additionally, patients should be advised that medications may cause drowsiness, and they should report any signs of sore throat, fever, headache, jaundice, bleeding, or bruising.

Osteoporosis Medication: Calcitonin

Indications

Calcitonin is used to treat osteoporosis.

Mechanism of Action

Calcitonin is a calcitonin receptor agonist. Calcitonin is released by the thyroid gland. It acts primarily on bone and also has effects on the kidneys and the gastrointestinal tract.

Specific Administration Considerations

Calcitonin is administered via nasal spray with one spray in one side of the nose daily. See Figure 9.24 for an image of calcitonin nasal spray.[67] The nasal spray pump should be primed before the first administration. Unopened calcitonin can be stored in the refrigerator until opened, but should not be refrigerated between doses. Opened bottles stored at room temperature should be discarded after 30 days of initial dose.

Adverse effects include serious hypersensitivity reactions (bronchospasm, swelling of the tongue or throat, anaphylaxis and anaphylactic shock), hypocalcemia, nasal mucosa adverse events, and malignancy.

Pregnancy: Calcitonin should not be used during pregnancy.

Patient Teaching and Education

Patients should be advised to take medications as directed. They should report any signs of hypercalcemia or an allergic response. Patients should receive instruction on the process of self-injection. They should also be advised that they may experience flushing and warmth following injection. Post-menopausal women should adhere to a diet high in calcium and vitamin D, and should be educated regarding the importance of exercise for reversing bone loss.[68]

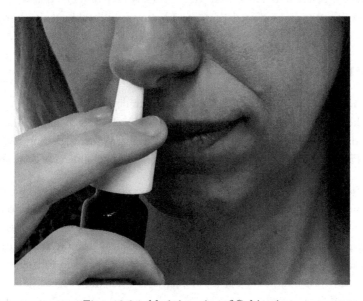

Figure 9.24 Administration of Calcitonin

Indications

Alendronate is used for the prevention and treatment of osteoporosis in postmenopausal women, to increase bone mass in men with osteoporosis, and for glucocorticoid-induced osteoporosis.

---

67   "Nasal Spray" by NIAID is licensed under CC BY 2.0.

68   uCentral from Unbound Medicine. https://www.unboundmedicine.com/ucentral.

Mechanism of Action

Alendronate is a bisphosphonate that inhibits osteoclast-mediated bone resorption. By preventing the breakdown of bone and enhancing the formation of new bone, alendronate assists in reversing bone loss and decreases the risk of fractures.

Specific Administration Considerations

Check dosages carefully because some formulations are administered daily, whereas others are administered one weekly. Alendronate should be taken upon arising for the day, but should be administered at least one-half hour before the first food, beverage, or medication of the day with plain water only. Other beverages (including mineral water), food, and some medications are likely to reduce the absorption of alendronate. Patients should not lie down for at least 30 minutes and until after their first food of the day. Patients may also require calcium and vitamin D supplementation, especially if concurrently taking glucocorticoids.

Alendronate is contraindicated in the following conditions: pregnancy, hypocalcemia, the inability to sit or stand for 30 minutes after swallowing, esophageal abnormalities that delay emptying, and patients at risk for aspiration. Alendronate is not recommended for patients with kidney disease with creatinine clearance less than 35 mL/min.

Discontinue alendronate if severe musculoskeletal pain occurs. A bone mineral density measurement should be made at the initiation of therapy and repeated after 6 to 12 months of combined alendronate and glucocorticoid treatment.

Patient Teaching and Education

Patients should take medication as directed at the same time each day, first thing in the morning. Patients should remain upright after they take medication for 30 minutes to minimize stomach and esophageal irritation. Patients should eat a balanced diet and may seek advice from the healthcare provider regarding supplementation with calcium and vitamin D. Patients should participate in regular exercise to help increase bone strength.[69]

Now let's take a closer look at the medication grid comparing thyroid and osteoporosis medications in Table 9.5.[70] Medication grids are intended to assist students to learn key points about each medication. Because information about medication is constantly changing, nurses should always consult evidence-based resources to review current recommendations before administering specific medication. Basic information related to each class of medication is outlined below. Detailed information on a specific medication can be found for free at *Daily Med* at https://dailymed.nlm.nih.gov/dailymed/index.cfm. On the home page, enter the drug name in the search bar to read more about the medication. Prototype/generic medications listed in the grids below are also hyperlinked directly to a *Daily Med* page.

---

69   uCentral from Unbound Medicine. https://www.unboundmedicine.com/ucentral.

70   This work is a derivative of *Daily Med* by U.S. National Library of Medicine in the public domain.

Table 9.5: Medication Grid Comparing Thyroid and Osteoporosis Medications

Class	Prototype/ Generic	Administration Considerations	Therapeutic Effects	Adverse/Side Effects
Thyroid replacement	levothyroxine	Take levothyroxine sodium tablets with a full glass of water as the tablet may rapidly disintegrate Administer levothyroxine as a single daily dose, on an empty stomach, one-half to one hour before breakfast Administer levothyroxine at least 4 hours before or after drugs known to interfere with levothyroxine sodium tablets absorption Anticipate lower dosages in elderly patients with pre-existing cardiac disease May interact with several medications so read drug label thoroughly on initial administration for potential effects	Increases T4 levels in hypothyroidism	Hypersensitivity reactions Cardiac dysrhythmias
Antithyroid	propylthio- uracil (PTU)	Usually administered every 8 hours May cause hypothyroidism so TSH and T4 levels should be monitored If a patient becomes pregnant, immediately notify health care provider because it can cause fetal harm	Inhibit production of T4	Hypothyroidism Liver failure Agranulocytosis Vasculitis Fetal harm
Calcium regulator	calcitonin	Administer nasal spray with one spray in one side of the nose daily Contraindicated during pregnancy Discard unrefrigerated bottle after 30 days of opening May store unopened bottles in refrigerator until expiration date	Treats osteoporosis	Serious hypersensitivity reactions (bronchospasm, swelling of the tongue or throat, anaphylaxis, and anaphylactic shock) Hypocalcemia Nasal mucosa adverse effects Malignancy
Bisphosphonates	alendronate	Administered upon arising and at least one-half hour before the first food, beverage, or medication of the day with plain water only The patient should sit or stand for 30 minutes after administration Contraindicated in pregnancy, hypocalcemia, and kidney disease Concurrent calcium and vitamin D supplements may be required	Enhances bone mineral density in osteoporosis	Upper GI tract adverse events Severe musculoskeletal pain Risk of osteonecrosis of the jaw

Critical Thinking Activity 9.5

A patient has been diagnosed with hypothyroidism and receives a prescription for levothyroxine.

What patient education should the nurse provide regarding taking this medication?

Note: Answers to the Critical Thinking activities can be found in the "Answer Key" sections at the end of the book.

9.6   MODULE LEARNING ACTIVITIES

Interactive Activities

 An interactive or media element has been excluded from this version of the text. You can view it online here: https://wtcs.pressbooks.pub/pharmacology/?p=1791

GLOSSARY

A1C: A lab test used to assess long-term blood glucose levels over 3 months. The general A1C target level is less than 7%.

Adrenal cortex: A component of the hypothalamic-pituitary-adrenal (HPA) axis that produces the steroid hormones important for the regulation of the stress response, blood pressure and blood volume, nutrient uptake and storage, fluid and electrolyte balance, and inflammation.

Adrenal medulla: Neuroendocrine tissue composed of postganglionic sympathetic nervous system (SNS) neurons that are stimulated by the autonomic nervous system to secrete hormones epinephrine and norepinephrine.

Aldosterone: A mineralocorticoid released by the adrenal cortex that controls fluid and electrolyte balance through the regulation of sodium and potassium.

Antidiuretic hormone (ADH): ADH is released by the posterior pituitary in response to stimuli from osmoreceptors indicating high blood osmolarity. Its effect is to cause increased water reabsorption by the kidneys. As more water is reabsorbed by the kidneys, the greater the amount of water that is returned to the blood, thus causing a decrease in blood osmolarity. ADH is also known as vasopressin because, in very high concentrations, it causes constriction of blood vessels, which increases blood pressure by increasing peripheral resistance.

Basal insulin: Long-acting (insulin glargine or insulin detemir) or intermediate-acting (NPH) insulin.

Basal Metabolic Rate: The amount of energy used by the body at rest.

Blood osmolarity: The concentration of solutes (such as sodium and glucose) in the blood.

Diabetes insipidus (DI): A disease characterized by underproduction of ADH that causes chronic dehydration.

Endocrine gland: Gland that secretes hormones that target other organs.

Exocrine gland: Gland that secretes digestive enzymes.

General adaptation syndrome (GAS): The pattern in which the body responds in different ways to stress: the alarm reaction (otherwise known as the fight-or-flight response,) the stage of resistance, and the stage of exhaustion.

Glycolysis: Stimulated by insulin, the metabolism of glucose for generation of ATP.

Goiter: A visible enlargement of the thyroid gland when there is hyperstimulation of TSH due to deficient levels of T3 and T4 hormones in the bloodstream or an autoimmune reaction in which antibodies overstimulate the follicle cells of the thyroid gland, causing hyperthyroidism.

Hormones: Chemical signals sent by the endocrine organs and transported via the bloodstream throughout the body where they bind to receptors on target cells and induce a characteristic response.

Humoral stimuli: Changes in blood levels of non-hormone chemicals that cause an endocrine gland to release or inhibit a hormone to maintain homeostasis. For example, high blood sugar causes the pancreas to release insulin.

Hyperglycemia: Elevated blood glucose levels.

Hyperparathyroidism: A disorder caused by an overproduction of PTH that results in excessive calcium resorption from bone, causing significantly decreased bone density and spontaneous fractures, decreased responsiveness of the nervous system, and calcium deposits in the body's tissues and organs, impairing their functioning.

Hyperthyroidism: Abnormally elevated blood level of thyroid hormones T3 and T4, often caused by a pituitary tumor, thyroid tumor, or autoimmune reaction in which antibodies overstimulate the follicle cells of the thyroid gland.

Hypoglycemia: A blood glucose level below 70 mg/dL; severe hypoglycemia refers to a blood glucose level below 40.

Hypoparathyroidism: Abnormally low blood calcium levels caused by parathyroid hormone deficiency, which may develop following thyroid surgery. Low blood calcium can cause muscle twitching, cramping, spasms, or convulsions; severe deficits can paralyze muscles, including those involved in breathing, and can be fatal.

Hypothalamic-pituitary-adrenal (HPA) axis: The hypothalamus stimulates the release of ACTH from the pituitary, which then stimulates the adrenal cortex to produce the hormone cortisol and steroid hormones important for the regulation of the stress response, blood pressure and blood volume, nutrient uptake and storage, fluid and electrolyte balance, and inflammation.

Hypothalamus–pituitary complex: The "command center" of the endocrine system that secretes several hormones that directly produce responses in target tissues, as well as hormones that regulate the synthesis and secretion of hormones of other glands. In addition, the hypothalamus–pituitary complex coordinates the messages of the endocrine and nervous systems.

Hypothyroidism: Abnormally low blood levels of thyroid hormones T3 and T4 in the bloodstream.

Insulin: A hormone that facilitates the uptake of glucose into skeletal and adipose body cells.

Mineralocorticoids: Hormones released by the adrenal cortex that regulate body minerals, especially sodium and potassium, that are essential for fluid and electrolyte balance. Aldosterone is the major mineralocorticoid.

Negative feedback loop: Characterized by the inhibition of further secretion of a hormone in response to adequate levels of that hormone.

Neural stimuli: Released in response to stimuli from the nervous system. For example, the activation of the release of epinephrine and norepinephrine in the fight-or-flight response is stimulated by the sympathetic nervous system.

Osmoreceptors: Specialized cells within the hypothalamus that are sensitive to the concentration of sodium ions and other solutes in the bloodstream.

Parathyroid hormone (PTH): The hormone released by parathyroid glands and is involved in the regulation of blood calcium levels.

Prandial insulins: During or relating to the eating of food.

Tropic hormones: Hormones that turn on or off the function of other endocrine glands, including ACTH, FSH, LH, and TSH.

Type 1 diabetes: An autoimmune disease that affects the beta cells of the pancreas so they do not produce insulin; thus, synthetic insulin must be administered by injection or infusion.

Type 2 diabetes: A condition where the body's cells become resistant to the effects of insulin. Over time, the beta cells become exhausted and if blood glucose levels cannot be controlled through a healthy diet and exercise, then oral diabetic medication must be implemented and eventually insulin administration may be required.

Chapter X

Analgesic and Musculoskeletal

10.1   ANALGESICS AND MUSCULOSKELETAL INTRODUCTION

Learning Objectives

- Cite the classifications and actions of analgesics

- Cite the classifications and actions of musculoskeletal system drugs

- Give examples of when, how, and to whom analgesics and musculoskeletal system drugs may be administered

- Identify the side effects and special considerations associated with analgesics

- Identify the side effects and special considerations associated with musculoskeletal system drugs

- Identify the considerations and implications of using analgesics across the life span

- Identify the considerations and implications of using musculoskeletal system medications across the life span

- Apply evidence-based concepts when using the nursing process

Complaints of pain are one of the most common reasons individuals seek out medical care. The pain signal indicates that something in the body is not quite right! Whether it be a headache, a broken bone, labor pain, chest pain, or other condition, pain assessment and treatment will become an important part of your daily work.

As a nurse, you will care for patients experiencing various types of pain manifestations and responses. It will be important for you to understand the various pharmacological and non-pharmacological treatment methods available for your patients.

10.2 REVIEW OF BASIC CONCEPTS

Before we learn about the medications that are used to treat analgesic and musculoskeletal conditions in our patients, we must first review the physiology of pain and the anatomy of the musculoskeletal system.

Analgesic System

Physiology of Pain

Pain occurs when there is tissue damage in the body. Tissue damage activates pain receptors of peripheral nerves. **Nociceptors**, the nerve endings that respond to painful stimuli, are located in arterial walls, joint surfaces, muscle fascia, periosteum, skin, and soft tissue. Nociceptors are barely present in most internal organs.[1]

The cause of tissue damage may be physical (e.g., heat, cold, pressure, stretch, spasm, and ischemia) or chemical (pain-producing substances are released into the extracellular fluid surrounding the nerve fibers that carry the pain signal). These pain-producing substances activate pain receptors, increase the sensitivity of pain receptors, or stimulate the release of inflammatory substances (e.g., **prostaglandins**).[2]

For a person to feel pain, the signal from the nociceptors in peripheral tissues must be transmitted to the spinal cord and then to the hypothalamus and cerebral cortex of the brain. The signal is transmitted to the brain by two types of nerve cells (A-delta and C fibers). The dorsal horn of the spinal cord is the relay station for information from these fibers. In the brain, the thalamus is the relay station for incoming sensory stimuli, including pain. From the thalamus, the pain messages are relayed to the cerebral cortex where they are perceived.[3] See Figure 10.1 for an illustration of how the pain signal is transmitted from peripheral tissues to the spinal cord and then to the brain.[4]

1 Frandsen, G. and Pennington, S. (2018). *Abrams' clinical drug: Rationales for nursing practice (11th ed.).* (pg. 305, 310, 952–953, 959–960). Wolters Kluwer.

2 Frandsen, G. and Pennington, S. (2018). *Abrams' clinical drug: Rationales for nursing practice (11th ed.).* (pg. 305, 310, 952–953, 959–960). Wolters Kluwer.

3 Frandsen, G. and Pennington, S. (2018). *Abrams' clinical drug: Rationales for nursing practice (11th ed.).* (pg. 305, 310, 952–953, 959–960). Wolters Kluwer.

4 "Sketch colored final.png" by Bettina Guebeli is licensed under CC BY-SA 4.0.

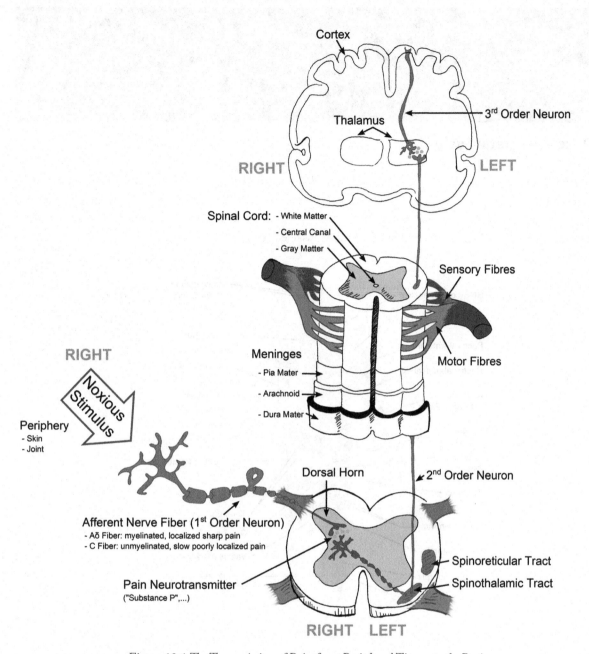

Figure 10.1 The Transmission of Pain from Peripheral Tissues to the Brain

Endogenous Analgesia

The CNS has its own endogenous analgesia system for relieving pain. The CNS suppresses pain signals from peripheral nerves. Opioid peptides interact with opioid receptors to inhibit perception and transmission of pain signals. These opioid peptides are endorphins, enkephalins, and dynorphins.[5]

See the video below for more information about how pain relievers work.

---

5   Frandsen, G. and Pennington, S. (2018). *Abrams' clinical drug: Rationales for nursing practice (11th ed.)*. (pg. 305, 310, 952–953, 959–960). Wolters Kluwer.

How Do Pain Relievers Work? by George Zaidan[6]

A YouTube element has been excluded from this version of the text. You can view it online here:
https://wtcs.pressbooks.pub/pharmacology/?p=2448

Musculoskeletal System

In the musculoskeletal system, the muscular and skeletal systems work together to support and move the body. The bones of the skeletal system serve to protect the body's organs, support the weight of the body, and give the body shape. The muscles of the muscular system attach to these bones, pulling on them to allow for movement of the body.[7] See Figure 10.2 for an illustration of the musculoskeletal system.[8]

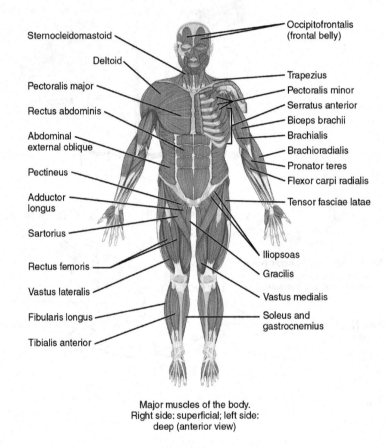

Major muscles of the body.
Right side: superficial; left side:
deep (anterior view)

Figure 10.2 The Musculoskeletal System

6   Ted-Ed. (2012, June 26). *How Do Pain Relievers Work? – George Zaidan* [Video]. YouTube. https://youtu.be/9mcuIc5O-DE.

7   Khan Academy. (n.d.). *The musculoskeletal system review.* https://www.khanacademy.org/science/high-school-biology/hs-human-body-systems/hs-the-musculoskeletal-system/a/hs-the-musculoskeletal-system-review.

8   This image is a derivative of "1105 Anterior and Posterior Views of Muscles.jpg" by CFCF is licensed under CC BY 4.0.

Muscles

The body contains three types of muscle tissue: skeletal muscle, smooth muscle, and cardiac muscle. See Figure 10.3 for images of different types of muscle.[9]

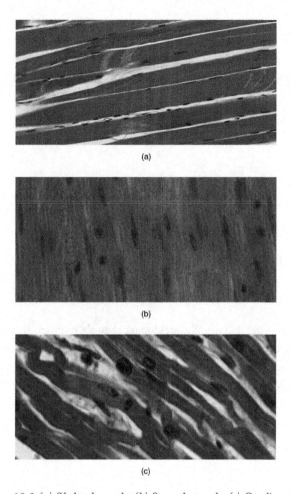

Figure 10.3 (a) Skeletal muscle; (b) Smooth muscle; (c) Cardiac muscle

Skeletal muscle is voluntary and striated. These are the muscles that attach to bones and control conscious movement. Smooth muscle is involuntary and non-striated. It is found in the hollow organs of the body, such as the stomach, intestines, and around blood vessels. Cardiac muscle is involuntary and striated. It is found only in the heart and is specialized to help pump blood throughout the body.[10]

When a muscle fiber receives a signal from the nervous system, myosin filaments are stimulated, pulling actin filaments closer together. This shortens sarcomeres within a fiber, causing it to contract.[11]

---

9   "414 Skeletal Smooth Cardiac.jpg" by OpenStax College is licensed under CC BY 4.0.

10   Khan Academy. (n.d.). *The musculoskeletal system review.* https://www.khanacademy.org/science/high-school-biology/hs-human-body-systems/hs-the-musculoskeletal-system/a/hs-the-musculoskeletal-system-review.

11   Khan Academy. (n.d.). *The musculoskeletal system review.* https://www.khanacademy.org/science/high-school-biology/hs-human-body-systems/hs-the-musculoskeletal-system/a/hs-the-musculoskeletal-system-review.

10.3 CONDITIONS AND DISEASES

Several conditions can cause pain or inflammation that require the use of analgesics or musculoskeletal medication. Common disorders are briefly reviewed below.

Acute Pain

Acute pain usually comes on suddenly and is caused by something specific. It is sharp in quality. Acute pain usually does not last longer than six months. It goes away when there is no longer an underlying cause for the pain. Causes of acute pain include:

- Surgery
- Broken bones
- Dental work
- Burns or cuts
- Labor and childbirth

After acute pain goes away, a person can go on with life as usual.[12]

Chronic Pain

Chronic pain is pain that is ongoing and usually lasts longer than six months. This type of pain can continue even after the injury or illness that caused it has healed or gone away. Pain signals remain active in the nervous system for weeks, months, or years. Some people suffer chronic pain even when there is no past injury or apparent body damage. Chronic pain is linked to conditions including:

- Headache
- Arthritis
- Cancer
- Nerve pain
- Back pain
- Fibromyalgia pain

People who have chronic pain can have physical effects that are stressful on the body. These include tense muscles, limited ability to move around, a lack of energy, and appetite changes. Emotional effects of chronic pain include depression, anger, anxiety, and fear of reinjury. Such a fear might limit a person's ability to return to their regular work or leisure activities.[13]

---

12   Cleveland Clinic. (2017, January 26). *Acute v. chronic pain.* https://my.clevelandclinic.org/health/articles/12051-acute-vs-chronic-pain.

13   Cleveland Clinic. (2017, January 26). *Acute v. chronic pain.* https://my.clevelandclinic.org/health/articles/12051-acute-vs-chronic-pain.

Fibromyalgia

Fibromyalgia is a condition that causes pain all over the body (also referred to as widespread pain), sleep problems, fatigue, and often emotional and mental distress. People with fibromyalgia may be more sensitive to pain than people without fibromyalgia. This is called abnormal pain perception processing. Fibromyalgia affects about 4 million US adults, about 2% of the adult population. The cause of fibromyalgia is not known, but it can be effectively treated and managed.[14]

The most common symptoms of fibromyalgia are the following:

- Pain and stiffness all over the body
- Fatigue and tiredness
- Depression and anxiety
- Sleep problems
- Problems with thinking, memory, and concentration
- Headaches, including migraines

Other symptoms may include:

- Tingling or numbness in hands and feet
- Pain in the face or jaw, including disorders of the jaw known as temporomandibular joint syndrome (TMJ)
- Digestive problems, such as abdominal pain, bloating, constipation, and even irritable bowel syndrome (IBS)

Known risk factors include:

- Age. Fibromyalgia can affect people of all ages, including children. However, most people are diagnosed during middle age
- Lupus or Rheumatoid Arthritis. Patients diagnosed with lupus or rheumatoid arthritis (RA) are more likely to develop fibromyalgia

Other factors that have been weakly associated with onset of fibromyalgia include:

- Sex. Women are twice as likely to have fibromyalgia as men
- Stressful or traumatic events, such as car accidents or post-traumatic stress disorder (PTSD)
- Repetitive injuries. Injury from repetitive stress on a joint, such as frequent knee bending
- Illness (such as viral infections)
- Family history
- Obesity

---

14   Centers for Disease Control and Prevention. (2017, October 11). *Arthritis, Fibromyalgia.* https://www.cdc.gov/arthritis /basics/fibromyalgia.htm.

My Notes

Doctors usually diagnose fibromyalgia using the patient's history, physical examination, X-rays, and blood work.[15]

Gout

Gout is a common form of inflammatory arthritis that is very painful. It usually affects one joint at a time (often the big toe joint). There are times when symptoms get worse, known as flares, and times when there are no symptoms, known as remission. Repeated bouts of gout can lead to gouty arthritis, a worsening form of arthritis.

There is no cure for gout, but you can effectively treat and manage the condition with medication and self-management strategies.

Gout flares start suddenly and can last days or weeks. These flares are followed by long periods of remission (weeks, months, or years) without symptoms before another flare begins. Along with the big toe, joints commonly affected are the lesser toe joints, the ankle, and the knee.[16]

Symptoms in the affected joint(s) may include:

- Pain, usually intense
- Swelling
- Redness
- Heat

Gout is caused by a condition known as hyperuricemia, where there is too much uric acid in the body. The body makes uric acid when it breaks down purines, which are found in your body and the foods you eat. When there is too much uric acid in the body, uric acid crystals (monosodium urate) can build up in joints, fluids, and tissues within the body. Hyperuricemia does not always cause gout, and hyperuricemia without gout symptoms does not need to be treated.

The following make it more likely that you will develop hyperuricemia, which causes gout:

- Being male
- Being obese

Having certain health conditions can also increase your chances of developing hyperuricemia. These conditions include the following:

- Congestive heart failure
- Hypertension (high blood pressure)
- Insulin resistance
- Metabolic syndrome
- Diabetes
- Poor kidney function

---

15   Centers for Disease Control and Prevention. (2017, October 11). *Arthritis, Fibromyalgia.* https://www.cdc.gov/arthritis /basics/fibromyalgia.htm.

16   Centers for Disease Control and Prevention. (2019, January 28). *Arthritis, Gout.* https://www.cdc.gov/arthritis/basics /gout.html.

Additional factors may increase your chances of developing hyperuricemia:

- Using certain medications, such as diuretics (water pills)

- Drinking alcohol. The risk of gout is greater as alcohol intake increases

- Eating or drinking food and drinks high in fructose (a type of sugar)

- Having a diet high in purines, which the body breaks down into uric acid. Purine-rich foods include red meat, organ meat, and some kinds of seafood, such as anchovies, sardines, mussels, scallops, trout, and tuna.

A medical doctor diagnoses gout by assessing your symptoms and the results of your physical examination, X-rays, and lab tests. Gout can only be diagnosed during a flare when a joint is hot, swollen, and painful and when a lab test finds uric acid crystals in the affected joint.[17]

Muscle Spasm

Spasms of skeletal muscles are most common and are often due to overuse and muscle fatigue, dehydration, and electrolyte abnormalities. The spasm occurs abruptly, is painful, and is usually short-lived. It may be relieved by gently stretching the muscle.[18] Diseases such as multiple sclerosis can also cause chronic muscle spasms.

Multiple Sclerosis

Multiple sclerosis (MS) involves an **immune-mediated disease process** in which an abnormal response of the body's immune system is directed against the central nervous system (CNS). The CNS is made up of the brain, spinal cord, and optic nerves.

Within the CNS, the immune system causes inflammation that damages myelin (the fatty substance that surrounds and insulates the nerve fibers), as well as the nerve fibers themselves and the specialized cells that make myelin. When myelin or nerve fibers are damaged or destroyed in MS, messages within the CNS are altered or stopped completely. Damage to areas of the CNS may produce a variety of neurological symptoms that will vary among people with MS in type and severity. The damaged areas develop scar tissue that gives the disease its name – multiple areas of scarring or multiple sclerosis. The cause of MS is not known, but it is believed to involve genetic susceptibility, abnormalities in the immune system, and environmental factors that combine to make MS symptoms variable and unpredictable. No two people have exactly the same symptoms, and each person's symptoms can change or fluctuate over time. One person might experience only one or two of the possible symptoms, while another person might experience several symptoms of the disease.

Symptoms include:

- Fatigue

- Numbness or tingling

- Weakness

- Dizziness or vertigo

---

17   Centers for Disease Control and Prevention. (2019, January 28). *Arthritis, Gout*. https://www.cdc.gov/arthritis/basics/gout.html.

18   Wedro, B. (2019, July 18). *Muscle spasms*. https://www.medicinenet.com/muscle_spasms/article.htm.

- ■ Walking difficulties
- ■ **Muscle spasticity**
- ■ Blurred vision

At this time, there are no symptoms, physical findings, or laboratory tests that can, by themselves, determine if a person has MS. Several strategies are used to determine if a person meets the long-established criteria for a diagnosis of MS and to rule out other possible causes of whatever symptoms they are experiencing. These strategies include a careful medical history, a neurologic exam, and various tests including magnetic resonance imaging (MRI), spinal fluid analysis, and blood tests.[19]

Myasthenia Gravis

Myasthenia Gravis (MG) is an autoimmune disease that occurs when the immune system attacks the body's own tissues. In MG, the attack interrupts the connection between nerve and muscle called the neuromuscular junction. Myasthenia gravis is characterized by autoantibodies against the acetylcholine receptor or against a receptor-associated protein called muscle-specific tyrosine kinase. You can read more details about acetylcholine receptors in the "Autonomic Nervous System" chapter.

MG causes weakness in muscles that control the eyes, face, neck, and limbs. Symptoms include partial paralysis of eye movements, double vision and droopy eyelids, as well as weakness and fatigue in neck and jaws and problems chewing, swallowing, and holding up the head. MG is treatable with drugs that suppress the immune system or boost the signals between nerve and muscle.[20] The group of drugs used to control MG are called acetylcholinesterase (ACh) inhibitors. They inhibit the action of the enzyme acetylcholinesterase so that more acetylcholine (ACh) is available to activate cholinergic receptors and promote muscle contraction. ACh inhibitors are classified as parasympathomimetics. Pyridostigmine is an example of an ACh inhibitor.

Overdosing with ACh inhibitors can cause a complication called cholinergic crisis, which is an acute exacerbation of symptoms. A cholinergic crisis usually occurs 30-60 minutes after taking cholinergic medication with severe muscle weakness that can lead to respiratory paralysis and death.[21]

---

19 National Multiple Sclerosis Society. (2018, March 8). *What is MS?* [Video]. YouTube. All Rights Reserved. https://youtu.be/geQP_zYS-6s.

20 Muscular Dystrophy Association. (n.d.). *Myasthenia gravis.* https://www.mda.org/disease/myasthenia-gravis.

21 McCuistion, L., Vuljoin-DiMaggio, K., Winton, M, and Yeager, J. (2018). *Pharmacology: A patient-centered nursing process approach.* pp. 268–270, 324, 332. Elsevier.

10.4 NURSING PROCESS FOR ANALGESICS AND MUSCULOSKELETAL MEDICATIONS

Now that we have reviewed basic concepts related to pain and several disorders requiring analgesic or musculoskeletal medication, let's consider the nursing process and how it applies to these types of medications.

Assessment

Although there are numerous details to consider when administering medications, it is important to always first think about what you are giving and why?

First, let's think of why?

Analgesic medications are given to alleviate pain. An important piece of your nursing assessment should be to assess the patient's pain level. The patient's pain level is what the patient says it is. This is accomplished by using a pain scale. Always find out the acceptable pain level for your patient. See Figure 10.5[22] for common nursing mnemonics for pain assessment.

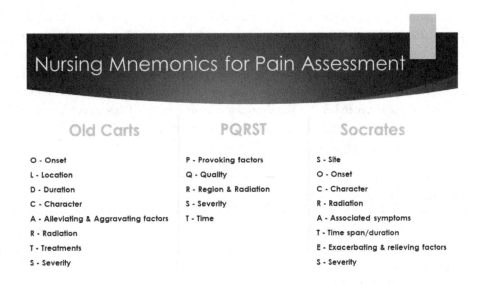

Figure 10.5 Mnemonics for Pain Assessment

Visual pain scales have been developed as a tool of communication about pain with children through patients at end of life. See Figure 10.6 for the FACES Pain Rating Scale. To use this scale, use the following evidence-based instructions. Explain to the patient that each face represents a person who has no pain (hurt), some, or a lot of pain. "Face 0 doesn't hurt at all. Face 2 hurts just a little. Face 4 hurts a little more. Face 6 hurts even more. Face 8 hurts a whole lot. Face 10 hurts as much as you can imagine, although you don't have to be crying to have this worst pain." Ask the person to choose the face that best represents the pain they are feeling.

Additional baseline information to collect prior to administration of any analgesic or musculoskeletal medication includes any history of allergy or previous adverse response.

---

22 "Mnemonics for Pain Assessment" by Julie Teeter is licensed under CC BY-SA 4.0.

My Notes

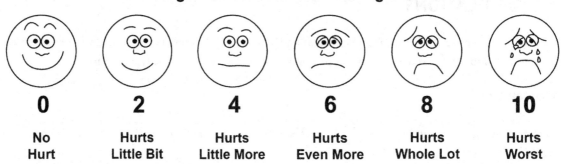

Wong-Baker FACES® Pain Rating Scale

0	2	4	6	8	10
No Hurt	Hurts Little Bit	Hurts Little More	Hurts Even More	Hurts Whole Lot	Hurts Worst

©1983 Wong-Baker FACES Foundation. www.WongBakerFACES.org
Used with permission. Originally published in *Whaley & Wong's Nursing Care of Infants and Children*. ©Elsevier Inc.

Figure 10.6. The Wong-Baker FACES Pain Rating Scale. Used with permission from http://www.WongBakerFACES.org.

Implementation of Interventions

With the administration of analgesic or musculoskeletal medications, it is important to always perform the five rights (right patient, medication, dose, route, and time) and to check for allergies prior to administration. Prior to administration, it is important to consider the best route of administration for this patient at this particular time. For example, if the patient is nauseated and vomiting, then an oral route may not be effective. See Figure 10.7 for a list of common opioid medications ranging from use for moderate to severe pain.[23] When administering opioid medications, it is important to remember that these medications are controlled substances with special regulations regarding storage, auditing counts, and disposal or wasting of medication. See more information about controlled substances in the "Legal/Ethical" chapter.

Common Opioid Analgesics

Generic Name	Trade Name(s)	Route	Adult
codeine/acetaminophen	Tylenol #3	PO	30 mg/300 mg
fentanyl	Duragesic Sublimaze	Transdermal IM IV	12 mcg-100mcg/h 0.5-1 mcg/kg 0.5-1 mcg/kg
hydrocodone/ acetaminophen	Lortab Norco Vicodin	PO PO PO	5 mg/300mg or 325 mg 10 mg/320mg or 325 mg

---

23   Vallerand, A. and Sanoski, C. A. (2019). *Davis's Drug Guide for Nurses* (16th ed.). F.A. Davis Company.

hydromorphone	Dilaudid	PO	4-8 mg
		Rectal	3 mg
		SubQ, IM & IV	1.5 mg (may be increased)
morphine	Duramorph, MS Contin, Oramorph SR, & Roxanol-T	PO & Rectal	30 mg (may be increased)
		SubQ, IM, & IV	4-10 mg (may be increased)
oxycodone	Oxy IR, Oxycontin & Oxy-FAST	PO	5 mg-10 mg (may be increased)
oxycodone/acetaminophen	Percocet & Roxicet	PO	5 mg/325 mg

Figure 10.7 Table of Common Opioid Analgesics

A general rule of thumb when administering analgesics is to use the least invasive medication that is anticipated to treat the level of pain reported by the patient. The WHO ladder was originally developed for selection of analgesics for patients with cancer but illustrates the concept that pain control should be based on the level indicated by the patient. See Figure 10.8[24] for an image of the WHO ladder. For example, if a patient reports a pain level of "2," then it is appropriate to start at the lowest rung of the ladder and administer a non-opioid. However, it may be clinically indicated to start at "Level 3" on the WHO ladder for patients who present with severe, difficult pain.

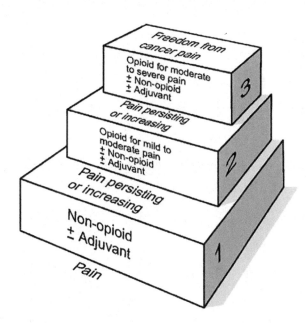

Figure 10.8 The WHO Pain Ladder. This diagram below shows the step–wise approach to cancer pain management recommended by the World Health Organization (WHO)

It is important to anticipate any common side effects and the expected outcome of the medication, as well as considerations regarding what to teach the patient and their family regarding the medications.

---

24   World Health Organization. *Cancer pain relief*. 2nd ed. Geneva: WHO; 1996.

My Notes

Evaluation

It is important to always evaluate the patient's response to the medication. With analgesic medications, the nurse should assess for decrease in pain 30 minutes after IV administration and 60 minutes after oral medication. If the patient's pain level is not acceptable, the nurse should investigate alternate treatment modalities. These modalities may include, but not limited to, aromatherapy, repositioning the patient, hot or cold treatments, and listening to music. As the nurse is the patient advocate, the healthcare provider may have to be informed if the patient's pain is not being controlled by analgesics. One of the adverse effects of opioid analgesics is respiratory depression. The nurse should evaluate the respiratory rate and pulse oximetry after administration of the medication. Other common side effects of opioid analgesic medications are constipation or nausea. The nurse may need to consider administering other medications that treat the side effects of analgesic medication.

10.5   ANALGESIC AND MUSCULOSKELETAL MEDICATIONS

As illustrated in the WHO ladder in Figure 10.8, analgesics used to treat pain are categorized as nonopioid, opioid, and adjuvant medications. Nonopioid medications include acetaminophen and nonsteroidal anti-inflammatory drugs (NSAIDs). There are several types of opioids, as listed previously in Figure 10.7. **Adjuvant analgesics** are defined as drugs with a primary indication other than pain that have analgesic properties in some painful conditions. This group includes numerous drugs in diverse classes such as gabapentin (an anticonvulsant), amitriptyline (a tricyclic antidepressant), or muscle relaxants.[25] Each of these classes will be discussed in more detail along with antigout medications and a brief overview of anesthetic medication.

Analgesic and Musculoskeletal Medication Classifications

Let's take a closer look at different classes of analgesics and musculoskeletal medications with specific administration considerations, therapeutic effects, adverse/side effects, and teaching needed for each class of medications. Analgesic and musculoskeletal medications are available in many different forms, such as oral tablets, oral liquids, injections, inhalation, and transdermal. Some products contain more than one medicine (for example, oxycodone and acetaminophen) to enhance pain relief.

---

25   Lussier, D., Huskey, A., and Portenoy, R. (2004). Adjuvant analgesics in cancer pain management. *Oncologist, 9*(5); 571–91. https://www.ncbi.nlm.nih.gov/pubmed/15477643.

10.6 NON-OPIOID ANALGESICS

Non-opioid analgesics include acetaminophen and nonsteroidal antiinflammatory drugs (NSAIDS).

Acetaminophen

Mechanism of Action

Acetaminophen inhibits the synthesis of prostaglandins that may serve as mediators of pain and fever primarily in the CNS.[26]

Indications for Use

Acetaminophen is used to treat mild pain and fever; however, it does not have anti-inflammatory properties.

Nursing Considerations Across the Life Span

Acetaminophen is safe for all ages and can be administered using various routes.

Geriatric populations should not exceed 3,000 mg in 24 hours, and chronic alcoholics should not exceed 2,000 mg in 24 hours due to the risk for hepatoxicity.

Adverse/Side Effects

Adverse effects include skin reddening, blisters, rash, and hepatotoxicity. Severe liver damage may occur if a patient:

- takes more than 4,000 mg of acetaminophen in 24 hours (3,200 mg for geriatric adults, 2,000 mg for chronic alcoholics)
- takes with other drugs containing acetaminophen
- consumes 3 or more alcoholic drinks every day while using this product.[27]

Some medications are combined with acetaminophen and are prescribed "as needed," so the nurse must calculate the cumulative dose of acetaminophen over the previous 24-hour period. For example, Percocet 5/325 contains a combination of oxycodone 5 mg and acetaminophen 325 mg and could be ordered 1-2 tablets every 4-6 hours as needed for pain. If 2 tablets are truly administered every 4 hours over a 24-hour period, this would add up to 3,900 mg of acetaminophen, which would exceed the recommended guidelines for a geriatric patient and could cause liver damage.

If overdose occurs, the antidote is acetylcysteine.

Patient Teaching and Education

Medications should be taken as directed and the dosing schedule should be adhered to appropriately. Patients should not take the medication for greater than 10 days. Additionally, patients should avoid taking alcohol while using these medications. If a rash occurs, this should be reported to the healthcare provider and the medication

---

26   Frandsen, G. and Pennington S. (2018). *Abrams' clinical drug: Rationales for nursing practice* (11th ed.). (pg.305, 310, 952–953, 959–960) Wolters Kluwer.

27   Vallerand, A., and Sanoski, C. A. (2019). *Davis's Drug Guide for Nurses* (16th ed.). F.A. Davis Company.

should be promptly stopped. Use of medications may interfere with blood glucose monitoring. If a fever lasts longer than three days or exceeds 39.5 C, this should be reported to the healthcare provider.[28]

Now let's take a closer look at the medication grid on acetaminophen in Table 10.6a.[29, 30] Medication grids are intended to assist students to learn key points about each medication. Because information about medication is constantly changing, nurses should always consult evidence-based resources to review current recommendations before administering specific medication. Basic information related to each class of medication is outlined below. Detailed information on a specific medication can be found for free at *Daily Med* at https://dailymed.nlm.nih.gov/dailymed/index.cfm. On the home page, enter the drug name in the search bar to read more about the medication. Prototype/generic medications listed in the grids below are also hyperlinked directly to a *Daily Med* page.

Table 10.6a: Acetaminophen Medication Grid

Class/ Subclass	Prototype-generic	Administration Considerations	Therapeutic Effects	Adverse/Side Effects
Nonopioid analgesic Antipyretic	acetaminophen	Can be given orally, rectally, and IV Assess pain prior to and after administration Administer with a full glass of water Maximum dose over 24-hour period: -4,000 mg for adults, -3,200 mg for geriatric patients -2,000 mg for patients with chronic alcoholism	Relief of mild pain and fever	Skin reddening Blisters Rash Hepatic failure (liver damage)

Critical Thinking Activity 10.6a

Your patient is admitted to the hospital with acute liver failure due to acetaminophen toxicity. Your patient reveals that they have had a cold for several days and have been taking over-the-counter cold medications and acetaminophen for a headache. They also mention that every night after work they drink a "few" beers.

What patient education about acetaminophen should be provided?

Note: Answers to the Critical Thinking activities can be found in the "Answer Key" sections at the end of the book.

---

28   uCentral from Unbound Medicine. https://www.unboundmedicine.com/ucentral.

29   Vallerand, A., and Sanoski, C. A. (2019). *Davis's Drug Guide for Nurses* (16th ed.). F.A. Davis Company.

30   Drugs.com [Internet]. *Aspirin*; © 2000–2019 [updated 1 December 28; cited 20 November 2019]. https://www.drugs.com/aspirin.html.

Nonsteroidal Antiinflammatories (NSAIDs)

Nonsteroidal antiinflammatories have an analgesic effect, as well as antipyretic and antiinflammatory actions. Some, such as aspirin, also have an antiplatelet effect. Aspirin and other NSAIDs relieve pain by inhibiting the biosynthesis of prostaglandin by different forms of the COX enzyme. COX2 inhibitors are selective and only inhibit the COX-2 enzyme. As a result of the inhibition of COX1 by an NSAID, there is decreased protection of the stomach lining and gastric irritation and bleeding may occur. This section will discuss the following NSAIDs: aspirin, ibuprofen, ketorolac, and celecoxib.[31]

Aspirin

Mechanism of Action

Aspirin produces analgesia and reduces inflammation and fever by inhibiting the production of prostaglandins. It also decreases platelet aggregation.

Indications for Use

Aspirin is used for the treatment of mild pain and fever. Once daily dosages are also used to reduce the risk of heart attack and stroke.

Nursing Considerations Across the Life Span

Aspirin is safe for adults and children older than 12 years of age.

Adverse/Side Effects

Adverse effects include GI upset, GI bleed, and tinnitus (ringing of the ears).

Allergy alert: Aspirin may cause a severe allergic reaction, which may include:

- hives
- facial swelling
- shock
- asthma (wheezing)

Stomach bleeding warning: This product contains an NSAID, which may cause severe stomach bleeding. The chance for bleeding is higher if a patient:

- takes a higher dose or takes it for a longer time than directed
- takes other drugs containing prescription or nonprescription NSAIDs (aspirin, ibuprofen, naproxen, or others)
- has had stomach ulcers or bleeding problems
- takes a blood thinning (anticoagulant) or steroid drug
- is age 60 or older

---

31 McCuiston, L., E., Vuljoin-DiMaggio, K., Winton, M., B., and Yeager, J. (2018) *Pharmacology: A patient centered nursing process approach.* (pp. 268–270, 324, 332) Elsevier.

■ has 3 or more alcoholic drinks every day while using this product

Aspirin is contraindicated if the patient has a bleeding disorder such as hemophilia or a recent history of bleeding in the stomach or intestine.

Patient Teaching and Education

Patients should avoid concurrent use of alcohol while taking medication to avoid gastric irritation. Additionally, they should report tinnitus, unusual bleeding, or fever lasting greater than 3 days to the healthcare provider.

Black Box Warning

Children or teenagers should not take aspirin to treat chickenpox or flu-like symptoms because of the risk of Reye's Syndrome. Reye's Syndrome primarily occurs in children in conjunction with a viral illness; it can cause symptoms such as persistent vomiting, confusion or loss of consciousness and requires immediate medical attention.

Now let's take a closer look at the medication grid on aspirin in Table 10.6.b.[32, 33, 34, 35]

Table 10.6b: Aspirin Medication Grid

Class/Subclass	Prototype-generic	Administration Considerations	Therapeutic Effects	Adverse/Side Effects
Nonopioid analgesic (NSAID) Antipyretic	aspirin	Give orally Assess pain prior to and after administration Children under 12 years: do not use unless directed by a provider Take with a full glass of water and sit upright for 15-30 minutes after administration Take with food if the patient reports that aspirin upsets their stomach Do not crush, chew, break, or open an enteric-coated or delayed-release pill; it should be swallowed whole The chewable tablet form must be chewed before swallowing Should be stopped 7 days prior to surgery due to the risk of postoperative bleeding	Treatment of mild pain and fever Reduces the risk of heart attack and stroke	GI upset GI bleeding Tinnitus

32   Frandsen, G. and Pennington S. (2018). *Abrams' clinical drug: Rationales for nursing practice* (11th ed.). (pg.305, 310, 952–953, 959–960) Wolters Kluwer.

33   Vallerand, A. and Sanoski, C. A. (2019). *Davis's Drug Guide for Nurse (*16th ed.). F.A. Davis Company.

34   Drugs.com [Internet]. *Aspirin*; © 2000–2019 [; updated 1 December 28; cited 20 November 2019]. https://www.drugs.com/aspirin.html.

35   Centers for Disease Control and Prevention. (2019, August 28). *Opioid overdose, CDC guideline for prescribing opioids for chronic pain.* https://www.cdc.gov/drugoverdose/prescribing/guideline.html.

Critical Thinking Activity 10.6b

A patient asks why aspirin is given to prevent a heart attack or stroke.

What is the nurse's response?

Note: Answers to the Critical Thinking activities can be found in the "Answer Key" sections at the end of the book.

Ibuprofen

Mechanism of Action

Ibuprofen inhibits prostaglandin synthesis.

Indications for Use

Ibuprofen is used to treat mild to moderate pain and fever, inflammatory disorders including rheumatoid arthritis and osteoarthritis, and pain associated with dysmenorrhea.

Nursing Considerations Across the Life Span

Ibuprofen is safe for infants 6 months or older. It is especially important not to use ibuprofen during the last 3 months of pregnancy unless directed to do so by a doctor because it may cause complications during delivery or in the unborn child.

Adverse/Side Effects

Adverse effects include headache, GI bleed, constipation, dyspepsia, nausea, vomiting, Steven-Johnson syndrome, and renal failure.

Allergy alert: Ibuprofen may cause a severe allergic reaction, especially in people allergic to aspirin. Symptoms may include:

- hives
- facial swelling
- asthma (wheezing)
- shock
- skin reddening
- rash
- blisters

Patient Teaching and Education

Patients should consume the medication with a full glass of water and remain upright for 30 minutes following medication administration. They should avoid the use of alcohol while taking this medication. Patients should be advised to not take the medication for longer than 10 days. If the patient notices rash, visual changes, tinnitus, weight gain, or influenza-like symptoms, these should be reported to the healthcare provider immediately.[36]

Stomach bleeding warning:

This product contains a nonsteroidal anti-inflammatory drug (NSAID), which may cause severe stomach bleeding. The chance for bleeding is higher if the patient:

- is age 60 or older
- has had stomach ulcers or bleeding problems
- takes a blood thinning (anticoagulant) or steroid drug
- takes other drugs containing prescription or nonprescription NSAIDs (aspirin, ibuprofen, naproxen, or others)
- has 3 or more alcoholic drinks every day while using this product
- takes more or for a longer time than directed

Heart attack and stroke warning:

All NSAIDs, except aspirin, increase the risk of heart attack, heart failure, and stroke. These can be fatal. The risk is higher if the patient takes more than is directed or takes it for longer than directed.

Black Box Warning

Ibuprofen is contraindicated for the treatment of perioperative pain after coronary artery bypass graft.

Now let's take a closer look at the medication grid on ibuprofen in Table 10.6c.[37, 38]

---

36   uCentral from Unbound Medicine. https://www.unboundmedicine.com/ucentral.

37   Frandsen, G. and Pennington S. (2018). *Abrams' clinical drug: Rationales for nursing practice* (11th ed.). (pg.305, 310, 952–953, 959–960) Wolters Kluwer.

38   Vallerand, A. and Sanoski, C. A. (2019). *Davis's Drug Guide for Nurse* (16th ed.). F.A. Davis Company.

My Notes

Table 10.6c: Ibuprofen Medication Grid				
Class/Subclass	**Prototype-generic**	**Administration Considerations**	**Therapeutic Effects**	**Adverse/Side Effects**
Nonopioid analgesic NSAID Antipyretic	ibuprofen	Given parenterally and orally Assess pain prior to and after administration May take with food or milk if stomach upset occurs Stay well hydrated to prevent renal failure Assess patient for signs of GI bleed Assess for skin rash Monitor BUN, serum creatinine, CBC, and liver function test Do not administer to patients who are allergic to aspirin or other NSAIDs	To relieve mild pain and to reduce fever	Headache GI bleed Constipation Dyspepsia Nausea Vomiting Steven-Johnson syndrome Renal failure

Critical Thinking Activity 10.6c

A patient who is a chronic alcoholic asks if it is okay to take ibuprofen for knee pain.

What is the nurse's best response?

Note: Answers to the Critical Thinking activities can be found in the "Answer Key" sections at the end of the book.

Ketorolac

Ketorolac is an NSAID that is commonly used to treat "breakthrough" pain that occurs during the treatment of severe acute pain being treated with opioids.

Mechanism of Action

Ketorolac inhibits prostaglandin synthesis.

Indications for Use

Ketorolac is indicated for the short-term (up to 5 days in adults) management of moderate to severe acute pain that requires analgesia at the opioid level.

Nursing Considerations Across the Life Span

Ketorolac is safe for adults. This dose should be reduced for patients ages 65 and over.

Adverse/Side Effects

Adverse effects include drowsiness, headache, GI bleed, abnormal taste, dyspepsia, nausea, Steven-Johnson syndrome, edema, and renal failure.

Patient Teaching and Education

The use of ketorolac may cause dizziness of drowsiness. Patients should also avoid alcohol or other aspirin-containing products unless directed by their healthcare provider. If the patient notices rash, visual changes, tinnitus, weight gain, or influenza-like symptoms, these should be reported to the healthcare provider immediately.[39]

Gastrointestinal Risk

Ketorolac tromethamine (IV form) can cause peptic ulcers, gastrointestinal bleeding, and/or perforation of the stomach or intestines, which can be fatal. These events can occur at any time during use and without warning symptoms. Therefore, ketorolac tromethamine is contraindicated in patients with active peptic ulcer disease, in patients with recent gastrointestinal bleeding or perforation, and in patients with a history of peptic ulcer disease or gastrointestinal bleeding. Elderly patients are at greater risk for serious gastrointestinal events.

Cardiovascular Thrombotic Events

Nonsteroidal anti-inflammatory drugs (NSAIDs) cause an increased risk of serious cardiovascular thrombotic events, including myocardial infarction and stroke, which can be fatal. This risk may occur early in treatment and may increase with duration of use.

Ketorolac tromethamine is contraindicated for patients who have recently received coronary artery bypass graft (CABG) surgery.

Renal Risk

Ketorolac tromethamine is contraindicated in patients with advanced renal impairment and in patients at risk for renal failure due to volume depletion.

Risk of Bleeding

Ketorolac tromethamine inhibits platelet function and is, therefore, contraindicated in patients with suspected or confirmed cerebrovascular bleeding, hemorrhagic diathesis, incomplete hemostasis, and a high risk of bleeding. Ketorolac tromethamine is contraindicated as a prophylactic analgesic before any major surgery.

Hypersensitivity Reactions

Hypersensitivity reactions ranging from bronchospasm to anaphylactic shock have occurred and appropriate counteractive measures must be available when administering the first dose of ketorolac. Ketorolac tromethamine

---

39   uCentral from Unbound Medicine. https://www.unboundmedicine.com/ucentral.

My Notes

is contraindicated in patients with previously demonstrated hypersensitivity to ketorolac tromethamine or who have had allergic manifestations to aspirin or other nonsteroidal anti-inflammatory drugs (NSAIDs).

Now let's take a closer look at the medication grid on ketorolac in Table 10.6d.[40, 41]

Table 10.6d: Ketorolac Medication Grid

Class/Subclass	Prototype-generic	Administration Considerations	Therapeutic Effects	Adverse/Side Effects
Nonopioid analgesic NSAID	ketorolac	Given orally, parenterally and as an ophthalmic solution Assess pain prior to and after administration Therapy should always be given initially by the IM or IV route; then use the oral route as a continuation of parenteral therapy Stay well hydrated to prevent renal failure Assess patient for signs of GI bleed Assess for skin rash Monitor BUN, serum creatinine, CBC, and liver function tests Do not administer before any major surgery Do not administer to patients who are allergic to aspirin or other NSAIDs	To relieve moderate pain short term (not to exceed 5 days)	Drowsiness Headache GI bleed Abnormal taste Dyspepsia Nausea Steven-Johnson syndrome Edema Renal failure

Critical Thinking Activity 10.6d

Ketorolac IV was administered to a patient for severe pain (rated as "8") due to a back injury.

When should the effectiveness of the medication be evaluated?

Note: Answers to the Critical Thinking activities can be found in the "Answer Key" sections at the end of the book.

Celecoxib

Celecoxib is a COX-2 inhibitor.

Mechanism of Action

Celecoxib specifically inhibits the enzyme COX-2 that is required for the synthesis of prostaglandins.

---

40   Vallerand, A. and Sanoski, C. A. (2019). *Davis's Drug Guide for Nurse* (16th ed.). F.A. Davis Company.

41   This work is a derivative of by *Daily Med* and the U.S. National Library of Medicine in the public domain.

Indications for Use

Celecoxib is used to treat the pain associated with osteoarthritis, rheumatoid arthritis (including juvenile), and ankylosing spondylitis. It also relieves the pain associated with dysmenorrhea.

Nursing Considerations Across the Life Span

Celecoxib is safe for children 2 years or older. Dosage adjustment is required for patients with hepatic impairment (see Black Box Warning).

Adverse/Side Effects

Adverse effects include hypertension, peripheral edema, increased liver enzymes, abdominal pain, dyspepsia, gastroesophageal reflux disease, vomiting, and diarrhea.

There are Black Box Warnings for increased risk of cardiovascular (CV) events and gastrointestinal bleeding, ulceration, and perforation. See more information about each condition below.

Patient Teaching and Education

Patients should take medication as directed and use the lowest effective dose for the shortest period of time. If signs of GI toxicity occur, these should be reported immediately to the healthcare provider.[42]

Cardiovascular Thrombotic Events

Nonsteroidal anti-inflammatory drugs (NSAIDs) cause an increased risk of serious cardiovascular thrombotic events, including myocardial infarction and stroke, which can be fatal. This risk may occur early in the treatment and may increase with duration of use. Celecoxib capsules are contraindicated in patients who have recently received coronary artery bypass graft (CABG) surgery.

Gastrointestinal Bleeding, Ulceration, and Perforation

NSAIDs cause an increased risk of serious gastrointestinal (GI) adverse events including bleeding, ulceration, and perforation of the stomach or intestines, which can be fatal. These events can occur at any time during use and without warning symptoms. Elderly patients and patients with a prior history of peptic ulcer disease and/or GI bleeding are at greater risk for serious (GI) events.

---

42   uCentral from Unbound Medicine. https://www.unboundmedicine.com/ucentral.

Now let's take a closer look at the medication grid on celecoxib in Table 10.6e.[43, 44]

Table 10.6e: Celecoxib Medication Grid

Class/ Subclass	Prototype-generic	Administration Considerations	Therapeutic Effects	Adverse/Side Effects
NSAIDs COX-2 inhibitor	celecoxib	May be given with or without food May sprinkle capsules on applesauce and ingest immediately with water Monitor patients for signs and symptoms of Steven-Johnson syndrome Monitor for signs and symptoms of GI bleed, hypertension, and heart failure Monitor liver enzymes	To decrease pain and inflammation caused by arthritis or spondylitis	Hypertension Peripheral edema Increased liver enzymes Abdominal pain, dyspepsia, gastroesophageal reflux disease, vomiting, and diarrhea Cardiovascular thrombotic events GI bleeding, ulceration and perforation Hepatotoxicity Hypertension Heart failure and edema Renal toxicity and hyperkalemia Anaphylactic reactions Serious skin reactions Hematologic toxicity

Critical Thinking Activity 10.6e

A patient has been prescribed celecoxib for their arthritic pain.

What patient teaching does the nurse plan to provide?

Note: Answers to the Critical Thinking activities can be found in the "Answer Key" sections at the end of the book.

43   Vallerand, A. and Sanoski, C. A. (2019). *Davis's Drug Guide for Nurse (*16th ed.). F.A. Davis Company.

44   This work is a derivative of by *Daily Med* and the U.S. National Library of Medicine in the public domain.

10.7 OPIOID ANALGESICS AND ANTAGONISTS

Opioid analgesics are prescribed for moderate and severe pain. See Figure 10.8 in the "Nursing Process" section for a list of common opioid medications used to treat moderation pain to severe pain. As discussed in that section, morphine is at the top of the WHO ladder and is used to treat severe pain. It is also commonly used to treat cancer pain and for pain at end of life because there is no "ceiling effect," meaning the higher the dose, the higher the level of analgesia. Morphine is also commonly used in **patient controlled analgesia (PCA)**; other medications administered via PCA include hydromorphone or fentanyl. To receive the opioid using a PCA device, the patient pushes a button, which releases a specific dose but also has a lockout mechanism to prevent an overdose.[45]

Morphine

Morphine is an example of an opioid used to treat moderate to severe pain.

Mechanism of Action

Morphine binds to opioid receptors in the CNS and alters the perception of and response to painful stimuli while producing generalized CNS depression.

Indications for Use

Morphine is indicated for the relief of moderate to severe acute and chronic pain and for pulmonary edema.

Nursing Considerations Across the Life Span

Morphine is safe for all ages. Use cautiously with patients with liver and renal impairment.

Adverse/Side Effects

Adverse effects include respiratory depression, hypotension, light-headedness, dizziness, sedation, constipation, nausea, vomiting, and sweating.

Patient Teaching and Education

Patients should be advised regarding the risks associated with opioid analgesic use. Please see the outlined "Special Considerations" for usage below.[46]

---

45   McCuistion, L., Vuljoin-DiMaggio, K., Winton, M, and Yeager, J. (2018). *Pharmacology: A patient-centered nursing process approach.* pp. 268–270, 324, 332. Elsevier.

46   uCentral from Unbound Medicine. https://www.unboundmedicine.com/ucentral.

Black Box Warning

The risk of serious adverse reactions, including slowed or difficulty breathing and death, have been reported with the combined effects of morphine with other CNS depressants. Naloxone is used to reverse opioid overdose. There is also a risk of drug abuse and dependence with morphine.

Special Considerations

Respiratory Depression

Respiratory depression is the primary risk of morphine sulfate. Respiratory depression occurs more frequently in elderly or debilitated patients and in those suffering from conditions accompanied by hypoxia, hypercapnia, or upper airway obstruction, for whom even moderate therapeutic doses may significantly decrease pulmonary ventilation.

Use morphine with extreme caution in patients with chronic obstructive pulmonary disease or cor pulmonale and in patients having a substantially decreased respiratory reserve, hypoxia, hypercapnia, or pre-existing respiratory depression. In such patients, even usual therapeutic doses of morphine sulfate may increase airway resistance and decrease respiratory drive to the point of apnea. Consider alternative non-opioid analgesics, and use morphine sulfate only under careful medical supervision at the lowest effective dose in such patients.

Misuse, Abuse, and Diversion of Opioids

Morphine sulfate is an opioid agonist and a Schedule II controlled substance. Such drugs are sought by drug abusers and people with addiction disorders. Diversion of Schedule II products is an act subject to criminal penalty.

Morphine can be abused in a manner similar to other opioid agonists, legal or illicit. This should be considered when prescribing or dispensing morphine sulfate in situations where there is increased risk of misuse, abuse, or diversion. Morphine may be abused by crushing, chewing, snorting, or injecting the product. These practices pose a significant risk to the abuser that could result in overdose and death.

Interactions with Alcohol and Drugs of Abuse

Morphine has addictive effects when used in conjunction with alcohol, other opioids, or illicit drugs that cause central nervous system depression because respiratory depression, hypotension, profound sedation, coma, or death may result.

Use In Head Injury and Increased Intracranial Pressure

In the presence of head injury, intracranial lesions, or a preexisting increase in intracranial pressure, the possible respiratory depressant effects of morphine and its potential to elevate cerebrospinal fluid pressure may be markedly exaggerated. Furthermore, morphine can produce effects on pupillary response and consciousness, which may obscure neurologic signs of increased intracranial pressure in patients with head injuries.

Hypotensive Effect

Morphine may cause severe hypotension in individuals unable to maintain blood pressure who have already been compromised by a depleted blood volume or drug administration of phenothiazines or general anesthetics.

Administer morphine sulfate with caution to patients in circulatory shock, as vasodilation produced by the drug may further reduce cardiac output and blood pressure.

Gastrointestinal Effects

Do not administer morphine to patients with gastrointestinal obstruction, especially paralytic ileus because morphine diminishes propulsive peristaltic waves in the gastrointestinal tract and may prolong the obstruction.

The administration of morphine sulfate may obscure the diagnosis or clinical course in patients with an acute abdominal condition.

Use in Pancreatic/Biliary Tract Disease

Use morphine with caution in patients with biliary tract disease, including acute pancreatitis, as morphine sulfate may cause spasming and diminished biliary and pancreatic secretions.

Special Risk Groups

Use morphine with caution and in reduced dosages in patients with severe renal or hepatic impairment, Addison's disease, hypothyroidism, prostatic hypertrophy, or urethral stricture, and in elderly or debilitated patients. Exercise caution in the administration of morphine sulfate to patients with CNS depression, toxic psychosis, acute alcoholism, and delirium tremens.

All opioids may aggravate convulsions in patients with convulsive disorders, and all opioids may induce or aggravate seizures.

Driving and Operating Machinery

Caution patients that morphine sulfate could impair the mental and/or physical abilities needed to perform potentially hazardous activities such as driving a car or operating machinery.

Caution patients about the potential combined effects of morphine sulfate with other CNS depressants, including other opioids, phenothiazines, sedative/hypnotics, and alcohol.

Now let's take a closer look at the medication grid on morphine in Table 10.7a.[47, 48, 49]

Table 10.7a: Morphine Medication Grid

Class/Subclass	Prototype-generic	Administration Considerations	Therapeutic Effects	Adverse/Side Effects
Opioid analgesic	morphine	Given parenterally and orally Assess pain prior to and after administration Monitor respiratory status Monitor blood pressure Assess pediatric and geriatric patients frequently Assess bowel function Use cautiously with antidepressants and other CNS depressants Naloxone is used to reverse opioid overdose	Relieves moderate to severe pain	Respiratory depression Confusion Hypotension Light-headedness Dizziness Sedation Constipation Nausea and vomiting Sweating

Critical Thinking Activity 10.7a

Oral morphine was administered to a patient for rib pain (rated as "6") from metastatic lung cancer.

When should the effectiveness of the medication be evaluated?

Note: Answers to the Critical Thinking activities can be found in the "Answer Key" sections at the end of the book.

Concerns Related to Opioid Use

CDC Guidelines for Prescribing Opioids for Chronic Pain

Improving the prescription of opioids through clinical practice guidelines can ensure patients have access to safer, effective pain treatment while also reducing the number of people who misuse or overdose from these drugs.

The CDC developed and published the *CDC Guideline for Prescribing Opioids for Chronic Pain* to provide recommendations for the prescribing of opioid pain medication for patients 18 and older in primary care settings. Recommendations focus on the use of opioids in treating chronic pain (pain lasting longer than 3 months or past the time of normal tissue healing) outside of active cancer treatment, palliative care, and end-of-life care.[50]

---

47   Frandsen, G., Pennington, S. (2018). *Abrams' clinical drug: Rationales for nursing practice (11th ed.).* (pg. 305, 310, 952–953, 959–960). Wolters Kluwer.

48   Vallerand, A. and Sanoski, C. A. (2019). *Davis's Drug Guide for Nurses,* (16th ed.). F.A. Davis Company.

49   This work is a derivative of *Daily Med* by U.S. National Library of Medicine in the public domain.

50   Centers for Disease Control and Prevention. (2019, August 28). *Opioid overdose, CDC guideline for prescribing opioids for chronic pain.* https://www.cdc.gov/drugoverdose/prescribing/guideline.html.

The Need

Improving the way opioids are prescribed through clinical practice guidelines can ensure patients have access to safer, more effective chronic pain treatment while reducing the risk of opioid use disorder, overdose, and death.

- More than 11.5 million Americans aged 12 or older reported misusing prescription opioids in 2016.

- An estimated 11% of adults experience daily pain.

- Millions of Americans are treated with prescription opioids for chronic pain.

- Primary care providers are concerned about patient addiction and report insufficient training in prescribing opioids.

Guideline Overview

The *CDC Guideline* addresses patient-centered clinical practices including conducting thorough assessments, considering all possible treatments, closely monitoring risks, and safely discontinuing opioids. The three main focus areas in the guideline include:

1. Determining when to initiate or continue opioids for chronic pain

   - Selection of non-pharmacologic therapy, nonopioid pharmacologic therapy, opioid therapy
   - Establishment of treatment goals
   - Discussion of risks and benefits of therapy with patients

2. Opioid selection, dosage, duration, follow-up, and discontinuation

   - Selection of immediate-release or extended-release and long-acting opioids

3. Dosage considerations

3. Duration of treatment

4. Considerations for follow-up and discontinuation of opioid therapy

   - Assessing risk and addressing harms of opioid use
   - Evaluation of risk factors for opioid-related harms and ways to mitigate patient risk
   - Review of prescription drug monitoring program (PDMP) data
   - Use of urine drug testing
   - Considerations for co-prescribing benzodiazepines
   - Arrangement of treatment for opioid use disorder[51]

Understanding the Epidemic

Drug overdose deaths continue to increase in the United States. From 1999 to 2017, more than 700,000 people have died from a drug overdose. Around 68% of the more than 70,200 drug overdose deaths in 2017 involved an opioid. In 2017, the number of overdose deaths involving opioids (including prescription opioids and illegal

---

51   Centers for Disease Control and Prevention. (2019, August 28). *Opioid overdose, CDC guideline for prescribing opioids for chronic pain.* https://www.cdc.gov/drugoverdose/prescribing/guideline.html.

opioids like heroin and illicitly manufactured fentanyl) was 6 times higher than in 1999. On average, 130 Americans die every day from an opioid overdose.[52]

From 1999-2017, almost 400,000 people died from an overdose involving any opioid, including prescription and illicit opioids. This rise in opioid overdose deaths can be outlined in three distinct waves. See Figure 10.9 for a graphic representation of the waves of opioid deaths.[53]

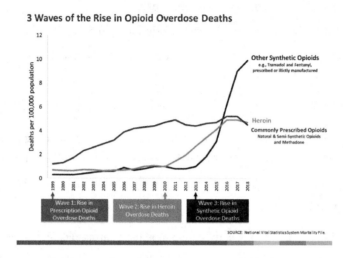

Figure 10.9 Three Waves of Opioid Overdose Deaths

The first wave began with increased prescribing of opioids in the 1990s, with overdose deaths involving prescription opioids (natural and semi-synthetic opioids and methadone). The second wave began in 2010 with rapid increases in overdose deaths involving heroin. The third wave began in 2013, with significant increases in overdose deaths involving synthetic opioids – particularly those involving illicitly-manufactured fentanyl.[54]

Combating the Opioid Overdose Epidemic

The CDC is committed to fighting the opioid overdose epidemic and supporting states and communities as they continue work to identify outbreaks, collect data, respond to overdoses, and provide care to those in their communities. CDC's Prevention for States and Data-Driven Prevention Initiative programs aims center around the enhancement of PDMPs within clinical and public health settings, insurer and community interventions, evaluation of state-level policies, and other innovative strategies that states can employ.

CDC's Enhanced State Opioid Overdose Surveillance program aims to support and build the capacity of states to monitor the epidemic by improving the timeliness and quality of surveillance data focusing on both fatal and nonfatal opioid overdose.[55]

---

52   Centers for Disease Control and Prevention. (2018, December 19). *Opioid Overdose, Understanding the Epidemic.* https://www.cdc.gov/drugoverdose/epidemic/index.html.

53   "3 Waves of the Rise of Opioid Overdose Deaths" by National Vital Statics System, CDC is licensed under CC0.

54   Centers for Disease Control and Prevention. (2018, December 19). *Opioid Overdose, Understanding the Epidemic.* https://www.cdc.gov/drugoverdose/epidemic/index.html.

55   Centers for Disease Control and Prevention. (2018, December 19). *Opioid Overdose, Understanding the Epidemic.* https://www.cdc.gov/drugoverdose/epidemic/index.html.

IV Drug Diversion and Impaired Health Care Workers

In every organization, drug diversion is a potential threat to patient safety. Risks to patients include inadequate pain relief and exposure to infectious diseases from contaminated needles and drugs, compounded by potentially unsafe care due to the health care worker's impaired performance. Furthermore, diversion may cause undue suffering to patients who don't receive analgesic relief, can be costly to an organization by damaging its reputation, and may lead to major civil and criminal monetary penalties[56] More information about surveillance programs, drug diversion, and impaired health workers is included in the "Legal/Ethical" chapter.

Download the PDF to read the full article by the Joint Commission.

Naloxone (Narcan)

Mechanism of Action

Naloxone reverses analgesia and the CNS and respiratory depression caused by opioid agonists. It competes with opioid receptor sites in the brain and, thereby, prevents binding with receptors or displaces opioids already occupying receptor sites.

Indications for Use

Naloxone is indicated for the complete or partial reversal of opioid depression, including respiratory depression induced by natural and synthetic opioids.

Nursing Considerations Across the Life Span

Naloxone is safe for all ages.

Adverse/Side Effects

Adverse effects include tremors, drowsiness, sweating, decreased respirations, hypertension, nausea, and vomiting.

Patient Teaching and Education

Patients should be advised regarding the risks associated with opioid analgesic use and the need for opioid antagonists. Please see the outlined "Special Considerations" for usage below.[57]

Special Considerations

Postoperative

The following adverse events have been associated with the use of naloxone hydrochloride injection in postoperative patients: hypotension, hypertension, ventricular tachycardia and fibrillation, dyspnea, pulmonary edema, and cardiac arrest. Death, coma, and encephalopathy have been reported as results of these events. Excessive doses of naloxone in postoperative patients may result in significant reversal of analgesia and may cause agitation.

---

56   The Joint Commission, Division of Healthcare Improvement. (2019). Drug diversion and impaired health care workers. *Quick Safety* (48).

57   uCentral from Unbound Medicine. https://www.unboundmedicine.com/ucentral.

Opioid Depression

Abrupt reversal of opioid depression may result in nausea, vomiting, sweating, tachycardia, increased blood pressure, tremulousness, seizures, ventricular tachycardia and fibrillation, pulmonary edema, and cardiac arrest, which may result in death.

Opioid Dependence

Abrupt reversal of opioid effects in persons who are physically dependent on opioids may precipitate an acute withdrawal syndrome, which may include, but not limited to, the following signs and symptoms: body aches, fever, sweating, runny nose, sneezing, piloerection, yawning, weakness, shivering or trembling, nervousness, restlessness or irritability, diarrhea, nausea or vomiting, abdominal cramps, increased blood pressure, and tachycardia. In the neonate, opioid withdrawal may also include convulsions, excessive crying, and hyperactive reflexes.

Now let's take a closer look at the medication grid on naloxone in Table 10.7b.[58, 59]

Table 10.7b: Naloxone Medication Grid

Class/ Subclass	Prototype- generic	Administration Considerations	Therapeutic Effects	Adverse/Side Effects
Opioid antagonist	naloxone	Given parenterally and inhaled Assess for reversal of opioid effect Assess for hypertension Assess for return of pain Naloxone has a shorter duration of action than opioids, and repeated doses are usually necessary	Blocks the effects of opioid CNS and respiratory depression	Agitation Tremors Drowsiness Sweating Decreased respirations Hypertension Nausea and vomiting

Critical Thinking Activity 10.7b

A post-operative patient just received naloxone for respiratory depression.

When should the patient's respiratory status be reassessed?

Note: Answers to the Critical Thinking activities can be found in the "Answer Key" sections at the end of the book.

---

58   Frandsen, G., Pennington, S. (2018). *Abrams' clinical drug: Rationales for nursing practice (11th ed.).* (pg. 305, 310, 952–953, 959–960). Wolters Kluwer.

59   This work is a derivative of *Daily Med* by U.S. National Library of Medicine in the public domain.

10.8 ADJUVANT ANALGESICS

Medications used as adjuvant analgesics have been developed for other purposes but were later found to be effective to treat pain. Examples of adjuvant medications include gapapentin (an anticonvulsant) and amitriptyline (a tricyclic antidepressant). Additional information about these specific medications can be found in the "Central Nervous System" chapter. Muscle relaxants are also considered an adjuvant analgesic and are used for various musculoskeletal disorders such as multiple sclerosis. Three different types of muscle relaxants will be discussed below: baclofen, cyclobenzaprine, and tizanidine.

Baclofen

Mechanism of Action

Baclofen inhibits reflexes at the spinal level.

Indications for Use

Baclofen is used to treat muscle symptoms, such as spasm, pain, and stiffness, caused by multiple sclerosis, spinal cord injuries, or other spinal cord disorders.

Nursing Considerations Across the Life Span

Baclofen is safe for patients 12 years and older.

Adverse/Side Effects

Adverse effects include drowsiness, dizziness or lightheadedness, confusion, nausea, constipation, and muscle weakness.

Abrupt Drug Withdrawal: Hallucinations and seizures have occurred on abrupt withdrawal of baclofen. Therefore, except for serious adverse reactions, the dose should be reduced slowly when the drug is discontinued.

Impaired Renal Function: Because baclofen is primarily excreted unchanged through the kidneys, it should be given with caution, and it may be necessary to reduce the dosage.

Signs and symptoms of overdose include vomiting, muscular hypotonia, drowsiness, accommodation disorders of the eye, coma, respiratory depression, and seizures.

Patient Teaching and Education

The medication should be taken as directed and abrupt withdrawal of the medication should be avoided. It may cause dizziness or drowsiness. Patients should be advised to change positions slowly because of the potential orthostatic changes that may occur. Additionally, patients should avoid concurrent use with alcohol or other CNS depressants.[60]

Now let's take a closer look at the medication grid on baclofen in Table 10.8a.[61, 62]

---

60   uCentral from Unbound Medicine. https://www.unboundmedicine.com/ucentral.

61   Vallerand, A., Sanoski, C. A. (2019). *Davis's Drug Guide for Nurses* (16th ed.). F.A. Davis Company.

62   This work is a derivative of *Daily Med* by U.S. National Library of Medicine in the public domain.

Table 10.8a: Baclofen Medication Grid

Class/Subclass	Prototype-generic	Administration Considerations	Therapeutic Effects	Adverse/Side Effects
Skeletal muscle relaxant and anti-spasticity agent	baclofen	Given parantally and orally Administer orally with milk or food to minimize gastric upset Assess for muscle spasticity before and during therapy Observe patient for drowsiness For intrathecal administration monitor patient closely during test dose and titration and have resuscitative equipment available	To relieve muscle spasms and spasticity	Drowsiness Confusion Dizziness or light-headedness Nausea Constipation Muscle weakness

Critical Thinking Activity 10.8a

A patient just started taking baclofen for muscle spasticity due to multiple sclerosis.

What teaching should the nurse provide?

Note: Answers to the Critical Thinking activities can be found in the "Answer Key" sections at the end of the book.

Cyclobenzaprine

Mechanism of Action

Cyclobenzaprine reduces tonic somatic muscle activity at the level of the brainstem. It is structurally similar to tricyclic antidepressants.

Indications for Use

Cyclobenzaprine is used to treat acute muscle spasms.

Nursing Considerations Across the Life Span

Cyclobenzaprine is safe for patients 15 years and older. Use cautiously with geriatric patients, patients with hepatic impairment, and those who take antidepressants and other CNS depressants.

In the elderly, the frequency and severity of adverse events associated with the use of cyclobenzaprine, with or without concomitant medications, are increased. In elderly patients, cyclobenzaprine should be initiated with a 5 mg dose and titrated slowly upward.

Adverse/Side Effects

Adverse effects include dizziness, drowsiness, dry mouth, urinary retention, serotonin syndrome with antidepressant use, or increased sedation with other CNS depressants.

Patient Teaching and Education

The medication should be taken as directed. It may cause dizziness or drowsiness. Patients should be advised to change positions slowly because of the potential orthostatic changes that may occur. Additionally, patients should avoid concurrent use with alcohol or other CNS depressants. Patients should be aware that constipation may occur as a side effect of medication therapy and increased fluid intake may assist in preventing complications.[63]

Serotonin Syndrome

The development of a potentially life-threatening serotonin syndrome has been reported with cyclobenzaprine hydrochloride when used in combination with other drugs, such as selective serotonin reuptake inhibitors (SSRIs), serotonin norepinephrine reuptake inhibitors (SNRIs), tricyclic antidepressants (TCAs), tramadol, bupropion, meperidine, verapamil, or MAO inhibitors (MAOIs). The concomitant use of cyclobenzaprine hydrochloride with MAO inhibitors is contraindicated.

Serotonin syndrome symptoms may include mental status changes (e.g., confusion, agitation, hallucinations), autonomic instability (e.g., diaphoresis, tachycardia, labile blood pressure, hyperthermia), neuromuscular abnormalities (e.g., tremor, ataxia, hyperreflexia, clonus, muscle rigidity), and/ or gastrointestinal symptoms (e.g., nausea, vomiting, diarrhea). Treatment with cyclobenzaprine hydrochloride and any concomitant serotonergic agents should be discontinued immediately if the above reactions occur, and supportive symptomatic treatment should be initiated. If concomitant treatment with cyclobenzaprine hydrochloride and other serotonergic drugs is clinically warranted, careful observation is advised, particularly during treatment initiation or dose increases.

General

Because of its atropine-like action, cyclobenzaprine hydrochloride should be used with caution in patients with a history of urinary retention, angle-closure glaucoma, increased intraocular pressure, and in those taking anticholinergic medication.

---

63   uCentral from Unbound Medicine. https://www.unboundmedicine.com/ucentral.

Impaired Hepatic Function

The plasma concentration of cyclobenzaprine is increased in patients with hepatic impairment.

Cyclobenzaprine, especially when used with alcohol or other CNS depressants, may impair mental and/or physical abilities required for performance of hazardous tasks, such as operating machinery or driving a motor vehicle.

Now let's take a closer look at the medication grid on cyclobenzaprine in Table 10.8b.[64, 65]

Table 10.8b: Cyclobenzaprine Medication Grid

Class/Subclass	Prototype-generic	Administration Considerations	Therapeutic Effects	Adverse/Side Effects
Skeletal muscle relaxant	cyclobenzaprine	May be administered with meals to minimize GI upset Assess patient for pain and muscle stiffness Use cautiously with antidepressants and other CNS depressants	Reduction of muscle spasms	Dizziness Drowsiness Dry mouth Urinary retention Serotonin syndrome

Critical Thinking Activity 10.8b

A patient asks if they can drive their car while taking cyclobenzaprine.

What is the nurse's best response?

Note: Answers to the Critical Thinking activities can be found in the "Answer Key" sections at the end of the book.

Tizanidine

Mechanism of Action

Tizanidine acts as an agonist at central alpha-adrenergic receptor sites. It reduces spasticity by increasing presynaptic inhibition of motor neurons.

64   Vallerand, A., Sanoski, C. A. (2019). *Davis's Drug Guide for Nurses* (16th ed.). F.A. Davis Company.

65   This work is a derivative of *Daily Med* by U.S. National Library of Medicine in the public domain.

Indications for Use

Tizanidine is used to treat increased muscle tone, spasms, and spasticity.

Nursing Considerations Across the Life Span

Tizanidine is safe for adults. Dosage adjustment may be required for the geriatric population.

Adverse/Side Effects

Adverse effects include somnolence, dry mouth, hypotension, bradycardia, dizziness, fatigue, weakness or asthenia, hallucinations, liver function test abnormality, and hepatotoxicity.

Patient Teaching and Education

The medication should be taken as directed. It may cause dizziness or drowsiness. Patients should be advised to change positions slowly because of the potential orthostatic changes that may occur. Additionally, patients should avoid concurrent use with alcohol or other CNS depressants.[66]

Now let's take a closer look at the medication grid on tizanidine in Table 10.8c.[67,68,69]

Table 10.8c: Tizanidine Medication Grid				
Class/Subclass	**Prototype-generic**	**Administration Considerations**	**Therapeutic Effects**	**Adverse/Side Effects**
Antispasticity	tizanidine	Given orally May be given with or without food Assess muscle spasticity before and during therapy Assess blood pressure and pulse Monitor for sedation Assess liver function	Reduction of muscle spasms and spasticity	Somnolence Dry mouth Hypotension Bradycardia Dizziness Fatigue Weakness or asthenia Hallucinations Liver function test abnormality and hepatotoxicity

66   uCentral from Unbound Medicine. https://www.unboundmedicine.com/ucentral.

67   Frandsen, G., and Pennington, S. (2018). *Abrams' clinical drug: Rationales for nursing practice* (11th ed.). pg. 305, 310, 952–953, 959–960. Wolters Kluwer.

68   Vallerand, A., Sanoski, C. A. (2019). *Davis's Drug Guide for Nurses* (16th ed.). F.A. Davis Company.

69   This work is a derivative of *Daily Med* by U.S. National Library of Medicine in the public domain.

Critical Thinking Activity 10.8c

A patient asks, "Why should I not drink alcohol with tizanidine?"

What is the nurse's best response?

Note: Answers to the Critical Thinking activities can be found in the "Answer Key" sections at the end of the book.

10.9 ANTIGOUT

Antigout medications are used to treat gout, a musculoskeletal disorder. Some antigout medications, such as colchicine, are classified as anti-inflammatory medication. Allopurinol is commonly used to prevent gout from recurring.

Allopurinol

Mechanism of Action

Allopurinol blocks the production of uric acid by inhibiting the action of xanthine oxidase.[70]

Indications for Use

Allopurinol is used for the prevention and treatment of gouty arthritis and nephropathy and for the treatment of secondary hyperuricemia.

Nursing Considerations Across the Life Span

Allopurinol is safe for all ages. For patients with renal impairment, the dose will be reduced.

Adverse/Side Effects

Adverse effects include hypotension, flushing, hypertension, drowsiness, nausea and vomiting, diarrhea, hepatitis, renal failure, or a drug rash with eosinophilia and systemic symptoms (DRESS) syndrome or drug hypersensitivity syndrome.[71]

Patient Teaching and Education

The medication should be taken as directed. An alkaline diet may be ordered for the patient, and they may be advised to increase fluid intake to prevent kidney stone formation. The medication may cause dizziness or drowsiness. Patients who consume large amounts of alcohol may increase uric acid concentrations and decrease the effectiveness of the medication. If patients develop a rash or blood in the urine, this should be reported promptly to the healthcare provider.[72]

Now let's take a closer look at the medication grid on allopurinol in Table 10.9.[73,74,75]

---

70   Vallerand, A., and Sanoski, C. A. (2019). *Davis's Drug Guide for Nurses* (16th ed.). F.A. Davis Company.

71   Cleveland Clinic. (2017, January 26). *Acute v. chronic pain.* https://my.clevelandclinic.org/health/articles/12051-acute-vs-chronic-pain.

72   uCentral from Unbound Medicine. https://www.unboundmedicine.com/ucentral.

73   Frandsen, G., and Pennington, S. (2018). *Abrams' clinical drug: Rationales for nursing practice* (11th ed.). pg. 305, 310, 952–953, 959–960. Wolters Kluwer.

74   Vallerand, A., and Sanoski, C. A. (2019). *Davis's Drug Guide for Nurses* (16th ed.). F.A. Davis Company.

75   Centers for Disease Control and Prevention. (2019, August 28). *Opioid overdose, CDC guideline for prescribing opioids for chronic pain.* https://www.cdc.gov/drugoverdose/prescribing/guideline.html.

Table 10.9: Allopurinol Medication Grid

Class/ Subclass	Prototype- generic	Administration Considerations	Therapeutic Effects	Adverse/Side Effects
Antigout agent	allopurinol	May be given with milk or meals to decrease stomach upset Give with plenty of water May be crushed Monitor patient's intake and output Monitor hematologic, renal, and liver functions before and during therapy If rash occurs, notify healthcare provider	Prevention and treatment of attacks of gouty arthritis and nephropathy Treatment of secondary hyperuricemia	Hypotension Flushing Hypertension Drowsiness Nausea and vomiting Diarrhea Hepatitis Rash Renal failure

10.10 ANESTHETICS

As a nurse, you may care for a patient prior to surgery (preoperative), during surgery (perioperative), or after surgery (postoperative). One of your roles is to monitor your patient's vitals signs, paying close attention to respiratory status (respiratory rate, depth, quality, and SpO2). You will also assess LOC (level of consciousness) and pain level. Below is a description of the types of anesthetics.

Local

Local anesthetic is when a medication (e.g., lidocaine) is injected into the skin at the site of the procedure to achieve numbness for procedures like suturing.

Conscious Sedation

Conscious sedation is a combination of medications that allow the patient to be relaxed (midazolam) and free of pain (e.g., fentanyl) during a medical procedure (e.g., colonoscopy). This allows the patient to remain awake and aware, without feeling discomfort. The patient may or may not be able to speak or respond in this state.

General Anesthesia

General anesthesia is a medication-induced reversible unconsciousness with loss of protective reflexes. Arousal, even to painful stimuli, cannot occur. General anesthesia requires the establishment and maintenance of airway control.[76] Propofol is an example of an intravenous general anesthetic. The intravenous (IV) injection of propofol induces anesthesia within 40 seconds from the start of injection.[77]

---

76   Frandsen, G., and Pennington, S. (2018). *Abrams' clinical drug: Rationales for nursing practice* (11th ed.). pg. 305, 310, 952–953, 959–960. Wolters Kluwer.

77   This work is a derivative of *Daily Med* by U.S. National Library of Medicine in the public domain.

10.11 MODULE LEARNING ACTIVITIES

Light Bulb Moment

Now let's apply what you have learned!

Your 82-year-old postoperative patient is hard to arouse 30 minutes after you administered IV morphine. Their BP is 102/72, respirations are 8 and shallow and SpO2 is 88% on room air. Which of the following (with health care provider orders) are priority nursing actions? Select all that apply.

a) Administer oxygen

b) Administer naloxone

c) Insert a foley catheter

d) Increase IV fluid rate

e) Raise the head of the bed

Note: Answers to the Light Bulb Moment can be found in the "Answer Key" sections at the end of the book.

Interactive Activities

An interactive or media element has been excluded from this version of the text. You can view it online here: https://wtcs.pressbooks.pub/pharmacology/?p=2465

GLOSSARY

Acute Pain: Pain that usually starts suddenly and has a known cause, like an injury or surgery. It normally gets better as your body heals and lasts less than three months.

Adjuvant analgesics: Drugs with a primary indication other than pain that have analgesic properties in some painful conditions. The group includes numerous drugs in diverse classes such as gabapentin (an anticonvulsant) or amitriptyline (a tricyclic antidepressant).

Chronic pain: Pain that lasts six months or more and can be caused by a disease or condition, injury, medical treatment, inflammation, or an unknown reason.

Immune-mediated disease process: Occurs when the body's immune system attacks the central nervous system.

Misuse: The use of illegal drugs and/or the use of prescription drugs in a manner other than as directed by a doctor, such as using in greater amounts, more often, or longer than told to take a drug or using someone else's prescription.

Muscle Spasticity: Condition in which certain muscles are continuously contracted. This contraction causes stiffness or tightness of the muscles and can interfere with normal movement, speech, and gait. Spasticity is usually caused by damage to the portion of the brain or spinal cord that controls voluntary movement.

Nociceptors: Nerve endings that selectively respond to painful stimuli and send pain signals to the brain and spinal cord.

Non-pharmacologic therapy: Treatments that do not involve medications, including physical treatments (e.g., heat or cold therapy, exercise therapy, weight loss) and cognitive-behavioral treatments (e.g., distractions/diversions and cognitive behavioral therapy).

Patient controlled analgesia (PCA): To receive the opioid, the patient pushes a button on the PCA device, which releases a specific dose but also has a lockout mechanism to prevent an overdose. Included with hydromorphone or fentanyl.

Prostaglandins: Produced in nearly all cells and are part of the body's way of dealing with injury and illness. Prostaglandins act as signals to control several different processes depending on the part of the body in which they are made. Prostaglandins are made at the sites of tissue damage or infection, where they cause inflammation, pain, and fever as part of the healing process.

Vertigo: A sense of spinning dizziness. It is a symptom of a range of conditions. It can happen when there is a problem with the inner ear, brain, or sensory nerve pathway.

Chapter XI

Answer Key

Answer keys for the critical thinking and light bulb activities
in each chapter are provided in the following sections.

1.   CHAPTER 1

Answer Key to Chapter 1 Critical Thinking Activities

You can review additional information regarding these answers in the corresponding section in which the Critical Thinking activities appear.

Critical Thinking Activity Section 1.5a

The biotransformations that take place in the liver are performed by the liver enzymes. Therefore, if the liver is damaged, metabolism and excretion are impacted, resulting in the need for lower dosages to avoid toxicity.

Critical Thinking Activity Section 1.6a

Kidney function is important because drugs and metabolites in the bloodstream are often filtered by the kidney. In the kidney tubules, a portion of the drug undergoes reabsorption back into the bloodstream, and the remainder is excreted in the urine.

Critical Thinking Activity Section 1.7a

Before administering a Beta-1 antagonist such as atenolol, the nurse should assess the patient's apical pulse and blood pressure to confirm they are within normal range. Atenolol causes a negative inotropic effect by weakening the contraction of the heart and thus, decreases the patient's blood pressure. It also causes a negative chronotropic effect and decreases the patient's heart rate.

Critical Thinking Activities Section 1.9

1. Nursing considerations when administering pain medication include efficacy, dose-response based on the dosage selected, onset, peak, duration, and half-life of the drug. The patient has physical therapy scheduled at 0900, so the nurse should administer acetaminophen now to relieve the pain and evaluate the effectiveness in 60 minutes. The nurse should also plan on reassessing the patient's pain and potentially administering a second dose of acetaminophen just prior to the physical therapy appointment because the half-life of acetaminophen is two to three hours. Additionally, acetaminophen has a 24-hour dose restriction, so the nurse should calculate how many total milligrams the patient has received over the past 24 hours prior to administering the medication.

2. Insulin is a high-alert medication due to severe side effects that can occur if administered incorrectly. The nurse should check the patient's blood sugar reading and consider withholding the medication if the patient continues to refuse food over the next few hours to avoid causing hypoglycemia. The provider may also need to be notified of the patient's change in condition and a change in the medication order may be required.

Critical Thinking Activity Section 1.10

The normal lab values of gentamicin are 5 to 10 mcg/mL (or 10.45 to 20.90 micromol/L), so 30 mcg/ml is too high. This abnormal result could indicate the patient has renal impairment affecting metabolism and excretion of this medication. The doctor and pharmacist should be notified to adjust the next dose of gentamycin before it is administered.

My Notes

Section 1.12 Light Bulb Moment

1. The nurse should select the rectal route due to the patient's difficulty swallowing to reduce the risk of aspiration.

2. The initial dose is less than the standard recommended dose based on the Mr. Johnson's age and the likelihood that his kidney functioning is decreased. Decreased kidney function affects the metabolism and excretion of gentamycin and could result in toxicities if the dose is too high.

3. Sara should wait to administer the medication until the patient's trough level is drawn. The trough level is required for the provider and the pharmacist to determine if the medication is within the range of the therapeutic window and to avoid the risk of toxicity to the patient.

4. Sam should evaluate the patient's vital signs, specifically the apical pulse and blood pressure, to be sure they are within normal range for this patient and the parameters prescribed by the provider. Atenolol has negative inotropic, chronotropic, and dromotropic effects. The negative inotropic effect weakens the contraction of the heart and lowers blood pressure. The negative chronotropic effect decreases the heart rate, and a negative dromotropic effect slows the conduction of the electrical charge in the heart. Understanding the effects of this Beta-1 antagonist medication allows Sam to anticipate expected actions of the medication and the patient's response.

5. Amiodarone is metabolized by the enzymes in the intestines to its active form. Grapefruit juice contains compounds that slow down this process and affect the levels of this medication in the blood. The nurse should educate Julia about this interaction and encourage other beverage choices in the future that do not cause this interaction.

6. The nurse anticipates that hydrocodone/acetaminophen will peak in approximately 1 hour. The patient will likely require another dose of medication for acute, severe pain that accompanies a knee replacement in approximately 4 hours.

2. CHAPTER 2

Chapter 2 Critical Thinking Activities

You can review additional information regarding these answers in the corresponding section in which the Critical Thinking activities appear.

Critical Thinking Activity Section 2.2a

Before administering the medications with similar mechanisms of action, the nurse should notify both providers to clarify the orders and advocate for patient safety.

Critical Thinking Activity Section 2.2b

The nurse should provide verbal education regarding when to take medication, side effects to watch for, and potential adverse effects. The patient should also be educated on any restrictions related to diet, over-the-counter medications, and herbal supplements.

Critical Thinking Activity Section 2.3a

The nurse should clarify the medication order with the provider before administration because pneumonia is not listed as an indication for levofloxacin in the Black Box Warning. Notification of the provider and the provider's response should be recorded in the patient's medical record.

Critical Thinking Activity Section 2.3b

1. The nurse should educate the patient that medications should never be shared with others. Sharing medications is not only illegal but also dangerous. The nurse should describe the dangers to the patient, including potential drug interactions, dietary interactions, loss of consciousness, or death if inappropriate drugs or dosages are used.

2. An impaired nurse may endanger the lives of their patients or harm themselves. It is a nurse's professional and ethical responsibility to report a colleague's suspected drug use to their nurse manager or supervisor and, in some states or jurisdictions, to the board of nursing.

Critical Thinking Activities Section 2.3c

1. The five rights the nurse checks before administering any medication include right patient, right medication, right dose, right route, and right time. Checking allergies and the expiration date of the medication are also included when checking the five rights.

2. Nurses confirm patient identification prior to administering medication by asking the patient their name and date of birth, checking the patient's identification band, and by scanning bar codes on the medication and patient's armband. In long-term care settings where patients don't wear armbands and may not be able to recall their name and date of birth, the nurse may use alternative methods of identification, such as using a patient's picture in the medication record or asking another staff member to confirm the patient's identity.

3. Prior to the administration of morphine, an opioid medication, the nurse should assess the patient's pain level, level of consciousness, respiratory rate, and oxygenation status. If the patient exhibits a decreased respiratory rate, decreased oxygenation level, or an increased sedation, the medication should be withheld and appropriate interventions implemented.

4. After administering an opioid medication, the nurse should evaluate the effectiveness of the medication in treating the pain, as well as continuing to monitor respiratory rate, oxygenation level, and sedation status.

5. The nurse should teach the patient about common side effects, such as constipation and drowsiness.

6. The shift handoff report should include the location of the patient's pain, the reported pain level, pain medications administered during the shift, the time of medication administration, and the patient's response to the medication.

Critical Thinking Activity Section 2.3d

The colleague can share information about the Professional Assistance Procedure in Wisconsin that provides support to nurses who are committed to their own recovery. It is important to emphasize that the nurse jeopardizes patient safety when practicing under the influence of a substance.

Critical Thinking Activity Section 2.4

The nurse should suggest the mother obtain an oral syringe from the pharmacist to ensure accurate measurement of the medication. Errors can occur when families use spoons in their home to administer medication.

Critical Thinking Activity Section 2.5a

The nurse can use alternative sources of medication information when the patient cannot recall their home medication and it is not available in the electronic medical health records. A common intervention is to ask the patient to bring all of their medications to their appointment, including prescribed medications, over-the-counter medications, vitamins, and herbal supplements. Family members, such as a spouse or adult children, can also provide valid information with the patient's permission. After determining the patient's current medications, the nurse should print a copy of the list of medications and instruct the patient to bring it with them to all of the heath care providers and update it as needed.

Critical Thinking Activity Section 2.5b

In addition to verifying the 5 rights of medication administration, the nurse should confirm the blood glucose level, insulin type, concentration, and the date the insulin vial was opened. The nurse should draw up the dose and confirm correct dosing with another RN prior to administration. The nurse should be aware of onset, peak, and duration of action and monitor for potential side effects such as hypoglycemia.

3.   CHAPTER 3

Critical Thinking Activities

You can review additional information regarding these answers in the corresponding section in which the Critical Thinking activities appear.

Critical Thinking Activity Section 3.2a

Patient education regarding the importance of adhering to the prescribed medication regimen is vital to help prevent drug resistance. During patient education, the nurse should emphasize the need to complete the full course of medication, in the dosages and frequencies prescribed, to treat the infection and prevent the dangers of drug resistance. In addition to patient education, another solution used to prevent drug resistance in high-risk medications is called directly observed therapy (DOT). DOT is the supervised administration of medications to patients. Patients are required to visit a health-care facility to receive their medications or a health-care professional administers medications in the patients' homes or other designated location. DOT has been implemented worldwide for the treatment of tuberculosis (TB), and research has been shown it to be effective in treating infections successfully and preventing additional drug resistance.

Critical Thinking Activity Section 3.5a

The administration of penicillin should be postponed for four hours because citrus juice can impede absorption of drugs like penicillin. The remaining doses of penicillin for the day should be rescheduled based on the time the breakfast dose was actually administered. Additionally, the patient should be educated about avoiding citrus juice while taking penicillin, and the dietary department should be notified to remove citrus juice from the meal choices.

Critical Thinking Activity Section 3.6a

The changes in the patient's renal labs demonstrate decreased renal function. The prescribing provider should be notified prior to administering additional doses of cefazolin because the medication or the dosage will likely need to be revised based on the patient's response.

Critical Thinking Activity Section 3.7a

The nurse should check the progress notes in the electronic medical record to determine if anything is documented about John's allergies and the decision to use imipenem. If nothing is documented, then the nurse should notify the prescribing provider of the patient's allergies to penicillin to confirm the appropriateness of this medication for John, document the provider's response in the medical record, and provide this information in the end-of-shift handoff report.

Critical Thinking Activity Section 3.8a

Monobactams are narrow-spectrum antibacterial medications used primarily to treat gram-negative bacteria like Pseudomonas aeruginosa. However, MRSA is a gram-positive bacteria, so aztreonam will not be effective in fighting this infection. The nurse should notify the prescribing provider of the results of the new culture report before administering the azotreonam.

Critical Thinking Activity Section 3.9a

The nurse should review the other medications the patient is taking.

Trimethoprim-Sulfamethoxazole has many significant drug interactions, including oral diabetics. This medication may increase hypoglycemic effects requiring closer monitoring of blood sugars. Additionally, the patient's renal status should be verified before administration of trimethoprim-sulfamethoxazole because dose adjustment may be required.

Critical Thinking Activity Section 3.10a

The nurse should immediately stop the medication and notify the provider regarding the new onset of tendon pain because this symptom indicates an adverse reaction of levofloxacin may be occurring.

Critical Thinking Activity Section 3.11a

The nurse should notify the provider of the patient's change condition because it may indicate an adverse effect of liver damage is occurring.

Critical Thinking Activity Section 3.12a

The nurse should not administer the medication until the trough levels have been drawn. The nurse should phone the lab and check on the status of the laboratory trough level.

Critical Thinking Activity Section 3.13a

The patient is under the age of six and is at risk for the adverse effect of teeth discoloration. The nurse should advocate for this patient by notifying the prescribing provider of this concern and requesting an alternate medication.

Critical Thinking Activity Section 3.14a

Oseltamivir should be administered within the first 24-48 hours of the onset of influenza symptoms. The patient may have already passed the window for maximum therapeutic effectiveness of oseltamivir. The provider should be notified regarding the onset of symptoms to clarify the prescription.

Critical Thinking Activity Section 3.15a

If there are no signs of improvement from the prescribed medication therapy, the nurse should notify the provider.

Critical Thinking Activity Section 3.16a

In order to prevent malaria, the CDC recommends patients should take antimalarial medications for four weeks after leaving the infected area. The nurse should provide additional patient education to the patient regarding this recommendation and evaluate for patient understanding.

Critical Thinking Activity Section 3.17a

Metronidazole is commonly used to treat C-diff. The medication must be given by mouth for the indication of a gastrointestinal infection like C-diff.

Critical Thinking Activity Section 3.18a

The nurse should provide education regarding the use of the medication, as well as ways to prevent re-infection. Methods to prevent reinfection include using proper handwashing, washing all fruits and vegetables, and wearing shoes in the barn or where animals and their feces are present.

Critical Thinking Activity Section 3.19a

The nurse should explain that directly observed therapy (DOT) means the administration of this medication will be supervised to ensure all doses are taken as prescribed to be sure the infection is treated properly and drug resistance does not develop. The patient will be required to visit a health-care facility to receive their medications or a health-care professional will administer the medication in the patient's home or other designated location.

Critical Thinking Activity Section 3.20a

The nurse should not administer the vancomycin until after the trough level is drawn. The nurse should call the lab to request prioritization of completing the trough level.

4.   CHAPTER 4

Section 4.16 Light Bulb Moment

1. A potential side effect of nicotine is the activation of the sympathetic nervous system that causes an increased heart rate. Nausea and weakness are potential side effects that can indicate nicotine overdose. The nurse should provide education to the patient regarding the avoidance of additional nicotine when using the nicotine patch. It may also be helpful to remove the patch at bedtime and reapply a new patch in the morning.

You can review additional information about nicotine administration in the "Nicotine" section.

2.a. The nurse should explain to the patient that tamsulosin relaxes muscles in the bladder and prostate to improve urine flow.

2.b. The nurse should monitor for hypotension and tachycardia, especially after administering the first dose of medication. The nurse should also advise the patient to change positions slowly in order to prevent falls that can occur due to hypotension.

You can review additional information about tamsulosin in the "Alpha-1 Antagonists" section.

3.a. Albuterol stimulates Beta-2 agonist receptors in the smooth muscle of bronchi and bronchioles to produce bronchodilation to ease the work of breathing.

3.b. Beta-1 receptors can also be inadvertently stimulated by albuterol and causes the side effect of tachycardia.

3.c. The nurse should educate the patient to take the medication as prescribed and avoid caffeine or other stimulants that can cause tachycardia.

You can review additional information about albuterol in the "Beta-2 Agonists" section.

4.a. Propranolol is a nonselective beta-blocker and inhibits both Beta-1 and Beta-2 receptors. Inhibiting Beta-1 receptors will decrease the heart rate and reduce the force of the heart's contraction, which will lower the patient's blood pressure.

4.b. Before administering propranolol, the nurse should always assess the patient's blood pressure and apical pulse. If the systolic blood pressure is less than 100 mm Hg or the apical heart rate is less than 60 beats per minute, the medication should be withheld and the provider notified unless other parameters are provided in the order.

4.c. Propranolol can inadvertently cause bronchoconstriction because it inhibits Beta-2 receptors in addition to Beta-1 receptors. Bronchocontriction causes wheezing.

4.d. When a nurse notices new wheezing, a focused respiratory assessment should be performed including assessing the patient's airway, respiratory rate, and oxygenation status. Depending on the urgency of the assessment findings, the nurse should also check the patient's medical record for a history of asthma or chronic obstructive pulmonary disease (COPD) and immediately notify the provider.

You can review additional information about propranolol in the "Beta-2 Antagonists" section.

5.a.   Before administering metoprolol, the nurse should always assess the patient's blood pressure and pulse.

5.b.   If the systolic blood pressure is less than 100 mm Hg or the apical heart rate is less than 60 beats per minute, the medication should be withheld and the provider notified unless other parameters are provided in the order.

5.c.   A new finding of edema can indicate that the adverse effect of worsening heart failure is occurring.

5.d.   The nurse should assess the patient for additional signs of worsening heart failure, such as fine crackles in the lungs and recent weight gain, and notify the provider regarding this change in patient condition.

You can review additional information about metoprolol in the "Beta-1 Antagonists" section.

6.a.   Dobutamine is a catecholamine and it will increase heart rate, the force of heart contraction, and speed of conduction between the SA to AV nodes. These actions will help to improve cardiac output for a patient experiencing an acute episode of heart failure.

6.b.   During administration of dobutamine, the nurse should continuously monitor the patient's heart rate, blood pressure, ECG, cardiac output, and urine output. Increased urine output will demonstrate the effectiveness of the medication in perfusing the kidneys.

You can review additional information about dobutamine in the "Alpha and Beta Receptor Agonists (Catecholamines)" section.

5. CHAPTER 5

Section 5.15 Light Bulb Moment

Asthma Scenario

1. The correct answer is c) Albuterol. Albuterol is a Beta-2 agonist that relaxes smooth muscle to cause bronchodilation and assist the patient with the work of breathing. It is a rapid-acting bronchodilator that is used during asthma attacks.

2. The nurse should instruct the patient to take the following steps to safely administer albuterol:

    - Insert the inhaler into the spacer and shake the canister

    - Breathe out all the way

    - Press down on the inhaler and breathe in slowly through the mouth

    - Breathe in for 10 seconds or as long as you can tolerate

    - Remove the inhaler from the mouth

    - Wait 30 seconds between doses

3. After administering the medication, the nurse should assess the patient's vital signs and lung sounds, paying special attention to the respiratory rate, pulse oximetry, and heart rate for signs of improvement, as well as for potential side effects such as tachycardia.

4. The nurse should educate the patient regarding the correct method to administer albuterol, potential side effects, and the signs and symptoms of an asthma exacerbation. The nurse should ensure the patient has a written copy of their asthma action plan and verify that the patient can explain the plan to ensure proper understanding. The nurse should also explain the importance of always having albuterol on hand and to help the patient make plans for refills so as to not run out of medication.

5. To ensure correct use of the inhaler, the nurse should ask the patient to provide a return demonstration.

You can review additional information about asthma in the "Diseases of the Respiratory System" section and albuterol in the "Beta-2 Agonist" section of this chapter.

Allergy Scenario

6. The correct answer is b) Epinephrine. Epinephrine is used to rapidly treat severe allergic reactions.

You can review additional information about epinephrine and the use of Epi-Pens in the "Alpha and Beta Receptor Agonists (Catecholamines)" section of the "Autonomic Nervous System" chapter.

6.   CHAPTER 6

Chapter 6 Critical Thinking Answers

You can review additional information regarding these answers in the corresponding section in which the Critical Thinking activities appear.

Critical Thinking Activity Section 6.7a

1. A nurse should assess the apical pulse for a full minute before administering digoxin due to its positive inotropic action (it increases contractility, stroke volume, and, thus, cardiac output), negative chronotropic action (it decreases heart rate), and negative dromotropic action (it decreases electrical conduction of the cardiac cells). These actions can lead to bradycardia. If the patient's heart rate is less than 60 beats per minute, the nurse should notify the provider before administering digoxin unless other parameters are provided.

2. The nurse evaluates the effectiveness of digoxin based on the patient's blood pressure, apical pulse, and decreased symptoms of heart failure for which it is indicated.

3. The nurse should monitor the patient's serum potassium level because a decreased potassium level places the patient at increased risk of digoxin toxicity. Normal potassium level is 3.5 to 5.0 mEq/L, and a result less than 3.5 should be immediately reported to the provider due the the risk for sudden dysrhythmias. Serum digoxin levels should also be monitored, with a normal therapeutic range being 0.8 to 2 ng/mL.

4. The nurse should assess the patient's apical pulse and withhold the administration of digoxin. The nurse should also check for current lab results related to the serum digoxin and potassium levels. The nurse should notify the provider of the patient's change in condition that could indicate digoxin toxicity and provide information regarding the patient's apical pulse and recent digoxin and potassium levels. An order for a serum digoxin level may be received from the provider. Based on the serum digoxin level, the patient may receive a new order for digibind. Digibind is used to treat digoxin toxicity.

Critical Thinking Activity Section 6.8

The nurse should monitor the patient's blood pressure and heart rate. After 5 minutes, the pain level should be reassessed and a second dose of nitroglycerin administered if the patient's chest pain continues. If there is no improvement in chest pain, emergency services should be obtained by calling 911 or the rapid response team.

Critical Thinking Activity Section 6.9

1. Before administering a diuretic, the nurse should assess blood pressure, the daily weight trend, serum potassium and other electrolyte levels, hydration status including 24-hour input/output, and current renal function.

2. Signs of toxicity include blurred vision, nausea, and visual impairment (such as seeing green and yellow halos). A low potassium level can increase the risk of digoxin toxicity. If a patient has digoxin toxicity, severe bradycardia and even death can occur if not treated promptly. The normal range for serum potassium is 3.5-5.0 mEq/L.

3. Furosemide (Lasix) is a loop diuretic.

4. Patients receiving loop diuretics are at high risk of dehydration. Loop diuretics work in the loop of Henle where a great deal of sodium and water are either reabsorbed or eliminated by the kidney tubules.

5. The nurse should assess for the development of dehydration in patients receiving diuretics by monitoring skin and mucus membranes for dryness, blood pressure for hypotension, heart rate for tachycardia, decreased urine output, concentrated urine, and increased serum sodium levels.

6. All electrolyte levels can be decreased in patients taking loop diuretics, but potassium in particular is at high risk for depletion due to the rapid water loss that occurs.

7. Furosemide can deplete potassium levels, which then increases the risk for developing digoxin toxicity.

Critical Thinking Activity Section 6.10

1. Metoprolol is a selective Beta-1 blocker that decreases the heart rate and force of contraction to reduce blood pressure. Lisinopril is an ACE inhibitor that reduces blood pressure through vasodilation and reduces fluid retention. Verapamil is a calcium channel blocker that causes vasodilation to reduce blood pressure. Hydro-chlorothiazide is a thiazide diuretic that reduces fluid retention. For this patient, all four medications may be required to maintain a blood pressure within normal range.

2. The nurse should explain that each medication works in different ways within the body to treat high blood pressure. It is vital to explain the importance of maintaining blood pressure within normal range to prevent additional complications such as a heart attack, heart failure, stroke, and kidney failure.

Critical Thinking Activity Section 6.12

1. Warfarin will not dissolve the existing clot, but it will help prevent additional clot formation.

2. When a patient is taking warfarin, the nurse should closely monitor INR and PT levels to verify they are in normal range to prevent bleeding complications. Specifically, the therapeutic range for INR is between 2.0 to 3.5 depending upon the indication.

3. Dietary instructions should be provided to maintain a consistent intake of foods high in vitamin K like leafy green vegetables. Daily changes in intake of foods that are high in vitamin K will influence the effectiveness of warfarin, as well as the patient's INR levels used to maintain the warfarin levels in therapeutic range.

4. Patient education should emphasize bleeding precautions, avoidance of NSAIDs and aspirin, the need for routine therapeutic monitoring, and when to call the provider with signs of increased bleeding or clotting.

5. The reversal agent for warfarin is vitamin K.

7.   CHAPTER 7

Chapter 7 Critical Thinking Activities

You can review additional information regarding these answers in the corresponding section in which the Critical Thinking activities appear.

Critical Thinking Activity Section 7.3

Postoperative patients often require a proton pump inhibitor due to the stress response that occurs during surgery and hospitalization. Pantoprazole suppresses the secretion of hydrochloric acid and prevents the formation of a stress ulcer.

Critical Thinking Activity Section 7.4a

1. The patient may be experiencing increased heart rate as a symptom of dehydration associated with water loss from the diarrhea. Additionally, a Black Box Warning for loperamide is abnormal heart rhythm. The nurse should assess the patient's heart rate and rhythm and notify the provider.

2. The nurse can recommend providing over-the-counter probiotics, which are also found in yogurt, for the prevention of diarrhea associated with antibiotic use or to assist in decreasing the symptoms of diarrhea.

Critical Thinking Activity Section 7.4b

1. A postoperative patient has many risk factors for constipation, including side effects of anesthesia and opiates, sedentary levels of activity, and decreased fluid and food intake after surgery. In addition to administering docusate or other laxatives as needed, the nurse should educate the patient about nonpharmacological interventions to relieve constipation, such as increased fluid and fiber intake and walking.

2. Docusate softens the stool and improves the regularity of bowel movements.

3. Docusate usually works within 12-72 hours. If it is not effective in creating a bowel movement with soft stool, the patient should be instructed to notify the nurse and additional laxatives can be administered.

4. Preventative measures for constipation include increasing fluid and fiber intake, ambulating, and using the least amount of opiates needed to effectively treat the pain.

5. Bowel protocols usually include a step-wise approach to constipation. Docusate or polyethylene glycol 3350 are often used preventively, but if a bowel movement does not occur within the expected timeframe, additional laxatives such as bisacodyl or an enema may be added. A bisacodyl suppository generally produces a bowel movement within one hour whereas a mineral oil enema usually works within 15 minutes of administration.

Critical Thinking Activity Section 7.5

1. The nurse assesses for dehydration by monitoring blood pressure for hypotension, heart rate for tachycardia, urine output for decreased level, skin for tenting, and mucus membranes for dryness.

2. The dissolving tablets eliminate the risk of vomiting the medication before it is absorbed. If the patient can't tolerate the dissolving tablets, the nurse can request the provider to change the route of ondansetron to the intravenous route.

3. The nurse should plan to proactively administer medications before meals to prevent nausea. The patient can also be instructed to follow a bland diet to prevent feelings of nausea that can be stimulated by spicy food or strong flavors. Fluids should be encouraged to prevent dehydration, but if fluids increase the patient's feelings of nausea, the patient can be instructed to take frequent sips of fluid or suck on ice chips.

8.   CHAPTER 8

Chapter 8 Critical Thinking Activities

You can review additional information regarding these answers in the corresponding section in which the Critical Thinking activities appear.

Critical Thinking Activity Section 8.5

Lorazepam is a benzodiazepine, which is a CNS depressant. The riskiest side effects associated with the use of lorazepam are respiratory depression and oversedation. Other central nervous system depressants, such as scopolamine and alcohol, can cause additive effects and should be avoided when taking lorazepam. Sedation, drowsiness, respiratory depression, hypotension, and unsteadiness may occur when taking lorazepam, so these side effects should be considered when participating in activities on the cruise.

Critical Thinking Activity Section 8.6

Patient and parent education about methylphenidate should include taking the medication in the morning and not after 4 p.m. It is important to monitor the child's growth and weight and to provide food and snacks that the child likes if weight loss is a concern. Methylphenidate has a Black Box Warning due to its high abuse potential, and signs of misuse should be reported to the provider. The risks of drinking alcohol while taking this medication should also be discussed.

Critical Thinking Activity Section 8.7

1. A patient taking an SSRI medication like fluoxetine is at risk for developing serotonin syndrome if they have liver dysfunction or are taking other CNS medications. SSRIs are contraindicated with MAOIs due to the risk of developing serotonin syndrome. Symptoms of serotonin syndrome include confusion, elevated temperature, and rapidly changing levels of blood pressure.

2. The nurse should advise the patient of the potential for suicidal thoughts with this medication and advise her to notify her provider if she has any thoughts of self-harm.

3. Common side effects of SSRIs that the nurse should discuss with the patient include sedation, low blood pressure that can cause dizziness, suicidal thoughts, heart palpitations, sexual dysfunction, and anticholinergic side effects such as dry mouth. Patients should be advised to avoid drinking alcohol when taking an SSRI.

4. The nurse should advise the patient that it may take up to 12 weeks to reach therapeutic levels of this medication where they feel better.

Critical Thinking Activity Section 8.8

1. The nurse should explain symptoms of manic episodes include rapid speech, hyperactivity, reduced need for sleep, poor judgment, hostility, aggression, decreased impulse control, and risky behaviors. For more information about mania and bipolar disorder, review the "Disorders of the CNS System" section.

2. Symptoms of lithium toxicity include diarrhea, vomiting, drowsiness, muscular weakness, and a lack of coordination. At higher lithium levels, giddiness, ataxia, blurred vision, tinnitus, and a large output of dilute urine may be seen. Lithium toxicity is prevented by regularly monitoring serum lithium levels to maintain a therapeutic range between 0.8 to 1.2 mEq/L.

My Notes

3. The nurse should advise the patient that lithium reaches therapeutic range within 1 to 3 weeks.

Critical Thinking Activity Section 8.10

1. Gabapentin is classified as an anti-seizure medication, but it is also used to help relieve neuropathic pain that patients with diabetes often describe as a "burning" or "tingling" sensation in their lower extremities.

2. Gabapentin is a CNS depressant and can cause sedation, dizziness, and ataxia that increase a patient's risk for falls.

3. The nurse should plan to monitor for worsening depression, suicidal ideation, fever, rash, lymphadenopathy, dizziness, sleepiness, stumbling, and a lack of coordination. Development of any of these signs should be reported to the provider; suicidal ideation requires urgent notification.

Critical Thinking Activity Section 8.11

1. Levodopa, the metabolic precursor of dopamine, crosses the blood-brain barrier and is then converted to dopamine in the brain. Carbidopa is combined with levodopa to help prevent the breakdown of levodopa before it is able to cross the blood-brain barrier.

2. Patients taking carbidopa and levodopa have reported suddenly falling asleep without prior warning of sleepiness while engaged in activities of daily living, including operation of motor vehicles. Patients should be advised to exercise caution while driving or operating machines during treatment with carbidopa and levodopa.

3. Dyskinesia is involuntary muscle movements including tics. If a patient develops dyskinesia while taking carbidopa-levodopa, dosing adjustment or alternate drug therapy is required.

9.   CHAPTER 9

Chapter 9 Critical Thinking Activities

You can review additional information regarding these answers in the corresponding section in which the Critical Thinking activities appear.

Critical Thinking Activity Section 9.3

1. The patient is at risk for a fracture due to a previous history of osteoporosis that weakens the bones and increases the risk for a fracture when injury occurs. Corticosteroids can cause muscle weakness that can lead to falls and fractures.

2. Alendronate, a bisphosphonates class of medication, is often used to treat osteoporosis and reduce the patient's risk of fracrures. Other preventative measures can be implemented such as weight-bearing exercise and calcium/ vitamin D supplementation.

3. The patient should be instructed to avoid getting up without assistance. The room should be well-lit without loose rugs that can cause tripping. If the patient uses assistive devices like a cane or walker, these devices should be readily available.

4. The use of glucocorticoids can increase glucose levels. Although the patient has no history of diabetes, the increased blood glucose levels may require the temporary use of insulin.

5. Signs of adrenal suppression include severe fatigue, gastrointestinal upset, and a suppressed immune response that places the patient at risk for developing infections.

Critical Thinking Activity Section 9.4

1. Type 1 diabetes is an autoimmune disease affecting the beta cells of the pancreas so they do not produce insulin; synthetic insulin must be administered by injection or infusion.

   Type 2 diabetes is acquired, and lifestyle factors such as poor diet and inactivity greatly increase a person's risk for developing this disease. In type 2 diabetes, the body's cells become resistant to the effects of insulin. In response, the pancreas increases its insulin secretion, but over time, the beta cells become exhausted. In many cases, type 2 diabetes can be reversed by moderate weight loss, regular physical activity, and consumption of a healthy diet. However, if blood glucose levels cannot be controlled with these measures, oral diabetic medication is implemented and eventually insulin may be required.

2. Surgery and hospitalization often stimulate a patient's stress response, which includes the release of cortisol. Cortisol increases blood glucose levels, so the patient may require insulin to control blood sugar levels while hospitalized.

3. The nurse should administer 12 units of Humalog insulin along with the scheduled 20 units of Humulin-N insulin at breakfast.

4. Metformin may be discontinued because it is contraindicated in patients with kidney disease (e.g., serum creatinine levels ≥1.5 mg/dL [males] or ≥1.4 mg/dL [females]).

5. The patient is displaying signs of hypoglycemia. A supplementary carbohydrate, such as 4 ounces of orange juice, should be administered as soon as possible. However, if the patient seems confused or unable to swallow, glucagon should be administered.

6. The patient has hypoglycemia because the peak effect of Humulin-N is about 6 hours. Because the medication is peaking between meal times, the patient's blood sugar continues to decrease. On the other hand, the onset of Humalog insulin is 15-30 minutes, with the peak effect in 1-3 hours, so the food eaten during meal time maintains a normal blood sugar as long as the meals and the insulin administration are matched.

7. The hemoglobin A1C test indicates the patient's average level of blood sugar over the past 2 to 3 months. It is also referred to as HbA1c, glycated hemoglobin test, or glycohemoglobin. Normal hemoglobin A1C is less than 5.7%. In patients with diabetes, the goal is to maintain hemoglobin A1C levels less than 7%. The patient's recent lab result of 10% indicates the need for additional diabetes medication, as well as patient education regarding diabetes management, to avoid the development of long-term complications of diabetes.

8. Lantus is a long-acting insulin that has a duration over 24 hours. It does not have a peak and should be administered once daily at the same time each day. Lantus should only be administered subcutaneously and should not be mixed with other insulin.

Critical Thinking Activity Section 9.5

The patient should be advised to take levothyroxine at the same time every morning, before eating or drinking. It should not be taken with other medications that may interfere with its absorption and should be taken at least 30 minutes before eating or 2 hours after eating. The patient should monitor for signs of hypothyroidism from too low of a dose of levothyroxine, such as constipation, weight gain, and fatigue. It is also important to watch for signs of too high of a dose of levothyroxine such as rapid or irregular heart rate.

10.   CHAPTER 10

Chapter 10 Critical Thinking Activities

You can review additional information regarding these answers in the corresponding section in which the Critical Thinking activities appear.

Critical Thinking Activity Section 10.6a

The patient should be advised that acetaminophen can cause acute liver damage when taken in excessive amounts or when used with alcohol. Many over-the-counter medications contain acetaminophen, so daily amounts must be monitored carefully. Recommended daily restrictions for acetaminophen include less than 4,000 mg of acetaminophen in 24 hours for an adult, less than 3,200 mg for geriatric adults, and less than 2,000 mg for patients with alcoholism. Fewer than three alcoholic drinks should be consumed daily while using acetaminophen.

Critical Thinking Activity Section 10.6b

The patient should be advised that aspirin has an anti-platelet effect, in addition to reducing pain, fever, and inflammation. By preventing the platelets from sticking together, clots that can cause heart attacks and strokes are prevented from forming.

Critical Thinking Activity Section 10.6c

Ibuprofen is a nonsteroidal anti-inflammatory drug (NSAID), which can cause severe and life-threatening stomach bleeding and must be taken cautiously. The patient should be advised that the risk for bleeding is higher if the patient:

- is age 60 or older
- has had stomach ulcers or bleeding problems
- takes a anticoagulant or steroid medication
- takes other drugs containing NSAIDs (such as aspirin, ibuprofen, or naproxen)
- consumes three or more alcoholic drinks every day while using this product
- takes ibuprofen in higher doses, more frequently, or for a longer time than directed

Critical Thinking Activity Section 10d

The nurse should evaluate the effectiveness of ketorolac IV in relieving the patient's pain 30 minutes after administration.

Critical Thinking Activity Section 10e

The nurse should provide the following patient education to a patient who has been prescribed celecoxib:

- It may be taken with or without food
- You can sprinkle capsules on applesauce and ingest it immediately with water
- You may experience heartburn, vomiting, or diarrhea with this medication
- Notify the provider immediately if you have abdominal pain, vomit blood or have blood in your stool, develop swelling in your hand or feet, or notice yellowing of your skin

Critical Thinking Activity Section 10.7a

Oral drops of morphine, commonly used for patients with metastatic cancer, should be effective within 1 hour of administration.

Critical Thinking Activity Section 10.7b

Naloxone immediately reverses the effects of respiratory depression and oversedations caused by opioids. After a patient receives naloxone, the nurse should continue to evaluate the patient's respiratory status at least every 15 minutes because naloxone has a shorter duration of action that many opioids, and repeated doses are usually necessary.

Critical Thinking Activity Section 10.8a

The nurse should educate the patient to take baclofen with milk or food to minimize gastric upset. Advise the patient that baclofen may cause dizziness or drowsiness, so they should change positions slowly and avoid driving and operating machines. Patients using baclofen should avoid using alcohol or taking other CNS depressants.

Critical Thinking Activity Section 10.8b

Cyclobenzaprine is a muscle relaxer and may cause drowsiness. If used with alcohol or other CNS depressants, it can impair mental or physical abilities, so the patient should be advised to not drive when taking cyclobenzaprine.

Critical Thinking Activity Section 10.8c

The patient should be advised that tizanidine can cause drowsiness and dizziness, and concurrent use with alcohol can worsen these effects.

Tizanidine can damage the liver so alcohol should be avoided to prevent additional damage.

Critical Thinking Activity Section 10.11

The correct answers are a), b), and e). Based on the patient's respiratory status, the nurse should immediately raise the patient's bed and apply oxygen to rapidly increase their oxygenation level. The nurse should ask for help from a team member and/or call the rapid response team while obtaining naloxone to administer for sedation and respiratory depression.

The nurse should continue to monitor the patient's respiratory status after naloxone is administered because repeated doses may be required.